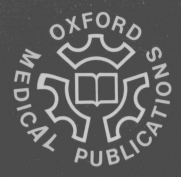

Primary
Child Care

A manual for health workers

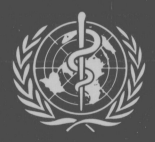

Maurice King
Felicity King
Soebagio Martodipoero

SOME FIGURES TO REMEMBER

A newborn baby weighs between 3 and 3·5 kg (26·4).

A one year old child weighs about 10 kg (inside back cover).

A healthy baby gains about half a kilo a month during the first six months of his life (26–19b, 26·21).

The normal temperature is between 36 and 37·5°C (10·1).

A child is anaemic if his haemoglobin is below 10 g/dl (22·2).

An artificially fed baby needs 150 ml/kg of milk a day (26·15).

An older child needs 120 ml/kg of fluid a day (15·6).

A severely dehydrated child needs 20 ml/kg of intravenous fluid fast (9·28).

Make 'salt-and-sugar-water' with eight level teaspoons of sugar, one level teaspoon of salt, and one litre of water (9·22).

A quiet child who breathes more than 60 times a minute probably has pneumonia (8·9).

A standard teaspoon holds 5 ml (3-1).

A cup holds about 200 ml (3-2).

There are about 20 drops in 1 ml (3-3).

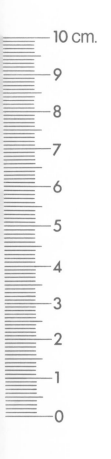

OXFORD MEDICAL PUBLICATIONS

Primary child care
A manual for health workers

Primary child care
A manual for health workers

MAURICE KING

M.D. (Cantab.), F.R.C.P. (Lond.)
Lately WHO Staff Member, the Puslitbang Pelayanan
Kesehatan, Surabaya, Indonesia; Professor of Social Medicine in
the University of Zambia, and Visiting Professor in Johns
Hopkins University.

FELICITY KING

B.M. (Oxon.), M.R.C.P. (Lond.)

SOEBAGYO MARTODIPOERO

M.D. (Airlangga)

Director of Basic Health Care Research, Puslitbang Pelayanan
Kesehatan, Surabaya, Indonesia.

Illustrated by Soenarto Timoer

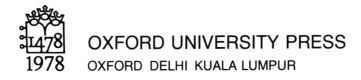

1478
1978

OXFORD UNIVERSITY PRESS
OXFORD DELHI KUALA LUMPUR

Oxford University Press, Walton Street, Oxford OX2 6DP

OXFORD LONDON GLASGOW NEW YORK
TORONTO MELBOURNE WELLINGTON CAPE TOWN
IBADAN NAIROBI DAR ES SALAAM LUSAKA
KUALA LUMPUR SINGAPORE JAKARTA HONG KONG TOKYO
DELHI BOMBAY CALCUTTA MADRAS KARACHI

Published on behalf of the World Health Organization

British Library Cataloguing in Publication Data
King, Maurice
Primary child care. – (Oxford medical publications).
1. Pediatrics 2. Underdeveloped areas – Medical
care
I. Title II. King, Felicity; Martodipoero, Soebagyo
III. World Health Organization IV. Series
615'.542'091724 RJ52 77–30455

ISBN 0–19–264229–4

The opinions in this book are those of the authors,
and do not necessarily reflect the opinions and
policies of the World Health Organization.

*Phototypeset in V.I.P. Times by
Western Printing Services Ltd, Bristol*

*Printed in Great Britain
by J. W. Arrowsmith Ltd., Bristol*

Preface

To all the children of our world for their year—1979

This is a system of primary child care. It is intended for adaptation and translation, in whole or in part, without royalty or credit, as part of WHO's contribution to International Children's Year—1979. It is also a manifestation of WHO's determination to see that the essential knowledge of primary child care is in the languages of all the world's health workers. As such it is but one of the ways in which the Organization can contribute to the improvement of maternal and child care. The promotion of such care is a contribution to our global multisectoral struggle, not only to improve the health of the citizens of our planet, but also to assist development and so to help lift them out of poverty.

We have called our system of primary child care a 'microplan'. It is concerned with many details—hence the term 'micro'. After adaptation it is intended to form the basis of a nationally-planned system of appropriate technology for primary child care—therefore the word 'plan'. If you do adapt this microplan, you will merely be adapting your own property—it was produced by WHO in response to needs expressed by its Member States. It contains a selection of the most appropriate technologies for primary child care taken from all over the world. As its designers, our task has merely been to assemble them in the most effective form in which they could contribute to the whole of primary health care.

But, why a *system* of primary care? The fundamental property of a system is that 'the whole is more then the sum of its parts'. Thus, although this manual may be useful by itself, it is likely to be much more useful now that it is integrated with a number of other components most of which are in a companion volume—'A Guide for the Community Leader, Manager, and Teacher', which is also available from Oxford University Press. These include a wide variety of evaluation instruments, management targets, and teaching aids. The latter are available from TALC (Teaching Aids at Low Cost, Institute of Child Health, Guildford Street, Great Ormond Street, London WC1N 1EH). The equipment lists for the microplan are coordinated with those of UNICEF. Another component in the 'Manager's Guide' is a program for implementing the microplan in a district and so improving the quality of primary child care there. These varied components promise to be useful as they are, but, when used together, their combined effect is likely to be more than merely additive. We hope therefore that you will adapt it as a system, rather than as fragments, because it is as a system that it promises to be most useful. This does not mean that it should be taken exactly as it is. You can, for example, readily add or remove any drug or disease, or improve on any technology or instrument, and so adapt it to your own needs.

Who is this microplan for? Many of the procedures in primary care are common to all levels of worker, so we have deliberately addressed it to any 'health worker' who can read this manual and who provides primary care, usually with little opportunity to refer children for help. It is the outcome of an attempt to answer the question 'What could a health worker reasonably do for the children who come to him, be they well or sick?' Since there is more to say about what he can do for a sick child than for a healthy one, this has inevitably occupied most of our pages.

Many kind, industrious, and devoted people have contributed to this endeavour, particularly Julie Sulianti Saroso, Ken Newell, Henry Pardoko, David Morley, Jon Rohde, Robert Northrup, Dilip Mahalanabis, Norbert Hirschorn, John Biddulph, Jim Smith, Ed Margulies, Katie Murtagh, Jack Bryant, Otto Wolff, Angel Petros-Barvazian, Alessandro Rossi-Espagnet, Michael Luck, Barbara Pumfrey, and Peter Godwin. Not for the first time and perhaps not the last, we have but provided thread for the pearls of others. We should also like to thank OXFAM, MISEREOR, and the Swedish Government (SIDA) for their help. Finally our labours would never have ended had not Mrs Marlinah Soetardji cheerfully and painstakingly typed out much of the manuscript twenty-five times.

Our task has been a great joy. We look forward to helping anyone who wants to prepare an adaptation, and we will be delighted to share your experience in implementing it. We demand no other recompense than to know that the children in your country are getting the care they need.

Maurice and Felicity King
Soebagio Martodipoero

Contents

for a healthy child on later visits. **4.14** When should he come to the clinic again?

for a child with a sore throat.   **18.14** The child who has stopped eating.
18.15 Caring for a child who is not eating.   **18.16** Tetanus.   **18.17** Caring
for a child who cannot open his mouth.

newborn baby. **26.7** Breast-feeding. **26.8** Expressing breast-milk. **26.9** Flat nipples. **26.10** Engorged breasts. **26.11** Sore nipples. **26.12** Septic breast infection. **26.13** Empty breasts. **26.14** Not enough milk. **26.15** Artificial feeding. **26.15b** 'How much milk does my bottle-fed baby need?' **26.16** Extra water. **26.17** 'Not enough money to buy milk.' **26.18** Eight ways of feeding a baby. **26.19** The baby who does not start to suck. **26.20** The baby who has stopped sucking. **26.21** Not gaining weight. **26.22** The baby who weighs less than 2 kg. **26.23** Jaundice. **26.24** Septicaemia. **26.25** Hypothermia. **26.26** Abnormal breathing. **26.27** Posseting and vomiting. **26.28** Vomiting blood. **26.29** Normal faeces. **26.30** 'Hard faeces.' **26.31** 'Not passing faeces.' **26.32** Diarrhoea. **26.33** Blood in the faeces. **26.34** The sticky cord. **26.35** The umbilicus which does not heal. **26.36** Cellulitis round the umbilicus. **26.37** Umbilical tetanus. **26.38** Umbilical bleeding. **26.39** Conjunctivitis. **26.40** Gonococcal conjunctivitis. **26.41** Dacrocystitis. **26.42** Tetanus, fits, and hypoglycaemia. **26.43** Nappy rash. **26.44** Peeling skin. **26.45** Erythema neonatorum. **26.46** Congenital marks on the skin. **26.47** Septic skin infections. **26.48** Paronychia. **26.49** The abnormally shaped head. **26.50** Abnormalities in the fontanelle. **26.51** Cleft lip or palate. **26.52** Talipes. **25.53** Tongue tie. **26.54** Extra fingers and toes. **26.55** Thrush. **26.56** Breast enlargement. **26.57** Not passing urine. **26.58** Red urine. **26.59** Hydrocoele. **26.59b** No testes. **26.60** Paralysis of the face. **26.61** Erb's palsy. **26.62** Broken clavicle. **26.63** Broken arm or leg. **26.65** Crying. **26.66** TB and leprosy in a child's mother. **26.67** Some help for the mother of a newborn child.

1 Introduction

1.1 The child, the family, and the community

In many countries about a quarter of all the children die before they are five years old. In some districts half of them die. Many of the living children are sick. We can prevent (stop) much of this disease and death. We can care for children in the way this book describes. It explains how we can prevent them becoming ill, and how we can cure them when they are ill.

This book is only about child care. But a child is only healthy when he is part of a healthy happy family. So we must not forget his family, and especially his mother. When she comes to see you, ask her if she wants antenatal (before birth) care? Or help with family planning? Is anyone else in the family sick?

A sick child is unhappy, and his death is a serious loss to his family. So the health of every child is important. But we must keep children healthy for another reason also. Many parents want very big families because they are frightened that some of their children will die. Because parents want big families, too many children are being born. So the number of people in the world is growing too fast. There is not enough land, or schools, or jobs for all the children who grow up each year. Many of them cannot have a good life. Also, if a mother has too many children, she cannot feed and care for them well. If children are born close together, they are less healthy than children born three or more years apart. So we must teach parents to use family planning and have smaller, well-spaced families. But parents will only want smaller families if we stop their children dying. So family planning needs good child care, and good child care needs family planning. This is why we have made family planning the ninth step in caring for a child (5.25).

DON'T FORGET THE REST OF THE FAMILY

A community is a group of people who live and work together, such as the people in a village. A family is part of a community. A good community makes sure that as many families as possible have jobs or land, enough food, and clean water. Plenty of good food, clean water, and loving care are more important for the health of a child than medicine. So a child's family and his community are most important for his health.

A HEALTHY COMMUNITY HAS HEALTHY CHILDREN

Our job as health workers is to work for the people of our community. So we must work with them and their leaders. We must help them to provide the health care they need and want. If the community wants better health care, it may give money to buy drugs, or a place to have a clinic. It may also give us helpers we can train to care for children. We must ask people what they think about the care we give. What do they think is good about it? In what ways is it bad? How do they think we could make it better?

1.2 Quality, and coverage

Often, we can cure sick children and save their lives. Each child we care for is as important to his parents as our own children are to us. Each sick child waiting to see us might be our child. His mother or father might be ourself. An empty cot and a dead child would be as sad for them as they would be for us. So we must care for the children who come to us as if they were our children.

THAT SICK CHILD IS OUR CHILD—HIS PARENTS ARE OURSELVES

We have two objectives (things we must try to reach) in caring for children. Both are difficult. Our first objective is to make the care we give as good as possible – this is its **quality.** Our second objective is to make our care cover ALL the children in a community – this is its **coverage.**

Quality. This book describes how we should care for children. It shows us how a child should be examined, diagnosed, managed, and treated. Giving good quality care like this helps children and their mothers. It also makes our work much more interesting. Sometimes we cannot do all we want to. We may not have all the

1

Don't forget the rest of his family!

What can you do for each of them?

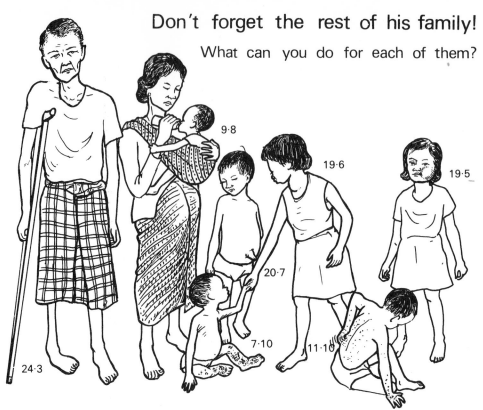

Fig. 1–1 Care for the whole family.

supplies, the equipment, or the time that we need. But there are always many things that we can do. Quality means doing everything as well as possible. Quality is difficult to measure, but we can measure part of it with the quality score (6.8).

Kindness is an important part of quality of care—kindness to a child and to his mother. If he is sick, and she is worried, he needs gentleness and she needs a careful explanation. Kindness is difficult to measure. It is made of many small things.

KINDNESS

Know your mothers and children, recognize them and call them by name. If they are worried, frightened, or in pain, make this less. Don't touch a tender place more than you need to. Clean wounds carefully. Learn how to cause the least possible pain when you give injections (3.5).

If you have to do something painful to an older child, tell him what you are going to do. Explain that ths pain will soon be over. Show him the instruments you are going to use. Tell him to shut his eyes. Comfort him when it is finished.

Give an explanation (5.24) to every mother. Teach her how she can comfort her sick child. For example, explain how she should cool him and wash out his mouth when he has a fever (10.3).

If you have few drugs, keep some to save the lives of seriously ill children. Be ready to see seriously ill children at any time of the day or night.

A mother's time is precious to her, so don't keep her waiting longer than necessary.

Show a mother how to do things, such as making an oral rehydration fluid (9.22). Don't only tell her.

Don't become angry with mothers or tell them they are stupid. Be as kind to an unmarried mother as to any other mother. Her child probably needs special care (6.3).

Never send a child away if you have not seen him. Care for poor mothers with the same kind words that you use for richer mothers. The families who most need our care are often too poor or too frightened to come to us.

GIVE SOME CARE TO EVERYONE.
GIVE MORE CARE TO THOSE IN GREATEST NEED

Coverage. Our job is to care for all the children in our community. So we must know how many of them we care for. Coverage is difficult to measure. We can measure it partly by measuring the 'average yearly visits per child under five' (6.10).

THE FAMILIES WHO MOST NEED OUR CARE ARE OFTEN TOO FRIGHTENED TO COME

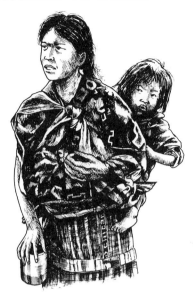

Fig. 1–2 The families who most need our help are often too frightened to come.

There are many sick children and few of us health workers. So the coverage of our care depends partly on the number of children we see each day—the quantity of care we give. This is how much work we do—our output. Quantity of care is easy to measure, and for this we use the 'patients per worker per day' score (6.9).

1.4 Teaching ourselves

Before you can use this manual, you must learn how to find things in it. To make this easier each chapter has many sections. For example, Section 9.3 is the third section in Chapter 9, and Section 4.12 is the twelfth section in Chapter 4. There is *one dot* in each section number, such as 9 dot 3, or 9.3. The figures are also numbered, but the numbers for them have a dash. So 9 *dash* 3 (9–3) is the third figure in Chapter 9. Some of the larger figures, such as Figure 9–18, are made of several smaller pictures. The tables (lists) have *two dots* in them, so 9:3 is the third table in Chapter 9. Sometimes, there are sections missing. For example, there is no Section 1.3. Sometimes there are extra sections. For example, there are Sections 2.2, and 2.2b. There is no Section 2.2a. These numbers showing other parts of the book are called **cross references**. They have been put in brackets like this—(9.3).

You will also need manuals on nutrition and on laboratory methods. The nutrition manual we have chosen is 'Nutrition for Developing Countries.' The laboratory manual is 'A Medical Laboratory for Developing Countries.' Both manuals are by ourselves and are pub-

lished by Oxford University Press. Cross references to the nutrition manual have an 'N' in front of them. N 8.6, for example, tells you how to make a cup-and-spoon feed. Cross references to the laboratory manual have an 'L' in front of them. Section L 11.11b shows you how to make a skin smear for leprosy.

Because this is a book to teach you how to do things, we have put the 'how to do it' parts in bold type like this—

HOW TO LEARN

Try to get a copy of this manual for yourself. Learn from it while you are in school. Look things up in it afterwards. Don't read it from the beginning to end. Don't learn it by heart. Instead, *learn how to use it*.

First read this chapter and be sure you know all the words in its last four sections. Then read Chapter 2 about the diseases of children. After that read about drugs in the first six sections only of Chapter 3. Then read Chapter 5 about caring for a sick child. After that read about malnutrition, cough, diarrhoea and fever (Chapters 8, 9, and 10). Learn about these common problems before you read the rest of the book. Look up the rarer ones. Learn the slogans. If there are any diseases which you will never see, cross them out.

Learn to use the vocabulary index. Read the rules at the beginning of the index carefully. If you cannot use it, this book will not help you much.

Don't go to every cross reference you come to. Go only to the references which will help you. When you go to another section, put a marker in the book, so that you don't lose your place.

Do the multiple choice questions in Booklets A, B and C of Book Two, the 'Guide for the Community Leader, Manager and Teacher.' There are special answer sheets for these which go red when you mark the right answer. There are 25 questions in each multiple choice instrument (question paper). There are three instruments for each

CROSS REFERENCES

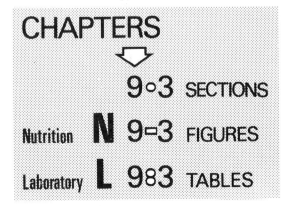

Fig. 1–3 Cross references.

chapter. One instrument from each chapter is in Booklet A, one in Booklet B, and one in Booklet C. Booklet A finds out how much you know at the beginning (pretest). Booklet B is for you to practise with and teach yourself. Booklet C finds out how much you have learnt (post-test). Write in your scores on the page you will find at the end of this manual. The multiple choice questions often tell you the ages and weights of children. Use the weight chart at the back of this book to find if these children are well or badly nourished.

Teach yourself how to do things using the skills check lists in Booklet B.

Find a friend who wants to learn the same chapter as you do. Both of you read it, and then ask each other questions about it. Learning is easier like this.

Write in the margins and empty pages of this book. Copy out parts that interest you. Make it 'your book'.

Try to see all the diseases the manual describes. When you have seen a disease, put a tick by it in the index.

When learning about parts of the body, feel for them in yourself and find them on a friend.

Don't be afraid to use this manual in front of a mother. Tell her you have a helpful book and you would like to look something up. If you don't want her to see you doing this, keep the manual in another room. Go and look at it there.

Different countries sometimes do things in different ways. For example, most countries give BCG on the right upper arm. Some countries give it on the left upper arm. If your country gives BCG on the *left* upper arm, change 'right upper arm' into 'left upper arm' all through this book. You may need to make other changes like this also.

DON'T BE AFRAID TO LOOK IN A BOOK

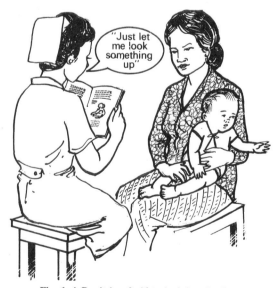

"Just let me look something up"

Fig. 1–4 Don't be afraid to look in a book.

When you do something in the manual, do what the manual says EXACTLY. If you have difficulty, read the manual again.

You will probably not be able to do all the things in this manual. Try to do everything you can.

Manuals are useful but they cannot teach us everything. The best way to learn something is for someone who knows to show us how to do it. So take every chance to learn from other people, and never be afraid to ask questions. Whenever you send a child to someone else for help, go with the child to watch when he is examined. If this is not possible, try to find out how the child was cared for.

LEARN HOW TO LEARN

Mothers bring their sick children to us with some symptom, such as a cough, fever, or a discharging ear. This first or most important symptom we call the **presenting symptom**. There is a chapter, or part of a chapter for each presenting symptom. All the presenting symptoms are in the vocabulary index. Let us take a discharging ear as an example. The causes of this are at the beginning of Section 17.8 like this—*Dolores has discharge (or pain) in her ear'*—acute otitis media, chronic otitis media, otitis externa, or foreign body. The sections which follow tell you about each of these diseases and describe their management and treatment. After this comes Section 17.14, which is called a '*Caring for . . .' section*. These 'Caring for . . .' sections help you to find out which disease is causing a child's symptoms. They are usually at the end of a chapter, and tell you what questions to ask his mother, and how to examine him. Near the end of a 'Caring for . . .' section you will see the word 'Diagnosis'. Under it is a list of all the diseases which can cause that presenting symptom. *The commonest disease comes first, and the rarest last.* Beside each disease is a reference to tell you where to read about its management and treatment.

What should you do if you cannot make a diagnosis? The 'Caring for . . .' sections tell you this also. Most of them end with a few lines called 'Management if diagnosis is difficult'.

KNOWING THIS MANUAL IS LESS IMPORTANT THAN KNOWING HOW TO USE IT

1.5 Teaching our helpers

Our job is to care for all the children in our community. But there are so many of them and so few of us that we need help. If our helpers are going to be useful, we must teach them. So teaching other people how to care for children may be even more important than caring for children ourselves. Our most important helper is a child's mother. This is why we have made explanation

SHOWING SOME TRADITIONAL MIDWIVES THE DANGER SIGNS OF DEHYDRATION

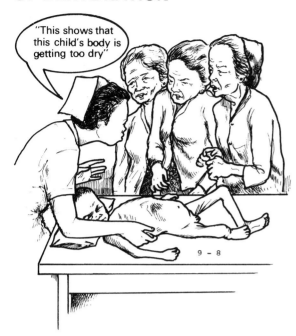

"This shows that this child's body is getting too dry"

9 – 8

Fig. 1–5 Showing some traditional midwives the danger signs of dehydration.

and education (teaching) one of the steps in caring for a sick child (5.24). We need other helpers also, both in the clinic and outside. Perhaps there are so many children to weigh that we should teach another person how to do this. Perhaps we can teach another person how to make some of the clinic records. We will then have more time to examine sick children. If we teach other people to do things, we must be sure they can do them well. So we must look at what they are doing.

If your district has village midwives, teach them a little about some important diseases. Teach them everything in Section 2.12 especially the danger signs to watch for when a child has a cough (8.20), or diarrhoea (9.31). Teach them how to make salt and sugar water (9.22) for a dehydrated child.

TEACHING OTHER PEOPLE MAY BE EVEN MORE IMPORTANT THAN DOING SOMETHING OURSELVES

Two hundred words

1.6 Language

English is not the first language of many readers. Because of this, we have tried to use as few difficult

words as possible. Most of the difficult words are in the vocabulary index. Some of the more common words are in the next few sections. Most of these words have other meanings, but the only meaning we use is the meaning we explain. Read the rest of this chapter carefully. Learn any words you do not know. Take a pencil and paper and describe what they mean in your own language. *If you already know them all, go on to the next chapter.*

1.7 Ordinary words   1.7

We need to know how often something happens. To describe this we use the words **always, usually, sometimes, occasionally, rarely** and **never**. Another word we use is **may**. May means that something can happen, but does not always happen. It is nearly the same as might. For example '. . . a child with a cold *may* have fever . . .'. This means that a cold sometimes causes fever but not always. **Usually** is a very useful word. It means that something happens very often, but not always. For example, 'Children usually walk before they are 18 months old'. This means that most children walk before they are 18 months old, but some do not.

Something happens **regularly**, if it always happens after about the same length of time, like the ticking (noise) of a watch. If something happens **irregularly**, it sometimes happens after a long time, and sometimes after a short time.

Fortunately means something happening which is good. **Unfortunately** means something happening which is bad.

A **substance** is something which is the same all through, and which can be cut up without being spoilt. Water, salt, earth, and blood are substances, but a cup and a shirt are not. They are **things**. Anything which flows, such as water, tea, or milk is a **fluid**. To **dilute** a fluid is to add more water to it. When salt or sugar are mixed with water, they **dissolve**, or make a **solution**. A solution of salt in water is called **saline**. Something which is **transparent** is clear like water, so that you can see through it. **Opaque** is the opposite of transparent. You cannot see through something which is opaque. A **turbid** fluid is cloudy. You cannot see through it clearly.

To **describe** something is to explain it or write it down. To **notice** something is to see it. To **recognize** something is to know what it is when you see it. To check something is to look at it to make sure it is normal. To **evaluate** something is to find out how good or how bad it is. To **increase** something is to make it larger, to **reduce** something is to make it smaller. To **harm** something means to spoil or break it. To **injure** is to harm a person.

Primary means first, **secondary** means second. **Intra-**   1.5
in front of a word means inside, so **intra-abdominal** means inside the abdomen. **Anti-** means against, so an **anti-septic** is against sepsis. **Hypo-** means too little, so **hypo-glycaemia** means too little sugar in the blood. **Hyper-** means too much, so **hyper-tonic** muscles have   1.6
too much tone. **Non-** means not, so a **non-immune** person is not immune to a disease.

De- means without and **hydr-** means water, so **dehy-**

5

drated means without water. The body of a dehydrated child is dry because it lacks water (9.17).

A **stage** is a step that something goes through. As we grow older we go through the stages of being babies, then children, and then adults. An **individual** is one person. A **community** is made of many people who live and work together.

A **decilitre** or **dl** is a tenth of a litre. A **millilitre** or **ml** is a thousandth of a litre. There are 100 ml in a dl. A **microlitre** is a millionth of a litre.

1.8 Nutrition words

Proteins are the substances in food which make or build our bodies (N 3.2). For example, beans, milk, and eggs, contain protein and are **body-building foods. Energy** is the ability to do work. Rice, maize, sugar, and oil are **energy foods** (N 4.2). They keep a child warm, and give him the energy to run about and play. We used to measure energy in calories. Now we measure it in **joules**. There are about four joules in a calorie (N 4.1b). A **vitamin** is a food substance which a child needs in very small amounts. Our bodies cannot make vitamins, so we have to eat them to stay healthy (N 4.4). A **staple food** is the most important food of a country, such as rice, maize, or cassava (N 4.3). **Porridge** is a soft food for young children made from a staple food. A **weight chart** is a special card for young children which shows us how well they are growing (7.1, N 1.3). A **growth-curve** is a line joining the dots for all the weighings on a child's weight chart (N 1.3). A **deficiency** of something is a lack of it, or not enough of it.

1.9 Words for parts of the body

Cells are the very small living 'bricks' from which the body is built. In most parts of the body cells join together to make solid **tissues**, such as muscle tissue, or skin tissue. Blood is a tissue, but it is fluid because the cells are not joined together. There are two kinds of cells in the blood. There are **red cells**, which are filled with a red substance called **haemoglobin**, and **white cells** which fight bacteria. Several kinds of tissue join together to make **organs**, such as the liver or the heart. When several organs work together to do the same job, they are called a **system**. The **respiratory system** is for breathing and the **urinary system** makes urine.

The wet 'skin' inside the mouth, the eyelids, the gut, and the tubes of the respiratory system is called **mucosa**. Any break in the skin or mucosa, which leaves the tissues under it uncovered, is called an **ulcer**. A **duct** is a tube. A **vessel** is a tube containing blood or lymph. **Lymph** is a clear fluid that is made in most tissues and goes back to the blood through lymph vessels. A **vein** is a tube taking blood to the heart. An **artery** is a tube taking blood from the heart to the other tissues.

The skin of the head is called the **scalp**. The brain is inside a box of bones called the **skull**. A thick nerve called the **spinal cord** joins onto the bottom of the brain. The spinal cord comes out through the bottom of the

SOME PARTS OF THE BODY

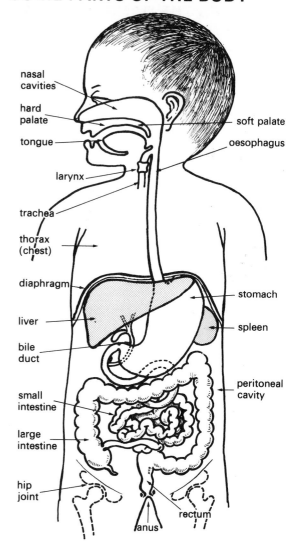

Fig. 1–6 Some parts of the body.

skull, and goes down inside the backbone. We call the backbone the **vertebral column** or **spine**. The **jaws** are the bones that hold the teeth. The **gums** are soft red tissues round the teeth.

The heart and lungs are in the chest or **thorax**. Below the thorax is the **abdomen** which has a soft front made of muscle. Between the thorax and the abdomen there is a thin layer (sheet) of muscle called the **diaphragm**. The diaphragm moves up and down during breathing. The **liver** is under the right side of the diaphragm. The **spleen** is under the left side of the diaphragm. The **umbilicus** is in the middle of the abdominal wall. The fold between the abdominal wall and the leg is called the **inguinal region** or **groin**. The side of the abdomen is called the

loin. The space under the arm, between the arm and the thorax is called the **axilla**. The parts of a child's body that he sits on are called his **buttocks**. The wide bone at the bottom of the spine and abdomen is called the **pelvis**. The **hip** joints are the joints between the legs and the pelvis. The palms are the fronts of the hands. The soles are the bottoms of the feet.

IF YOU CAN UNDERSTAND ALL THESE WORDS YOU CAN UNDERSTAND THE REST OF THE BOOK

The throat or **pharynx** is at the back of the mouth. **Nasal** means belonging to the nose. The **gut** is a tube which goes from the mouth to the **anus** (the hole faeces come out through). A tube called the **oesophagus** takes food from the mouth down through the thorax into a bag called the **stomach**. Food then goes through a tube several metres long called the **small intestine**. After this food goes through a shorter but wider tube called the **large intestine**. The last few centimetres of the gut before the **anus** is called the **rectum**. **Digestion** means breaking down food into very small pieces inside the gut. **Absorption** means taking these small pieces into the blood and lymph through the wall of the gut. **Excretion** means removing waste from the body.

Urine is a watery waste substance which is made in the **kidneys**. Urine goes down tubes called the **ureters** into a bag called the **bladder**. Urine is stored in the bladder until it is passed out through a tube called the **urethra**. The **scrotum** is the bag of skin which contains the **testes** (a boy's sex organs).

The white parts of the eyes are called the **sclera**. The thin wet mucosa over the sclera and the inside of the eyelids is called the **conjunctiva**.

1.10 Words for sick children

A child who has been born after nine months in the uterus is **full term**. If he is born too early he is **preterm**.

We use the word **well** in two ways. Well can mean good. Well also means healthy. The things which happen in healthy children are **normal**. Anything which should not happen to a healthy child is abnormal. For example, yellow urine is normal, red urine is abnormal. Something may be **mildly** (a little) abnormal or it may be **grossly** (very very) abnormal. There are two stages between mildly and grossly abnormal. For these we use the words **moderately** and **severely**. If we look for something and are sure it is not there, we say it is **negative**. If we are not sure about something, we say it is **doubtful**. These stages can be scored with 'plusses' like this: negative 0, doubtful ±, mildly abnormal +, moderately abnormal ++, severely abnormal +++, and grossly abnormal ++++. Sometimes, instead of saying grossly, we say very severely. These plusses are useful in making records. For example, if we are not sure that we can feel a child's spleen, we write 'spleen ±'. If he has a very very large spleen, we write 'spleen ++++'. We never write more than four plusses.

THE URINARY SYSTEM

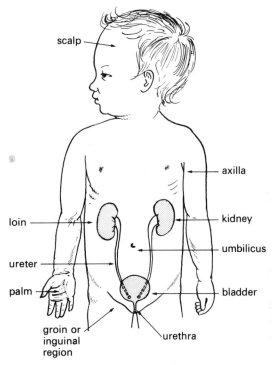

Fig. 1–7 The urinary system.

A child who throws food or fluid out of his stomach is **vomiting**. Sometimes the word sick is used to mean vomit, but here we use **sick** for any child who is not well. We use the word '**ill**' in a special way, for any child who is not well in the whole of himself and who shows the signs found in Table 5:2. To **treat** a child is to try to cure his disease. To **cure** him is to make him well again. To **recover** is to become well. A wound which **heals** cures itself. To **form** something is to make it. A child has a **deformity** if his body has an abnormal shape. Polio (24.4) and leprosy (12.1) cause deformities. They also cause **disability**. This means they stop a child doing

MILD, MODERATE, SEVERE AND GROSS

Negative ⊚   Moderate ✛✛

Doubtful ✛   Severe ✛✛✛

Mild ✛   Gross ✛✛✛✛

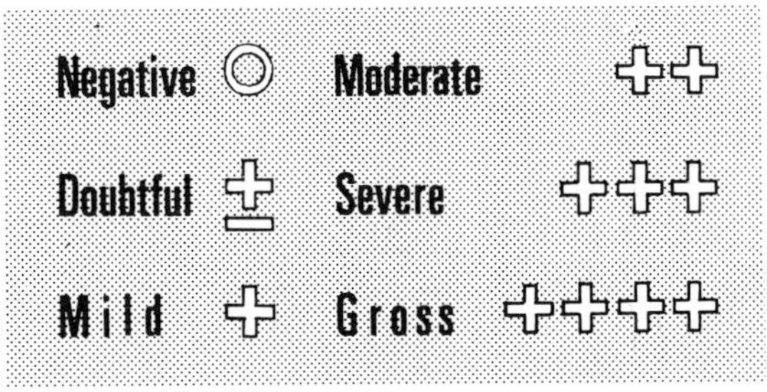

Fig. 1–8 Mild, moderate, severe, and gross.

1.8

1.9

1.10

things, such as walking or using his hands. A child with a disability may be unable to go to a normal school when he is young, or work when he is older. A **serious** disease is one which may kill a child or make him very ill, or cause deformity or disability. Both polio and leprosy can fix the tissues around a child's joint so that it does not move normally. A joint like this has a **contracture**.

A child who becomes suddenly sick with a disease has an **attack** of it. He is a **case** of that disease. If he goes to a clinic or hospital, he becomes a **patient**. When someone becomes ill, the things that he feels are wrong with himself, such as diarrhoea or pain, are called **symptoms**. Anything which a health worker sees, feels, or hears to be wrong with a patient, is called a **sign**. Pale lips, a stiff neck, a large spleen, or wheezing are all signs. Some things, such as a cough, can be both a symptom and a sign. A patient can say he has a cough, and a health worker can hear it. The difference between symptoms and signs is useful in adults. But a young child cannot tell us what he feels, so we do not know what his own symptoms are. So, in a young child we use the word symptom for anything which his mother says is abnormal. We use the word sign for anything that we find is abnormal.

Most children have several symptoms. But there are usually one or two important symptoms, for which a mother brings a child to see us. We call these his **presenting symptoms**. All common presenting symptoms are in the vocabulary index. To present means to show. 'Measles usually presents with fever and a cough' means that children with measles usually come to us because of fever or cough. **Local** means in one place in the body only. **General** means all over the body. So a **local** symptom such as a painful leg, is in one part of a child only. A general symptom, such as fever, is all over him.

A child becomes sick when part or all of his body has been harmed, and does not work normally. The abnormal place is called the **lesion**. Some lesions, such as boils or insect bites are local and small, and the rest of his body is normal. Other lesions, such as fever or dehydration, make the whole of his body abnormal, so the lesion is general. A child may have only one lesion, or he may have many lesions all over him, outside on his skin and inside him also. When he has many lesions on the skin he has a **rash**. Lesions which are the same on the right and left sides of the body are **symmetrical**. Lesions which are different on the right and left sides, are **asymmetrical**.

The word **disease** means much more than a lesion or a symptom. Disease means all the symptoms and lesions a child has, how they change, what causes them, and other things also. Measles, for example, is a disease. A virus causes measles (2.2). A child with measles has many lesions on his skin (the rash), in his eyes (red eyes), and inside his mouth (Koplik's spots). He usually recovers in two weeks, and does not become sick in the same way again. So, when we use the word 'measles', we mean all this.

Each disease has its own pattern ('picture') of signs and symptoms in time. In measles, for example, Koplik's spots come on about the third day of the fever, and the rash on about the fourth day. Whooping cough is another disease. It also causes a cough and fever, but there is no rash. The cough is different and lasts longer. So, measles and whooping cough have different patterns of signs and symptoms in time. If we can recognize different disease patterns, we can find out which disease a child has. When we do this we are diagnosing his disease or making the **diagnosis**.

Often, children have more than one disease, such as scabies and malnutrition. Sometimes, one disease causes another. The second disease is called a **complication**. For example, children with measles sometimes get pneumonia, so that pneumonia is a complication of measles. A severely ill child who needs treatment quickly is called an **emergency**.

A DEFORMED AND DISABLED CHILD

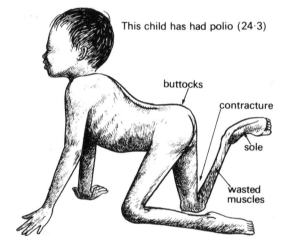

This child has had polio (24·3)

buttocks

contracture

sole

wasted muscles

Fig. 1–9 A deformed and disabled child.

We shall use the word **caring** to mean everything we do for a child. **Managing** him means deciding what to do for him (5.21). To **observe** a child means to watch carefully to see what happens to him. For example, we might ask his mother to bring him next day.

A child who is awake and interested in what is going on around him is **conscious**. If he seems to be asleep, but we cannot wake him, he is **unconscious** or in **coma**. If he is neither completely conscious, nor completely unconscious, he is **drowsy** (abnormally sleepy). If a child is **delirious**, he talks nonsense. He does not know where he is, and may not be able to recognize people. Fever often makes children delirious. If a child is always moving about abnormally, and will not stay still, he is **restless**. If he is unhappy, and easily becomes angry, he is **irritable**.

If a part of a child's body hurts when we touch it, it is **tender**. The opposite of tender is **painless**. If a skin lesion

itches, it feels as if it needs to be scratched. If something is larger than normal, it is **swollen** or **enlarged**. If it is half way between hard and soft, it is **firm**. A **lump** is an abnormal swelling which we can feel to be separate from the tissues round it. A swelling which feels as if it were filled with fluid is **fluctuant**. **Distended** means filled up more than normal, usually with a fluid.

A child's **faeces** or **stools** are the solid waste from his body, which he passes or **excretes** (throws away). The first stools of a newborn baby are called **meconium**. **Diarrhoea** means passing many liquid stools. **Constipation** means passing few stools, or none, or passing hard stools. **Frequency** means passing urine often. A **specimen** is some blood, or urine, or faeces which is to be examined in a laboratory. If an abnormal fluid comes out of a child's body anywhere, it is called a **discharge**. **Mucus** is the thick sticky fluid that comes from his nose when he has a cold. **Pus** is the yellow liquid inside a boil. A swelling filled with pus is called an **abscess**. **Pyogenic** organisms cause the body to make pus. **Purulent** means containing pus. If a child coughs up pus or mucus, we call it **sputum**.

To **spit** is to throw something out of the mouth. To **inhale** or **inspire** is to breathe air into the respiratory system. A child can also inhale fluid or vomit. To **expire** is to breathe out. Expire has a second meaning—a drug or vaccine **expires** when it becomes old and useless.

Waste substances are thrown away by the body in the urine or in the faeces. But the word **wasting** of the body means becoming thin. A child who goes yellow is **jaun-diced**. If he is pale because there is not enough haemoglobin in his blood, he is **anaemic** (22.1). If his lips and skin become blue, he is **cyanosed** (8.2).

Muscles are tissues which can **contract** (become shorter) or **relax** (become longer). Even when a child is quiet and not moving his arms and legs, his muscles are contracting a little. This kind of muscle contraction is called muscle **tone**. The muscle tone of a healthy child holds his arms and legs in their normal position when he is moved. When a child is 'ill' (5.15) they stop contracting and making this tone. When we move him or shake him, his arms and legs hang from him as if there was no muscle in them. He is **'floppy'** or **hypotonic** (too little muscle tone). Muscles which cannot contract are **paralysed**. Tetanus (18.16) and some other diseases make muscles contract too much, so that they have too much tone and are **hypertonic**. Very tight hypertonic muscles are in **spasm**.

There is another kind of muscle (smooth muscle) round the tubes inside the body. There is smooth muscle round the walls of the blood vessels, the gut, and the respiratory system. When this muscle relaxes (becomes longer), these tubes **dilate** (become wider). When this muscle contracts they become narrower.

If one of the tubes of the body becomes blocked, it is **obstructed**. Something which goes into an abnormal place in a child, such as a bead into his ear, is called a **foreign body**.

If you know these words you will probably be able to understand anything written in the rest of the book.

CHANGES NECESSARY IN THIS BOOK

Perhaps you are working in a country where BCG is given on the left arm, not the right arm (as in this book). Or perhaps there is no sickle cell anaemia in your country. If there are changes write them in here.

2 Disease in the child and the community

2.1 Children's diseases

The two most common kinds of disease in children are **malnutrition** and **infection**. A malnourished child does not eat enough of the right foods. An infected child has harmful organisms growing inside him. Many children are both malnourished and infected, and these two kinds of disease often make each other worse (7.5). All other kinds of disease are much less important than these two. Malnutrition is described in Chapter 7, so this chapter is mostly about harmful organisms and the infections they cause.

Sometimes, a child becomes sick because of an **accident** (14.1), such as falling out of a tree. Some diseases, such as bed-wetting, are abnormalities in what a child does, or how he behaves. They are called **behaviour diseases**. Occasionally, a child is born with an abnormality. This may be a **hereditary disease** like sickle cell anaemia, which he had when he was conceived. Or it may be a **congenital** disease, such as a cleft palate (26.51). Congenital diseases are caused by abnormal growth while a child is in the uterus. Occasionally, some tissue in a child's body grows too much, and he has a **tumour**.

These are the diseases of young children. They are different from the diseases of adults.

Some diseases last longer than others. Measles, cholera, and pneumonia, for example, last a short time. They come quickly and a child recovers quickly, or dies. Acute means for a short time, sudden and severe, so these are **acute** diseases. Other diseases, such as TB or leprosy, come more slowly and last much longer. They either kill a child slowly, or he recovers slowly, or he goes on being ill. Chronic means for a long time (months or years), so TB and leprosy are **chronic** diseases.

Some diseases are more common than others. Every day you will see children with colds. But you will only see a child with a club foot (26.52) once a year, or less often. Some diseases, such as diarrhoea, are common in every district. Other diseases, such as malaria, are common in some districts, but you never see them in other districts. Learn about the common diseases where you work. Don't learn about diseases which you will never see.

Some diseases are less serious than others. For example, colds and mild attacks of diarrhoea cure themselves. Other diseases, such as pneumonia, make a child very sick and may kill him. Purulent meningitis, always kills a child if you don't treat him.

Drug treatment helps some diseases more than others. For example, drugs don't help most kinds of diarrhoea (9.30), but they can cure pneumonia and save a child's life. When we treat a child, we must ask ourselves—What difference will our treatment make? Expensive drugs are wasted if we give them to children who are going to recover anyway. Most clinics have few drugs. So we must look for the children who need our drugs most. Our drugs can help these children most and save their lives. In later chapters you will learn who these children are.

We can fight diseases in different ways. Sometimes, we can stop or **prevent** a disease before it begins. But, if a child is already sick, we try to **cure** him. We must keep

Table 2:1   Children's Diseases

Common

not getting enough of the right food to eat	*MALNUTRITION	
harmful organisms living inside a child	*INFECTIONS	insects worms fungi protozoa bacteria viruses
injury or poisoning	*ACCIDENTS	
behaving in the wrong way	*BEHAVIOUR DISEASES	
given to a child by his parents	*HEREDITARY DISEASES	
mistakes in the way a child's body grows in the womb	*CONGENITAL DISEASES	

Less and less common

Uncommon

the abnormal growth of a tissue	*TUMOURS

children healthy, so prevention is better than cure. Prevention is usually cheaper than cure. Fortunately, we can prevent most serious children's diseases. The nutrition book tells you how to prevent malnutrition (N 10.1). Here you can learn how to prevent infectious diseases (2.7) and accidents (14.1).

2.2 Harmful organisms

All living things are called **organisms**. We are organisms, so are children and chickens. Trees and buffaloes are large organisms, and ants are small ones. There are also many organisms which are so much smaller than ants that we cannot see them. 'Micro-' means small, so we call them **micro-organisms**. We can only see them through a **microscope**. When you explain micro-organisms to mothers, call them 'very small plants and animals'.

Most micro-organisms live in the soil, or in water, and do not harm children. Many are useful and help the soil. There are micro-organisms almost everywhere. They are on this book, on our hands, in our mouths, and all over the clinic. We call the organisms that live in a place its **flora**. The soil has a flora of many kinds of organisms. A forest, a river, the skin, and a child's gut (9.2) all have a flora of organisms.

Some organisms are harmful. For example, an **insect** causes scabies (11.10), and several kinds of **worm** (helminth) live in the gut. Worms lay **ova** (eggs) which are passed in the stools and hatch into young worms called **larvae** (21–1).

The micro-organisms which cause malaria, amoebic dysentery, and giardiasis are very small animals called **protozoa**. The micro-organisms which cause thrush are like very small white plants, and are called **fungi**.

Bacteria are another kind of micro-organism. They are smaller than protozoa. They cause skin sepsis, boils, typhoid, TB, and some kinds of diarrhoea. The bacteria which cause boils are round, like small balls, and we call them **cocci**. The bacteria which cause TB and leprosy, are long like pencils, and we call them **bacilli**. Bacteria like snakes are called **spirochaetes**. They cause Vincent's stomatitis (18.7).

Viruses are the smallest micro-organisms. Viruses cause measles, polio (poliomyelitis), chickenpox, colds and herpes (11.15). Unfortunately, *we have no drugs to kill viruses*, but we do have drugs to kill all the larger organisms. Fortunately, most children with virus infections recover by themselves.

All the harmful organisms which live in a child and cause disease are called **parasites**. But we shall only use the word parasite for 'malaria parasite' (10.7).

When harmful organisms go into a child and live in him, he is **infected**. If they grow in him and make him sick, he has an **infectious disease**. We can diagnose an infectious disease. We can find the organisms that are causing it. Sometimes, a laboratory can help us to find them. A laboratory can find the ova of worms in the stool, or malaria parasites in the blood. A small health centre laboratory can find only the larger organisms. It

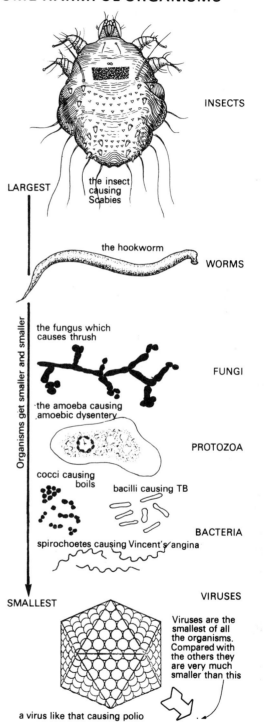

SOME HARMFUL ORGANISMS

2.2

2.1

INSECTS

the insect causing Scabies

LARGEST

the hookworm

WORMS

Organisms get smaller and smaller

the fungus which causes thrush

FUNGI

the amoeba causing amoebic dysentery

PROTOZOA

cocci causing boils

bacilli causing TB

BACTERIA

spirochoetes causing Vincent's angina

SMALLEST

VIRUSES

Viruses are the smallest of all the organisms. Compared with the others they are very much smaller than this

a virus like that causing polio

Fig. 2–1 Some harmful organisms.

cannot find viruses. A laboratory is so useful for diagnosis that every health centre should have one.

2.2b Killing organisms on things—sterilizing

We use drugs to kill organisms inside people. But organisms often leave infected people and go onto things, such as thermometers and syringes. We can kill these organisms with strong chemicals called **antiseptics** and **disinfectants** (3.11). We can also kill organisms by heat, either by boiling, or in the steam of a pressure cooker (6.13). Something such as a needle, on which all organisms have been killed, is **sterile**. We must sterilize instruments. This is very important.

Some parts of the body, such as the brain and CSF (15.2), have *no* organisms in them. Any organisms that go into them are harmful. So needles which go into the CSF must be completely sterile. They must have *NO organisms of any kind on them*. Other parts of the body, such as the mouth, already have many ordinary organisms in them. A few more ordinary organisms on a thermometer or spatula cause no harm. But harmful organisms from a sick child are dangerous if they get into the mouth of a healthy child. So, we must boil a spatula after we have used it. If we do not boil a spatula, it can carry harmful organisms from a sick child to a healthy child. But, if a few ordinary organisms get onto it, they cause no harm.

Cold does not kill organisms—it stops them growing and keeps them alive. So we keep live vaccines (4.3) in a refrigerator. If you put something in a refrigerator, it does *not* become sterile.

**HEAT KILLS ORGANISMS,
COLD KEEPS THEM ALIVE**

Infection in a child

2.3 The fight between a child and his organisms

When harmful organisms go inside a child his body fights them. If his body can fight them well he is **immune** to them. If he has a strong immunity, his body wins the fight. His body kills the organisms and he stays healthy. If his immunity is weak the organisms win and make him ill or kill him. When organisms make a child ill, they multiply (become many) until there are many millions of organisms inside him. Often, a child has some immunity but not enough to win the fight completely. The organisms can only grow slowly and he is mildly ill.

A strong healthy older child is immune to most harmful organisms. But children who are newborn, preterm (26.22), or malnourished, cannot fight organisms so well. These children have little immunity, so they lose the fight and infections easily kill them (26.24). So we must try to increase a child's immunity to infectious diseases.

Occasionally, harmful organisms live in a healthy immune person, but they do not make him sick. They live in his gut or on his skin or in his throat. Sometimes they spread and harm other people, especially young children. If healthy people carry harmful organisms in this way, we call them **carriers**.

A CHILD WITH A BOIL

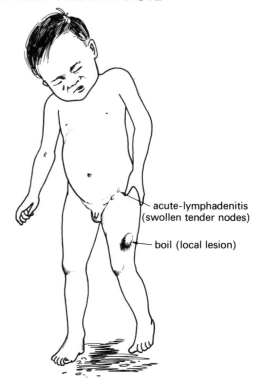

acute-lymphadenitis (swollen tender nodes)

boil (local lesion)

Fig. 2–2 A child with a boil.

2.4 Acute septic infection and acute inflammation

If harmful organisms are living in a child he has an **infection**. If organisms grow in his tissues, they cause signs such as swelling and redness. These are the signs of **inflammation**. Acute infection and inflammation can happen anywhere in the body. But we can see signs most easily in the skin, so we will describe them in the skin.

Local and general signs. The skin round an acute inflammatory lesion, such as a boil, becomes **red, swollen, warm,** and **painful** (2–2). These are the **local** (in one place) **signs** of acute infection. A boil is a **local lesion**. The top of a boil becomes yellow, it breaks open, and pus comes out. After this a crust forms, and the redness and swelling slowly go. A big boil leaves a scar.

**REDNESS, WARMTH, SWELLING, AND PAIN
ARE THE *LOCAL* SIGNS
OF ACUTE INFECTION**

Bacteria (cocci) cause boils. They grow in the skin. They make poisons which cause the blood vessels to become wider (dilate), so that there is more blood in them. This extra warm blood makes the lesion look red and feel warmer. Fluid and white cells come out of the blood vessels into the tissues. The fluid makes the tissues swell and the white cells attack the bacteria. If there are many white cells in the tissues they form **pus**. Pus is a mixture of dead white cells and millions of bacteria. The white cells in the lesion are called **pus cells**. A lesion full of pus is called an **abscess**. A boil is a small abscess.

Only some kinds of bacteria cause the tissues to make pus. We call these bacteria **pyogenic** (pus-making). If a lesion has pyogenic bacteria, acute inflammation, and pus, it is **septic**. Tonsillitis, otitis media, pneumonia, pyoderma, and injection abscesses are all septic infections caused by pyogenic bacteria.

A child with a strong immunity can fight bacteria which attack his tissues. He can keep the bacteria close to the place where they first came into him. They can only cause a small local lesion, and the rest of his body is healthy. But, if his immunity is less, his local lesion grows large. Harmful substances from it go into his body and make him 'ill' (5.15). He has fever, and a fast pulse. He becomes irritable and stops playing and eating. These are the **general** (all over the body) **signs** of a severe acute

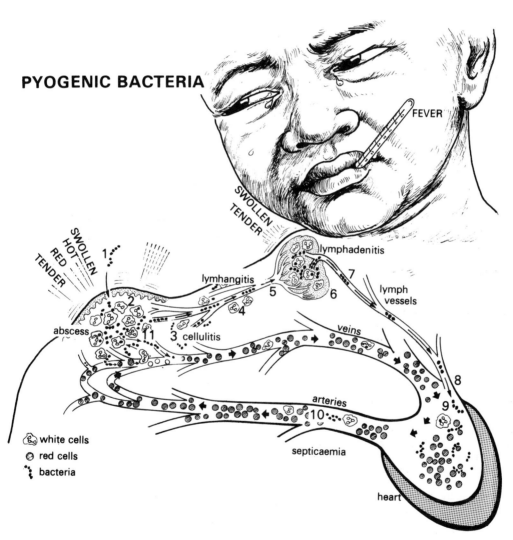

PYOGENIC BACTERIA

FEVER

SWOLLEN TENDER

SWOLLEN HOT RED TENDER

1

lymphadenitis

lymhangitis

5   6   7

lymph vessels

4

abscess

2   11   3 cellulitis

veins

8

9

arteries

10

septicaemia

heart

white cells
red cells
bacteria

2.3
2.4

Fig. 2–3 Pyogenic bacteria spreading in a child. Bacteria (1) go into a child through his skin and multiply. White cells come out of the blood and form an abscess (2) filled with pus. Some of the white cells eat bacteria. Bacteria spread in the tissues round the abscess and cause cellulitis (3). The bacteria go into the lymph vessels and cause lymphangitis (4). They go through the lymph vessels (5) to the lymph nodes and cause lymphadenitis (6). They get out of the lymph vessels (7) and back into the blood (8) and (9). Bacteria multiply in the blood and cause septicaemia (10). Sometimes bacteria go into the blood from the local lesion (11).

infection. If a child has no immunity he loses the fight with his bacteria completely. They spread through him, and grow in his blood. This is called **septicaemia** and is very serious. A child with septicaemia becomes cold and shocked (14.2), and may die.

FEVER, A FAST PULSE, AND AN 'ILL' CHILD ARE THE *GENERAL* SIGNS OF AN ACUTE INFECTION

Spreading septic infection on the skin. If bacteria start to spread through the tissues, the redness and swelling round a septic lesion become larger. Spreading inflammation like this is dangerous. We call it **cellulitis.**

Infection also spreads in the lymphatic system. Lymph is a clear fluid which is formed slowly in most healthy tissues. It goes back into the blood through small tubes called **lymph vessels** (19–1). These lymph vessels take lymph to small organs which are shaped like beans. We call these organs **lymph nodes** (2–4). These nodes can usually kill any bacteria in the lymph. Sometimes, bacteria grow in a node and cause inflammation. The node becomes swollen, painful, and *tender*—**acute septic lymphadenitis.** This is common, but it is not usually serious. Sometimes the infected lymph node swells, and an abscess full of pus forms. Because acute lymphadenitis is an important sign, you must know where to look for large tender lymph nodes. Lymph from each part of the body goes to special nodes. You can see these in Figures 19–1 and 19–1b. **Chronic septic lymphadenitis** (large firm *not* tender nodes) is very common but not serious (19.2).

Occasionally, bacteria grow and cause inflammation in the lymph vessels—**lymphangitis.** These inflamed lymph vessels make a red line on the skin. This line goes from the local lesion to the nearest lymph nodes. Lymphangitis is much *less* common and much *more* serious than acute lymphadenitis. It is difficult to see in children with dark skins. Lymphangitis is a sign of serious infection which is spreading quickly. Bacteria easily go from the infected lymph vessels into the blood and cause septicaemia.

Fortunately, most bacteria do not go beyond the local lesion. So most septic infections are not serious. But we must watch carefully for signs that a skin infection is spreading. We must watch for cellulitis, lymphangitis, and severe lymphadenitis, fever, and an 'ill' child. Organisms may go from his tissues and grow in his blood. He may die from septicaemia, so we must treat him *quickly.* Fortunately, this is usually easy. We can give him penicillin or sulphadimidine.

THE DANGER SIGNS OF SEPTIC INFECTION ARE SPREADING SWELLING AND REDNESS, LYMPHANGITIS, SEVERE LYMPHADENITIS, FEVER, AND AN 'ILL' CHILD

2.5 Other septic infections

Septic infections are common inside the body. The names of these infections usually end in '**-itis**'. A child can have bronchitis in his bronchi, otitis media in his ears, osteomyelitis in his bones, and meningitis in his meninges. These infections are deep inside him, so we cannot see inflamed lymph vessels (lymphangitis), or feel swollen tender lymph nodes (lymphadenitis). But we can see the general signs of an acute infection, such as fever, and an 'ill' child. There are also special local symptoms for infections in each part of the body. Ear infections cause pain and discharge. Gut infections cause diarrhoea. Infections in the bronchi cause coughing. These local symptoms help us to diagnose acute infections inside the body.

2.6 Other kinds of inflammation and infection

Chronic septic infection. Sometimes, a child does not have enough immunity to win the fight against his infecting organisms. So he does not recover. But he does not lose the fight completely. He does not die from septicaemia. Instead, the organisms stay inside his local lesion for a long time and his disease becomes chronic. This can happen if you do not give him enough drugs when you treat his acute infection. If you do not treat otitis media (17.10), or skin ulcers (11.7) carefully, they easily become chronic.

THE SIGNS OF ACUTE SEPTIC INFECTION

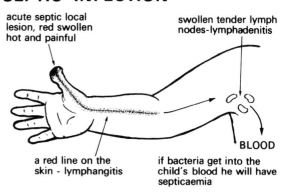

acute septic local lesion, red swollen hot and painful

swollen tender lymph nodes-lymphadenitis

a red line on the skin - lymphangitis

if bacteria get into the child's blood he will have septicaemia

BLOOD

Fig. 2–4 The signs of acute septic infection.

Primary and secondary infection. Organisms sometimes help one another to cause harm. The first kind of organism to go into a child causes a **primary infection.** It may be a virus (as in measles), or a fungus (as in ringworm), or an insect (as in scabies). Then pyogenic bacteria go into the harmed tissues and cause pus to form. This **secondary infection** is common in measles, ringworm, and scabies. It may cause more harm than the primary infection. Often, as in measles, we have no drug to kill the first organism. But we can kill the pyogenic bacteria which cause the secondary infection.

TB, viruses, and toxins. TB is a chronic disease and causes chronic inflammation. It does not usually cause pus to form. It does not cause septicaemia, but it may spread and cause lesions in many parts of the body (13–1).

Viruses cause a different kind of inflammation. They live inside the cells of the body and can harm or kill them. Viruses do not cause pus to form. But the general signs of infection are the same.

The bacteria which cause tetanus (18.16) and diphtheria (18.12) stay in the local lesion. They don't go into the blood and cause septicaemia. Instead, they stay in the local lesion and make poisons (toxins) which harm other parts of the body.

2.7 The paths of infection

Most harmful organisms can live only inside people. So they have to go from one person to another. They have to leave an infected person, move across, and go into a healthy person. They can go from one child to another, or from adults to children. When organisms go from person to person like this, they spread (are transmitted) in a community.

Organisms have found many paths for leaving an infected person, moving across, and going into a healthy person. Each organism has its own special path. If we can cut or block these paths, we can prevent infectious dis-

HOW HARMFUL ORGANISMS ARE SPREAD

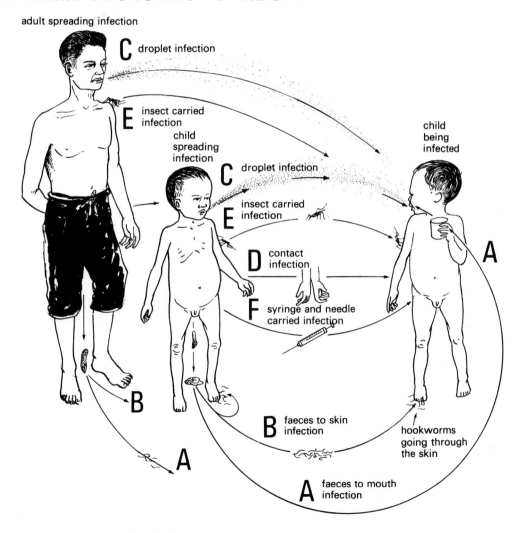

Fig. 2–6 How harmful organisms are spread.

eases spreading. Occasionally, we can stop organisms leaving people. Often we can stop them moving across to another person. Sometimes we can stop them going into another person. We can also make a child's body strong, so he can easily fight harmful organisms when they are inside him—we can increase his immunity.

Faeces-to-mouth infections (Path A). Many harmful organisms live in the gut, and leave the body in the faeces. Faeces may contain the ova of worms, the bacteria or viruses causing diarrhoea, or the viruses which cause hepatitis or polio. So, faeces are very dangerous. Organisms which come out of the body in faeces usually go into another person through his mouth. Organisms from faeces may get into a child's drinking water, or into his food. They can get into his food on dirty hands or on the feet of infected flies (9.8). They get onto his hands when he touches something dirty, and go into his mouth when he sucks his fingers.

We can prevent faeces-to-mouth infections. We can teach people to pass faeces into a latrine. Unfortunately, people sometimes cannot do this and they are difficult to teach. We can also boil a child's drinking water. His mother should wash her hands before she touches his food. She should teach him to wash his hands before he eats. She should cover his food, so that flies cannot walk on it (9–5).

Faeces-to-skin infections (Path B). Some worms go out of the body in the faeces, and come in again through the skin. Hookworm ova, for example, are passed in the faeces. They hatch into larvae on the ground. If a child walks or sits on these hookworms, they bite their way through his skin (21–2). Sometimes, a child with hookworms reinfects himself and infects other children (21–1). *Strongyloides* also spreads this way (21.6). Fresh faeces on the skin is not dangerous. Faeces is only dangerous after ova have had time to hatch and become larvae. This takes some days.

If people use latrines, and wear shoes, we can prevent this kind of infection.

Droplet infections (Path C). When a person with a respiratory infection coughs or sneezes, droplets (very small drops) of sputum go into the air. These droplets contain millions of bacteria and viruses. If a healthy child inhales them he may become infected. Children get TB, measles, pneumonia, whooping cough, and upper respiratory infections like this.

Droplet infections are difficult to prevent. The best way to prevent TB is to find all infectious adults and treat them. We can also teach TB patients to swallow their sputum and not to spit onto the floor.

Contact infections (Path D). Contact means touching. Organisms on the skin can spread if an infected person touches a healthy person. Scabies, skin sepsis, and ringworm spread like this. The pus from a child with a septic skin lesion contains millions of bacteria. These

bacteria easily spread to another person who touches him.

Colds too probably spread by contact. If a child touches his nose, he covers his hands with viruses. If another person touches the child's hand and then his own nose, he gets the cold.

If something has been used by another infected person it can infect a child. For example, organisms from an infected patient can go onto towels, thermometers, and forceps. Organisms from these things can infect the next patient they are used for. Organisms can also go onto tables and chairs, or onto a health worker's hands and infect them.

If we wash we can prevent contact infections. We should wash our hands each time we examine a child. We should also teach mothers and children to wash their hands more often. We can boil infected instruments, or sterilize them in the steam of a pressure cooker. If we cannot boil something, we can kill the organisms on it with a disinfectant, such as lysol.

Infections carried by insects (Path E). Malaria is an infection carried by an insect. A mosquito bites an infected person and drinks his blood. The blood contains malaria parasites. These parasites live and grow in the mosquito. If it bites a child, it infects him.

We can prevent malaria. We can kill mosquitoes with insecticides (insect-killing 'medicine'). We can also drain away the water from the places where mosquitoes lay eggs. A mother can put gauze (net) on the windows of her house, and a net over her sleeping child.

Infections carried by syringes and needles (Path F). If we don't sterilize needles and syringes, they can carry organisms from one child to another child. This is not a common way of spreading infection. But health workers *cause it* so we *must* prevent it. Injection abscesses (3.6) and syringe jaundice (22.10) are caused like this.

These are some of the ways harmful organisms spread. There are other ways. For example, the ova of a worm called *Schistosoma haematobium* (bilharzia) are passed in a child's urine. These ova hatch in water. The larvae go into a snail, and then out of the snail into another child through his skin (23–4)—'urine-to-skin infection'.

2.8 Helping a child to fight infections

If a child has a strong immunity, harmful organisms cannot easily infect him and make him ill. We can increase his immunity in two ways—better nutrition and immunization.

Better nutrition. This helps to prevent infections becoming severe. Measles and diarrhoea, for example, are much less severe in well-nourished children. Well-nourished children get diarrhoea less often than malnourished ones. So, improving a child's nutrition helps to prevent infection (7.5).

Immunization. We can give a child special medicines called **vaccines** (4.2). There are useful vaccines against measles, polio, tetanus, diphtheria, whooping cough, and TB. There are no vaccines against most other diseases, such as diarrhoea or pneumonia.

GOOD NUTRITION PREVENTS INFECTION

2.9 Beliefs (what people think) and customs (what people do)

We have used English words for diseases such as malaria and sepsis. We describe how we believe they are caused and how we treat them. But a sick child's mother, and especially his grandmother, may believe that his disease is caused in a different way. For example, she may think that worms cause kwashiorkor (7.10). She may want to treat it in the way her custom says is right. She may be frightened of our way. Her belief is important. If we don't make her want to do something our way, she will do it her way.

A GOOD CUSTOM

GOOD

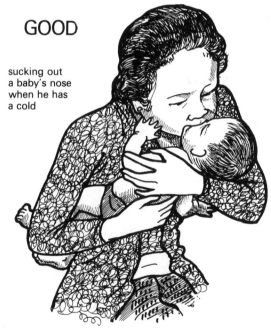

sucking out a baby's nose when he has a cold

Fig. 2–7 A good custom.

Mothers may have their own names for the diseases which we call measles and whooping cough. Their word for measles may mean exactly the same thing as our word, or it may not. For example, in some countries the same word is used for measles and chickenpox.

Sometimes, we use a word that was first used by the ordinary mothers of a country. Kwashiorkor, for example, is a word that was first used by mothers in Ghana. Some other languages also have their own word for this disease. But there is seldom a local word for meningitis, and never a word for septicaemia. Also, there may be special local words for which there is no English word. For example, the Javanese word 'sawan' means any disease causing fever and fits in babies. You must know the local names for diseases in your community, and what they mean, so ask about them. If there is a local word, it shows that the disease is common. Find out if they are different from the words for disease which we use in this book.

Each community has its own special beliefs about the causes of disease, and customs of treatment. For example, in some communities mothers think that they should cover a child's fontanelle. They think that if they don't cover it air may get into him through his fontanelle and make him ill. They do not know that air cannot get into a child this way. Mothers in other communities think that it is dangerous to treat a child with measles before his rash has come. They think that treatment may 'push his disease inside him' and make it worse. In another district people cut off a child's uvula (18–2) to cure a cough. If he has a fit they give him lemon juice, or cow's urine.

What a mother believes helps to decide what she does. So beliefs are important, because they are tied to customs. But customs are more important, because customs decide what a mother *does* for her child. When we teach mothers we try to change what they *do*. We try to change their *behaviour*. Changing their beliefs is less important.

Some customs are good. For example, the people of Madura pour water over a child with a fit. This is a good treatment, because a fit is often caused by high fever, and water cools him (10.4). In some communities mothers suck the mucus out of their babies noses with their mouths. This is also a good custom. Breast-feeding a child until he is three years old is another good custom. If mothers have good customs like this, tell them they are good, and let them do them.

Many customs make no difference to health. In one community mothers rub the chest of a sick child with a coin. In another community a mother takes a brush with her when she takes her newborn baby out of the house. In some communities a pregnant woman must not sew. These customs do not make a child's health better or worse, but they comfort his mother. So you do not need to say anything about them in your teaching.

Sometimes we do not know if a custom is helpful or harmful. Most traditional (due to custom) medicines are like this. They do not cure disease, and most of them do nothing. Some are useful placebo (3.1) treatment. They often *seem* to cure people because most diseases cure themselves without treatment. Some of these medicines may be harmful, but we do not know if they are harmful. Say nothing about them, except that they waste money.

A HARMFUL CUSTOM

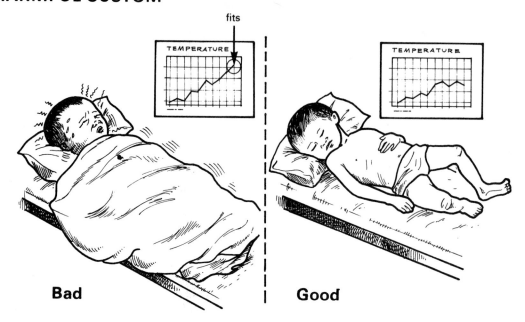

fits

Bad

Good

Fig. 2–8 A harmful custom—putting too many clothes on a child when he has a fever.

Some customs are harmful. For example, in some communities mothers put faeces from a cow on a baby's umbilicus. This contains tetanus bacteria, and often causes tetanus which kills him. So it is a very bad custom. In some communities mothers don't give food to a child with diarrhoea. This is another bad custom. Not giving him fluid is worse. Some mothers put too many clothes on a child with fever. This is a bad custom. It makes his fever worse and may cause hyperpyrexia (very high fever, 10.4) and fits. These customs are very dangerous for a child's health, so we must try to change them.

Every community has its own customs which help or harm health. We cannot describe them all here. In your community there will be special beliefs and customs for pregnancy, childbirth, food, disease, and the way to care for a young child. Learn about the beliefs and customs of the community where you are working. Encourage (help) the good customs. Try to stop the bad customs. Put something good in the place of something bad. Do nothing about the customs which make no difference.

HELP GOOD CUSTOMS, REPLACE BAD CUSTOMS, AND DO NOTHING ABOUT THE OTHERS

2.10 The community diagnosis

If possible, we must prevent disease, not in one child only, but in all the children in our community. We cannot do this completely, but we can do something.

A HARMLESS CUSTOM

Harmless

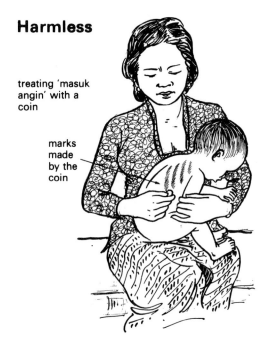

treating 'masuk angin' with a coin

marks made by the coin

Fig. 2–9 A harmless custom—rubbing a child with a coin.

Before we start to treat a child, we have to diagnose his disease. The community is the same. First we must make the **community diagnosis.** We must find out what diseases the children in our community have, and what people believe and do about them. The three most important kinds of disease in children are malnutrition, infection, and accidents. The other kinds of disease are serious for the few children who have them. But they are not common enough to be important for the whole community. The community diagnosis of malnutrition is in the nutrition book (N 9.1). So here we will only describe the community diagnosis of infectious diseases and accidents.

A DOUBTFUL CUSTOM

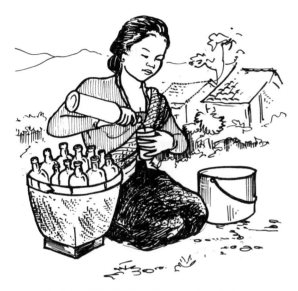

Fig. 2–10 A doubtful custom—local medicine.

When we make the community diagnosis we first need to know *how common* each disease is. We can find out how common each disease is in the clinic. We can look at our clinic records. But many children don't come to the clinic. So we need to know about diseases in the whole community. This is more difficult, but we can learn something about this. We can visit children at home.

We also need to know *how serious* diseases are. How much death and disability do they cause? Again, this is difficult. But while we care for children we come to know which diseases are killing and disabling them.

We must also ask families what they think about disease, and especially *how important* each disease is to them. If they think a disease is important, they are more likely to work hard to prevent it.

Next we must decide what we can *do* about these diseases—how *manageable* they are in the community. If possible, we want to prevent a disease. If we cannot prevent a disease, we want to cure it. So manageability means prevention and cure. Some diseases are much more manageable than others. For example, backward children (24.9) are difficult to prevent, and impossible to cure—they are not very manageable. But we can prevent and treat diarrhoea, so diarrhoea is more manageable than backwardness.

We can prevent disease in several ways. The two most useful ways in a children's clinic are immunization (4.2), and health education. Health education means changing people's behaviour (what they do) so as to make health better. For example, mothers may not start giving their children porridge when they are four months old. We may have to teach or educate them to do this. By educating mothers we can change their behaviour, and help them to care for their children better. When we decide how manageable a disease is we must ask ourselves—Can we prevent it by health education or immunization?

HEALTH EDUCATION MEANS HELPING TO CHANGE PEOPLE'S BEHAVIOUR SO AS TO MAKE THEIR HEALTH BETTER

The community diagnosis is made of all these things for each disease—how common, how serious, now important to the community, and how manageable. We can make a score for the community diagnosis like Table 2:2. Make the score in plusses, with up to four plusses in each column. 'Plusses' are not an exact way of measuring, but they are good enough to make a useful community diagnosis. There is a column for how important a disease is to the community. There are other columns for how serious it is, how common it is, and how manageable it is. *Multiply* the plusses to make the score. Diarrhoea, for example, comes to $3 \times 3 \times 2 \times 2 = 36$. Pneumonia comes to $2 \times 3 \times 2 \times 2 = 24$. The score tells us which are the best diseases to fight in our community. Diarrhoea comes first with pneumonia next. Your score will be different, because diseases differ from one district to another. They will differ in all the ways shown in the table. The community diagnosis for your district will be different from the community diagnosis in other places.

This is an easy way to start thinking about the community diagnosis. But it is only a beginning, and we must think deeper than this. We can try to prevent diarrhoea by making sure that all children are well-nourished, by breast-feeding, by boiling water, by using latrines, by washing hands, and by keeping flies away from food. A mother can prevent mild diarrhoea from becoming serious. She can give her child salt and sugar water. Which way prevents deaths from diarrhoea most easily? We cannot easily find out. But we must try all the ways we know—most of the ways are health education.

2.11 The seven steps to health education

We can teach each mother by herself when we see her child. This is **individual health education**. It is very

Table 2:2   The community diagnosis of infectious disease and accidents in children, for . . . . district July 1979

(1) Disease	(2) How common	(3) How serious medically	(4) How important to the community	(5) How manageable	(6) Score
Skin infections	+ + + +	+	+	+ + +	12
Colds	+ + + +	0	+	0	0
TB	+	+ + +	+ +	+ +	12
Diarrhoea	+ + +	+ + +	+ +	+ +	36
Hookworm	+ +	+ +	+	+ +	8
Pneumonia	+ +	+ + +	+ +	+ +	24
Poliomyelitis	+	+ + +	+	+	3
Accidents	+	+ +	+	+	2

important, so the eighth step in caring for every child is *explanation and education* (5.24). Usually, there is not time to teach every mother all that she needs to know by herself. So we must teach several mothers together in a class or group—**group health education**. We only say a little about this here, because you can read how to do it in Chapter 10 of the nutrition book. If you can teach a group of mothers about nutrition, you can teach them the rest of child care also. Here are the seven steps to health education that you will find in that chapter.

First step. Make the community diagnosis. We cannot begin to help people until we know about them, and about the diseases they have. So when we start, we must make the community diagnosis. Many families in a district have the same problems, but each mother also has special problems of her own. So we have to help each mother by herself whenever we can.

Second step. Make a health education plan. Make a list of the behaviour changes that your mothers need. Write a lesson for each change. Make each lesson about one behaviour change only. Give it a short name, such as 'Accidents'. Write out every lesson and make visual aids for it. Think of some questions to ask mothers later to evaluate it.

Third step. Make friends with the people you teach. If mothers think of you as a friend, they learn more. So be very kind to them, and say how pleased you are to see them. When the lesson is over thank them for coming.

Fourth step. Find people's wants. People change their behaviour most easily if this gives them something they want. So you must know what mothers want. All mothers want healthy children. For example, you can tell mothers that, if they add protein foods to porridge, their children will be healthy.

Fifth step. Show people that they can have what they want. Show mothers that they can have what they want if they change their behaviour. The behaviour change must be *possible*. For example, don't tell a mother to buy meat for her malnourished child if she cannot do this.

Sixth step. Record health education. This is necessary for evaluation. When mothers come to a clinic several times you will need to know what you have taught them on earlier visits. So, if a mother has heard a lesson, record the name of the lesson on her child's weight chart. This is why the names for lessons should be short.

Seventh step. Evaluate health education. Have mothers changed their behaviour, so that now they look after their children differently? This is difficult to find out. We can visit them at home and find out. We can also ask them questions about the talks which they have heard.

2.12 Some behaviour changes that might help your community

All communities are different, so health education plans must be different. You must decide which are the most necessary and the easiest behaviour changes for your mothers to make. If this is difficult, here are *some* behaviour changes that might help your community.

Use clinic services in the best way. Don't ask for an injection for every disease (3.5). Bring well children to the clinic for immunization (4.2). Keep a child's weight chart safely and bring it whenever he comes to a clinic (6.2). Breast-feed him until he is eighteen months or two years old (7.2). Start to give him porridge when he is four months old (7.2). Give him protective foods every day (7.2). Feed him when he is sick (7.2). Recognize the 'danger signs' when he has a cough (8.20) or diarrhoea (9.31). Use latrines to prevent diarrhoea and worm

TEACHING MOTHERS HOW TO CARE FOR THEMSELVES AND THEIR CHILDREN

Group health education

Using a flannelgraph to teach a group of mothers

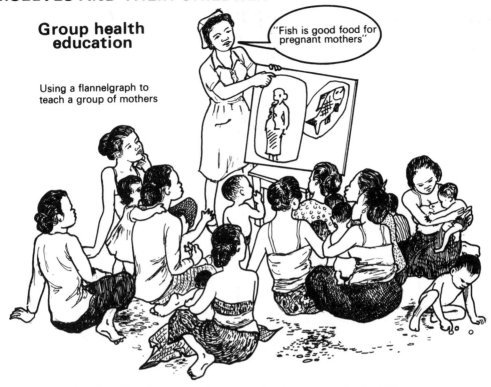

"Fish is good food for pregnant mothers"

Fig. 2–11 Teaching mothers how to care for themselves and their children.

infections (9.8). Boil a child's drinking water (9.8). Wash hands before you touch his food (9.8). Keep flies away from his food (9.8). Keep dirt out of his mouth (9.8). Make glucose–salt solution or salt and sugar water for him if he has diarrhoea (9.22). Don't put too many clothes on him if he has a fever (10.3). Put a mosquito net over his bed to prevent malaria (10.7). Wash him often to prevent skin (11.1) and eye disease. Care for his eyes if they are infected (16.8). Don't be frightened of leprosy, think of it as an ordinary disease (12.4). Prevent vitamin A deficiency—give children plenty of orange or yellow fruits and vegetables (16.14). Make a young child's home safe for him, so that he is not injured (14.1). Treat 'fever fits'—cool him with water (10.4). Care for a newborn baby in the right way (26.2).

2.13 Community health action

We can teach a mother how to prevent disease in her family. This is useful, but there are so many mothers that we cannot teach them all. We need to find and teach the important people in the community. These people can then lead and teach everyone else how to make their health better. When the community works together to make its health better, it takes **community health action** (11.1). Action means doing something. Perhaps we can talk to the district governor about how important healthy children are. He may want to help them. Help the community to help itself—this is the most important and the most difficult part of health education (N 11.1).

3 Supplies and equipment

DRUGS

3.1 Causal and symptomatic treatment

We must use drugs in the right way. This chapter tells you about drugs and how to give them. Other chapters tell you when to give them. We can use drugs to treat the cause of a disease or its symptoms.

Causal drugs. These drugs are the most important. They take away the cause of a disease. The two most common kinds of causal drug are **antimicrobials** and **nutrients**. Antimicrobials kill organisms which cause infections. For example, isoniazid kills TB bacilli, so it is a causal drug for TB. Nutrients such as iron and vitamins are substances which a child may lack in his food.

Symptomatic drugs. These stop a child's symptoms, such as fever or headache. But they do not cure the disease that is causing these symptoms. Aspirin is a drug like this. It makes a child's fever less, but it does not kill the malaria parasites that may be causing his fever. Here are some symptomatic drugs—
  —paracetamol and aspirin to stop pain and reduce fever.
  —phenobarbitone and paraldehyde to stop fits.
  —ephedrine and adrenaline to relax bronchial muscles.
Sometimes we give a child both a causal drug and a symptomatic drug. When he has pneumonia, for example, we can give him penicillin and aspirin.

Many of the children in a clinic do not need drugs. They are not very sick, and they recover without treatment. These are the children with colds, mild coughs, or fever. They will probably recover in a few days, even if they have no drugs. The best way to help these children is to teach their mothers how to care for them and feed them. But often a mother wants you to do something for her child. If you do nothing she will go home unhappy, and will not come to the clinic again. So you need to give her child something. If he does not need a drug, perhaps you can immunize him with a vaccine (4.2) such as DPT or tetanus toxoid. This is a good way to help a child and

please his mother. If a mother wants an injection, DPT is a good injection to give.

We can please and comfort mothers in other ways. We can give a child a cheap, harmless, pleasing medicine called a **placebo**. 'Placebo' means 'be pleased'. Children's cough mixture is a placebo because it does not contain any helpful drug. Yeast tablets are another placebo. But a mother does not know this, and she is pleased because she has something to give her child. Placebos are useful because they give comfort, which is very important. But they do not cure disease, so we must make sure that they are harmless. A cheap safe placebo is better than an expensive and unnecessary injection.

3.2 Side effects

We choose drugs so that they cause more harm to the disease than to the child. For example, we choose antimicrobial drugs so that they harm the micro-organisms in a child, but don't harm him. Unfortunately, most drugs harm children sometimes. We call this occasional harm the **side effects** of a drug. Usually, side effects are

THE DOSE OF LIQUID MEDICINES IS MEASURED IN 5 ML TEASPOONS

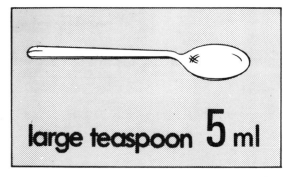

Fig. 3–1 The dose of liquid medicines is measured in 5 ml teaspoons.

not serious and they go when you stop the drugs. Occasionally, they are very serious.

Many drugs can cause fever, vomiting, jaundice, or rashes (11.25). Other side effects are special for a few drugs, or for one drug only. For example, chloramphenicol kills preterm babies (3.18). Tetracycline colours the teeth yellow (3.17). Dapsone sometimes causes pain, weakness, and fever (3.24). Remember: any drug can be harmful. So occasionally a drug may be *causing* a child's symptoms, and not curing them. If you give a child many drugs, there is a greater chance of harmful side effects. So give him as few drugs as possible.

Allergic reactions. Some drugs have a specially important side effect called an allergic reaction. For example, penicillin is completely harmless to most children, even in large doses. But occasionally a child's body does not like penicillin. Sometimes it causes an itchy rash (urticaria 11.24). Occasionally penicillin suddenly makes a child very ill with difficult breathing, wheezing, cyanosis, and shock (14.2). The child is allergic to penicillin. He must never have it again.

Tetanus antitoxin (18.16) causes the same kind of allergic reaction. Patients who are dangerously allergic to penicillin and antitoxin may have had symptoms before. So always ask a mother if an injection has ever made her child sick, before you give him either of these drugs. Penicillin allergy is rare, so we don't test for it before we give a child penicillin. Allergy to antitoxin is more common. So, before you give antitoxin, always test for an allergic reaction.

TESTING FOR ALLERGY TO ANTITOXIN
Inject one drop of antitoxin into the skin with a hypodermic needle (0.45 × 10 mm).
Wait half an hour.
If there is any redness of the skin or any symptoms, the child is allergic. Don't give him any more. It may kill him.
If nothing happens after half an hour, antitoxin is probably safe.

A severe allergic reaction is like asthma (8.13). Treat it in the same way.

TREATING AN ACUTE ALLERGIC REACTION
Always keep a sterile syringe and an ampoule of adrenaline ready. You may need them quickly.
Immediately symptoms start give subcutaneous adrenaline—for the dose see Figure 3–16, and Section 3.40.
If the drug has caused only a red itchy rash (urticaria 11.24), promethazine may help.
Write ALLERGIC TO PENICILLIN (or antitoxin) on his weight chart.

EXPLANATION **Explain to the child's mother what allergy means. Tell her that she must never let any health worker give him the same drug again.**

A CUP HOLDS ABOUT 200 ml

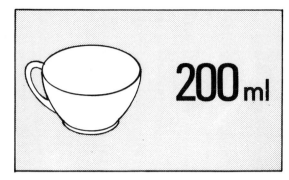

Fig. 3–2 A cup holds about 200 ml.

3.1

KEEP AN AMPOULE OF ADRENALINE READY FOR A SEVERE DRUG REACTION

3.3 Doses and courses

3.3

We use the word **dose** in two ways. (1) It is the amount of a drug that we give a child at any one time. (2) Or it is the amount we give him during a day. For example—20 mg/kg/day. Too little of a drug is always useless. Too much is usually dangerous. Sometimes we only need to give a drug once. Often, we must give several times a day for several days, or months. If we must give a drug for a special length of time, that time is called a **course**.

3.2

Give symptomatic drugs only when a child has symptoms. Always give causal drugs for the right course. A child may have to finish his course *after he seems to have recovered*. If he does not finish his course, some of the organisms inside him may stay alive. So the right course of a causal drug is as important as the right dose. For example, never give isoniazid for TB for less than a year. Never give iron mixture for anaemia for less than three months. One dose of iron mixture is useless, so is only a week's treatment with isoniazid. Sometimes there is only one length for a course, or courses can be different lengths. To help you, the dose figures (3–12 to 3–16) show both the longest and the shortest course for each drug. Always give a course that is between these two.

THE RIGHT COURSE OF A CAUSAL DRUG IS AS IMPORTANT AS THE RIGHT DOSE

The doses of solid drugs are measured in grams (g) or milligrams (mg). The dose of liquid drugs is measured in millilitres (ml). A 'ml' is the same as a 'cc'. There are about 20 drops of water in a ml. A *large* teaspoon holds about 5 ml of fluid or about 5 g of most powders. In this book a 'teaspoonful' always means 5 ml (3–1). This is a large, or standard teaspoon. Don't use small teaspoons. They only hold 3 ml. A cup holds about 200 ml of fluid.

A STANDARD TEASPOONFUL IS 5 ML

Mille means a thousand, so there are a thousand millilitres in a litre, and a thousand milligrams in a gram.

One-and-a-half grams is 1500 mg.

One gram is 1000 mg.

Half a gram (0·5 gm) is 500 mg.

A quarter of a gram (0·25 g) is 250 mg.

A tenth of a gram (0·1 g) is 100 mg.

A big child needs more of a drug than a small child. The dose of a drug depends on a child's weight, and so on how old he is. If possible work out doses by weight. Doses are sometimes written as the number of milligrams a child needs each day for every kilogram he weighs. For example, the dose of tetracycline is 25 mg/kg/day. This means 25 milligrams for each kilogram he weighs every day. When we write doses like this *a day means 24 hours* or a day and a night. Usually, we have to give a drug several times a day. All the doses for the day added together and divided by his weight should make 25 mg/kg.

DOSE DEPENDS ON WEIGHT

The number of doses of a drug each day is important. But exactly when a child takes them is not important. The doses should not be too close together, or too far apart. If a child must have four doses each day, he should have one dose early in the morning, and one dose late at night. He will need one dose about midday, and another dose in the afternoon.

Use the figures in this chapter and don't learn doses by heart. When you begin treating children, look them up. After you have treated many sick children, you will know what the right dose should be. If you are not sure of a dose, always look it up.

GIVE THE RIGHT DRUG IN THE RIGHT DOSE FOR THE RIGHT TIME

3.4 Ways of giving drugs

We can give drugs to children by mouth, or by injection. We can put drugs on a child's skin (ointments, lotions, or paints) or into his nose, eyes, or rectum. Drugs don't stay in his body. As soon as they get into a child they start to go away, either quickly, or slowly. Some drugs are destroyed by the body, others such as penicillin, are excreted in the urine. A few drugs, such as paraldehyde, are breathed out in the breath.

Drugs stay in the body for different times. Benzyl penicillin stays for a few hours only. Dapsone, stays for many hours. A drug only works when there is enough of it in the body. So drugs which leave the body quickly

THERE ARE ABOUT 20 DROPS IN ONE MILLILITRE

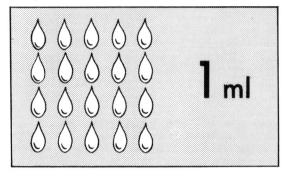

Fig. 3–3 There are about 20 drops in 1 ml.

must be given often. For example, we must give benzyl penicillin four times a day, but we only need to give dapsone once a day.

The cheapest and safest way to give a drug is to let the child eat it. We can give him drugs by mouth as **tablets**, or **capsules**, or as a fluid **mixture**. Mixtures are easiest for a child, especially if they contain sugar and taste good (syrups or elixirs). Some mixtures have small pieces of solid drug in them which fall to the bottom of the bottle. So always shake a mixture of this kind, before you give it. If you don't do this, the child who has mixture from the top will have too little drug. The child who has mixture from the bottom will have too much drug.

ALWAYS SHAKE THE BOTTLE

We put mixtures into bottles. So teach mothers to bring a *clean* empty bottle *with a lid* to the clinic. Show them the best kind to bring. If necessary, find someone who will sell bottles outside the clinic. Mixtures, such as cough mixture, which don't need shaking can be poured from a big bottle with a tap (3–7).

Tablets can be any size from 5 mg to 500 mg. Often, a drug is sold in tablets of several different sizes. Remember to look on the tin to find the size of a tablet. Phenobarbitone, for example, is sold in tablets of 15, 30, 60, and 100 mg.

We measure children's mixtures in 5 ml doses (one large teaspoonful). Some mixtures are made in two strengths, one for adults and older children, and another for babies and small children. An adult mixture can be dangerous to babies, so check carefully.

CHECK THE SIZE OF A TABLET AND THE STRENGTH OF A MIXTURE

If a child vomits a drug, give him another dose, or give him another drug by injection. If he is severely ill this is very important. He may die if the drug does not get into his body. For example, if a child with pneumonia vomits his sulphadimidine, stop giving it to him. Give him a course of penicillin by injection instead.

Keep all solid drugs in dark bottles, or in tins, because light harms some of them. Put labels on them with the name of the drug and the size of the tablet. Never use unlabelled drugs.

Many mothers cannot remember the doses of more than one or two drugs. So don't give too many drugs at the same time. For example, a child may need treatment for malaria, severe anaemia, and hookworms. Don't treat all these diseases at the same time. Instead, first treat his malaria with chloroquine. Later, give him iron and folic acid for his anaemia. Then give TCE (3.27) for his worms (22.5).

**DON'T GIVE TOO MANY DRUGS
AT THE SAME TIME**

Prepacked drugs. Counting each child's tablets wastes time in a busy clinic. Pack the most common tablets in small plastic bags, or paper envelopes, or pieces of paper. Keep some of these packets on your table (5–2).

SOME WAYS OF GIVING DRUGS

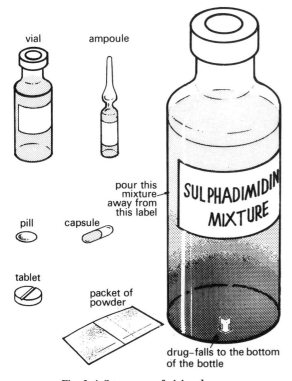

vial

ampoule

pour this mixture away from this label

SULPHADIMIDINE MIXTURE

pill

capsule

tablet

packet of powder

drug–falls to the bottom of the bottle

Fig. 3–4 Some ways of giving drugs.

THERE ARE DIFFERENT SIZES OF TABLET

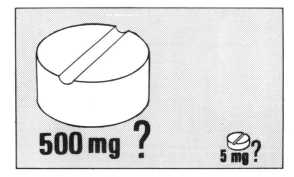

500 mg ?

5 mg ?

Fig. 3–5 There are different sizes of tablets.

Some fortunate clinics have enough small bottles to prepack mixtures also. In the dose figures you will see some numbers in circles. These are the amounts of each drug to prepack for each size of child. Pack the drug when the clinic is not busy, or teach a helper to do it. Label each packet with the name of the drug and write how often it should be taken.

Pack dapsone and isoniazid, which are given in long courses, in packets for one month. People soon stop coming to the clinic if they have to come every week for a year or more.

GIVING A CHILD DRUGS BY MOUTH

TABLETS. **Read the label on the tin. If a child needs half a tablet, cut it with a knife through the line across it. Some tablets such as sulphadimidine cut easily. Others break when they are cut, so give mothers some extra ones. If a child is too young to swallow a tablet, crush (break) it into powder. Mix it with a little water and sugar (or honey) and give it to him with a spoon.**

MIXTURES. **Shake the mixture. Take out the cork and put it topside down on the table. Pour some mixture into a clean 5 ml teaspoon. Pour the mixture out on the side of the bottle away from the label. If you do not do this, a drip may run down the label and spoil it. Watch the child while he is having his mixture, so that you are sure he drinks it.**

Show his mother the right kind of spoon to use. Have some different sizes to show her. Keep them together on a key ring (3–7).

EXPLANATION. **Tell the child's mother that a drug by mouth can be as helpful as an injection. Tell her when to give him his drug and explain how she must give it. *Show her how to give him his first dose in the clinic before he goes home.* Tell her anything else that she needs to know about using the drug. For example, a child who is having sulphadimidine must drink plenty of fluids (3.14). After you have explained, ask her to tell you what you have said.**

3.4

25

Prepacked drugs save time

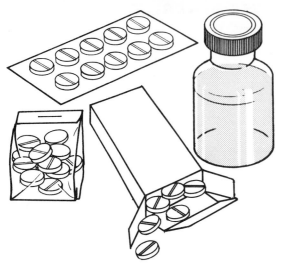

Fig. 3–6 Get drugs ready before the clinic starts.

If she can read, write on the bottle or packet how she is to give the medicines.

If he is having a causal drug, tell her that he *must* finish the course. She must *not* keep some of it for another illness.

Explain that the right dose of a drug is important. Explain that she must keep drugs in a safe place where children cannot reach them and poison themselves. Ferrous sulphate, pyrimethamine, and dapsone are especially dangerous (14.6). Tell her when she should come again.

RECORDING AND REPORTING. **Record the drug you have given.**

GIVE HIM HIS FIRST DOSE
BEFORE HE GOES HOME

3.5 Syringes, needles, and injections

Some drugs, such as streptomycin are not absorbed from the gut, so we must inject them. We can give injections to unconscious children, and they cannot be vomited. When we want to make sure a child has all his drug, we usually inject it.

We can give injections into the skin—**intradermally**, under the skin—**subcutaneously**, into the muscles —**intramuscularly**, or into the veins—**intravenously**. Drugs are slowly absorbed into the blood when we give them **subcutaneously**. They are absorbed slightly faster when we give them intramuscularly, and very fast indeed when we give them intravenously. The only intradermal injections we give are BCG vaccine for preventing TB (13.4), and antitoxin in testing for allergy (3.2). We give

chloroquine and adrenaline subcutaneously. Most other injections, especially penicillin are intramuscular. The only intravenous injections we give are intravenous quinine and Darrow's solution (9.27).

Injections are given with syringes. The outer part of a syringe is the **barrel**, the inner part is the **plunger**. The **graduations** are the marks on the barrel. Three sizes of syringe are useful, 5 ml, 2 ml, and 1ml. The 1 ml syringes are long and thin and break easily. We call them '**Microstat syringes**' (13.5). We use them for giving BCG vaccine, and for measuring the dose of drugs in babies.

EQUIPMENT FOR LIQUID MEDICINES

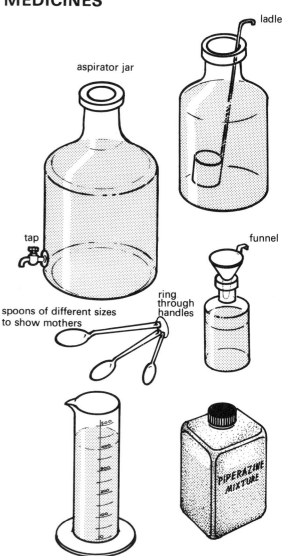

Fig. 3–7 Equipment for liquid medicines.

Keep one of these syringes for BCG only. Don't use it for anything else.

The **adaptor** is the part of a syringe that fits onto a needle. There are two kinds of needle and adaptor—**Record** and **Luer**. Luer adaptors are larger and will not fit Record needles. All the syringes and needles in the equipment list are Luer.

There are several kinds of plastic syringe. Plastic disposable syringes are sterile inside a packet. Usually, you cannot sterilize them again. SO USE DISPOSABLE SYRINGES ONCE ONLY AND THROW THEM AWAY.

You can sterilize some kinds of syringe by boiling, or in a pressure cooker. These are the best kind of syringes to use. Some plastic syringes have a Record adaptor on the end of a Luer adaptor. If you want to use one for Luer needles, you can cut off its Record adaptor.

A **stylet** is the wire that goes inside a needle. We measure the thickness of a needle in millimetres—'mm'. We use 0·7 mm needles for everything except intradermal injections. For these, we use thinner 0·45 mm needles. The length of needles is also measured in milli-metres. In this book we will use the word **hypodermic** for a thin short 0·45 × 10 mm needle, and **intramuscular** for a thicker longer 0·7 × 38 mm needle.

The **bevel** is the sloping part of the point of a needle. We use long bevel needles for injections. We use short bevel needles for lumbar punctures (15.3) and scalp vein transfusions (9–17). **Disposable** needles have a plastic cover and are already sterile. We use them only once and then throw them away. Sterility is very important for lumbar puncture (15.3), so there are some disposable short bevel 0·9 × 40 mm needles in the equipment list.

Sharpen needles when they become blunt (L 12.10). Learn how to give an injection with as little pain as possible—use a sharp needle and go through the skin quickly.

SHARPEN BLUNT NEEDLES

We must sterilize syringes and needles between each injection, so that all the organisms in them are killed. If we do not do this, dangerous organisms can be carried

THE NEEDLES AND SYRINGES YOU WILL NEED

Syringes and needles

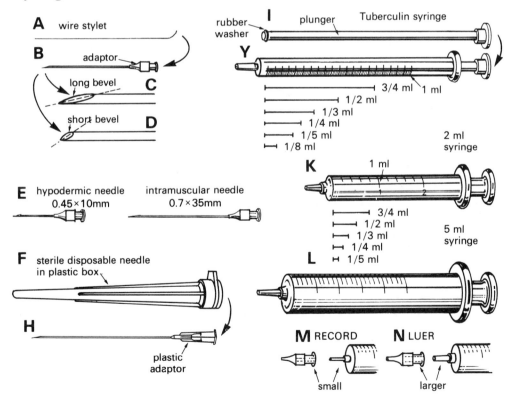

Fig. 3–8 The needles and syringes you will need.

from one child to another. Several diseases can spread in this way, especially virus hepatitis (Path F, 2–6, 22.11).

Every child *must* have a sterile needle for himself. If possible, he should have a sterile syringe for himself also. Often, there are not enough syringes in the clinic for this. If you only have a few syringes, try not to use the same syringe for more than ten children. If blood gets into a syringe, always sterilize it before you use it again.

If possible, use a pressure cooker (6.13). You can sterilize enough syringes and needles at one time in a pressure cooker to inject 200 children or more.

EVERY CHILD MUST HAVE A STERILE NEEDLE FOR HIMSELF

Injections are dangerous if you give them in the wrong place. A nerve called the **sciatic nerve** goes from the buttock into the leg (3–9). If you inject a drug into a child's sciatic nerve, you may paralyse his leg. The sciatic nerve is in the lower inner quarter of his buttock. Keep your needle away from it. Inject a child under five in the outer side of his thigh. Inject an older child or adult in the upper outer quarter of the buttock (3–9).

INJECTIONS

Tell an older child that he is going to have a 'prick'. Explain that it will soon be over and he can go home. Make the syringe ready where he cannot see it.

Fill two jars with pieces (swabs) of cotton wool. Make the swabs in one jar wet with spirit. Leave the others dry.

Wash your hands. Take a sterile needle and syringe. Read the label on the vial or ampoule carefully.

Vials. Clean the rubber top of the vial with a spirit swab. Draw some air into the syringe. Push the needle through the rubber top. Inject the same amount of air as the drug you are going to take out of the vial.

GIVING A YOUNG CHILD AN INTRAMUSCULAR INJECTION

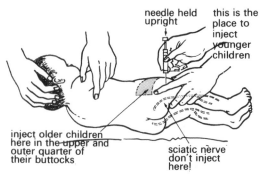

needle held upright

this is the place to inject younger children

inject older children here in the upper and outer quarter of their buttocks

sciatic nerve don't inject here!

Fig. 3–9 Giving a young child an intramuscular injection.

Ampoules. **Shake the drug down from the neck into the ampoule. Use a file to make *one* short scratch on its neck. Hold the top in a piece of gauze and break it off. Bend it away from the scratch.**
Fill the syringe and push out any air.

INTRADERMAL INJECTIONS. **Go to Section 13.5.**

SUBCUTANEOUS INJECTION. **Pinch up the skin on the outside of the child's upper arm. Clean the skin with a spirit swab. Push in the needle with the syringe sloping (45°). Pull back the plunger to see if blood comes. If it does, the needle is in a vein, so take it out and try in another place. If no blood comes, inject the drug slowly, then quickly take the needle out. Press the hole for a minute with a dry swab.**

INTRAMUSCULAR INJECTION. *Children under five years old.* **Clean the outer side of the child's thigh with a spirit swab. Hold the syringe with your right index finger on the adaptor of the needle, as if it were a pen. Make the skin tight with your left thumb and index finger. Hold the syringe upright (90°) and *quickly* push the needle through the skin. Push the syringe straight in—don't bend it. Don't let the needle go in more than 25 mm. Keep the last 10 mm outside the child. If the adaptor touches the child, and the needle breaks, the bottom end is difficult to take out. Pull back the plunger to see if blood comes. If it does, the needle is in a vein, so take it out, and inject in another place. If no blood comes, inject the drug slowly. Then quickly take out the needle and press over the hole with a dry swab to stop bleeding.**

INTRAVENOUS INJECTION. **See Figure 9–15. Put your needle into the skin, bevel uppermost. Put it in beside the vein. Then put it into the vein. Suck before you inject. If the needle is in the vein, blood will come. Inject slowly during 10 minutes. Don't inject the drug outside the vein, or you may cause an ulcer.**
Comfort him. If he needs two drugs by injection, give them in different syringes. If a needle breaks inside a child, send him for help.

Injections frighten children and can be dangerous, so only give them if they are necessary. Don't give them as a placebo (3.1). Many mothers want injections for their children, so we must explain to them very carefully why an injection is not necessary.

GIVE AS FEW INJECTIONS AS POSSIBLE DON'T GIVE PLACEBO INJECTIONS

3.6 'There is a painful swelling at the place where you gave Ijebu his injection'—injection abscess

The bacteria on a dirty needle or syringe can grow at the place of an injection. They cause a painful tender swelling called an injection abscess. Prevent these abscesses. *Always* use a sterile syringe and needle. Don't touch the end of needle before you use it. Treat an injection abscess like any other abscess (11.5). Rarely, an injection abscess is sterile and contains no bacteria (3.44). Often, the bacteria in it are resistant to penicillin.

DON'T TOUCH THE END OF A NEEDLE BEFORE YOU GIVE AN INJECTION

Expendable Supplies

3.7 The 'important fifty'

Expendable supplies are such things as penicillin, or bandages, which are used up. They are listed in Table 3:1. They are different from equipment, such as torches or spatulae which we can use again many times. This equipment is in Table 3:2 at the end of the chapter. The fifty most important supplies are in heavy type in Table 3:1. We *must* try to have these things. Sometimes there are several things which we could use, but we only need one of them. For example, sulphadimidine can be a mixture, or tablets. Both are useful, but we only need one or the other.

We need some of the 'important 50' supplies, such as penicillin, every day. Other drugs, such as adrenaline, are seldom wanted, but they can save lives, so we must have them. Most of the fifty are needed in every district. But some, such as chloroquine are only needed in districts which have malaria.

Vaccines, soap, disinfectant, drip sets, and weight charts are among the 'important 50.' They are as necessary as most of the drugs. Try to keep all the important 50, and to get more before they are finished. For example, if new supplies take a month to come, keep an extra

INJECTION ABSCESSES ARE OUR FAULT

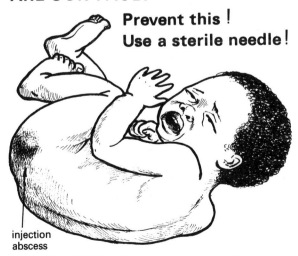

Prevent this !
Use a sterile needle !

injection
abscess

Fig. 3–10 Injection abscesses are our fault.

THE IMPORTANT 50 SUPPLIES

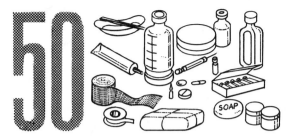

Fig. 3–11 The important 50 supplies.

3.7

month's supply in store. If you do this, and your new supply is late, your drugs will not be finished immediately.

3.9 Using drugs in the right way

3.9

Some drugs have several names, because each firm gives a drug a different name. Use the names we give here. Always buy drugs by these names, because drugs are often much cheaper when you buy them like this.

Save money. Buy only useful medicines or cheap placebos. Don't buy tonics, because we do not use them in modern medicine. Don't waste money on unnecessary vitamins and mineral mixtures. A child can get vitamins in his food. If you give him more vitamins than he needs, they do no good and he excretes them in his urine. If you have to give something to a child, immunizations are better than vitamins.

UNNECESSARY VITAMINS MAKE EXPENSIVE URINE

Don't give antipyretic (fever-lowering) injections, because they can cause serious blood diseases. Instead, cool a child with water and give him paracetamol tablets. This is cheaper and safer (10.4). Don't use steroids, because these can be dangerous, unless they are necessary to prevent death. *Never* give anabolic (body building) steroids to malnourished children. They don't work. These children need food, not steroids. There is an anti-histamine drug called promethazine in the list, but it is one of the least useful drugs. There is no need for anti-histamine injections. Many drugs for diarrhoea are also a 'bad buy' because they do not work (9.30). Buy only the cheapest cough mixture. Don't buy mixtures of drugs, especially mixtures of antibiotics. Lastly, only buy the drugs which you understand and know how to use.

3.6

ONLY BUY DRUGS YOU UNDERSTAND

Spend money on the life-saving drugs. Always have them. The life-saving drugs are, sulphadimidine, penicillin, chloramphenicol, tetracycline, streptomycin,

Table 3:1 Expendable supplies for child care

Septic infections

SULPHADIMIDINE, mixture 100 mg per ml, bottle 1000 ml $2·44, UNIPAC 1568020

SULPHADIMIDINE, tablets, 500 mg, tin of 1000 tablets $4·05, UNIPAC 1568025

BENZYL PENICILLIN (Penicillin G), injection, with 5 ml ampoule of diluent, 600 mg vial $0·08, UNIPAC 1557980

PROCAINE PENICILLIN, injection fortified BP (PPF), 300 mg of procaine penicillin, and 60 mg of benzyl penicillin, vial $0·08, UNIPAC 1558502

PROCAINE PENICILLIN injection, 300 mg per ml

BENZATHINE PENICILLIN (or benethamine), fortified injection, vials of about 1 g

AMPICILLIN, for injection, vials of 250 mg

AMPICILLIN, mixture, bottles of powder for dilution with water to make 60 ml of mixture with 125 mg in 5 ml

CHLORAMPHENICOL, mixture, 125 mg in 5 ml, 60 ml bottle $0·32, UNIPAC 1531010

CHLORAMPHENICOL, capsules, 250 mg, tin of 1000, capsules $14·52, UNIPAC 1531000

TETRACYCLINE, mixture, 125 mg in 5 ml, 60 ml bottle $0·27, UNIPAC 1569400

TETRACYCLINE, capsules 250 mg, bottle of 1000 capsules $10·29, UNIPAC 15690000

CHLORTETRACYCLINE, eye ointment, 1 per cent in tubes of 5 g $0·08, UNIPAC 1510000

SILVER PROTEIN, mild, 2·5 g bottle $2·02, UNIPAC 1564000

TB

STREPTOMYCIN, injection 1 g vials $0·06, UNIPAC 1565000

ISONIAZID (INH), tablets 100 mg, tin of 1000 tablets $1·82, UNIPAC 1554000

ISONIAZID, compound tablet, 133 mg with thiacetazone 50 mg

ISONIAZID, compound tablet 100 mg with thiacetazone 50 mg, tin of 1000 tablets $3·65, UNIPAC 1554003

AMINOSALICYLATE, sodium (PAS), tablet 500 mg, tin of 5000 tablets $40·12, UNIPAC 1556000

Leprosy

DAPSONE, tablets 100 mg, tin of 1000 tablets $1·94, UNIPAC 1542200

CLOFAZIMINE, capsules 100 mg

Malaria

CHLOROQUINE, tablets, containing 150 mg of chloroquine base, bottle of 1000 tablets $6·64, UNIPAC 1532000

CHLOROQUINE, injection, ampoules of 200 mg in 5 ml, box of 10 ampoules $1·39, UNIPAC 1531925

isoniazid (INH), chloroquine, tetrachlorethylene (or bephenium), glucose–salt solution, adrenaline, paraldehyde (or phenobarbitone injection), and the vaccines.

Many of the children in a clinic need no drugs. Most sick children need only one drug, some need two drugs, but very few need more than two. Don't give vitamin tablets to every child who comes to a clinic, or sulphadimidine to every child with diarrhoea (9.30). If you use drugs carefully you will have enough life saving-drugs for the very sick children.

UNICEF is given money by the richer governments of the world. UNICEF uses this money to help children everywhere. UNICEF *gives* drugs to sick children. Because UNICEF gives us drugs free, we must give these drugs free to poor mothers for their children. We must not sell UNICEF drugs.

CAUSAL DRUGS

Antimicrobials

3.11 Antibiotics, antiseptics, and disinfectants

The most common diseases of children are infections with harmful organisms. The most useful drugs are the **antimicrobials**. Some antimicrobials kill organisms. Other antimicrobials injure organisms, so that the tissues of the body can kill or remove them. **Antibiotics** kill bacteria. They are a special kind of antimicrobial. We use six antibiotics for killing the bacteria which cause septic infections—sulphadimidine, penicillin, ampicillin, tetracycline, chloramphenicol, and streptomycin. Sulphadimidine is not an antibiotic. But we use it in the same way as the other five antibiotics. So think of sulphadimidine as an antibiotic. We use several other antimicrobial drugs, which are not antibiotics, such as isoniazid (for TB), dapsone (for leprosy) and chloroquine (for malaria).

Antimicrobial drugs work *inside* a child's body. They don't harm him. There are other chemicals which kill micro-organisms, but they are harmful inside a child's body. We can only use them *outside* him, on his skin, We call these chemicals **antiseptics**. They are not drugs, and are dangerous to drink. Hypochlorite and iodine are antiseptics.

We use some chemicals, such as lysol, to kill organisms on dirty dressings, or on infected clothes. These chemicals burn skin, if they touch it. We call them **disinfectants**. You must not use them on the body, and you must not give them by mouth.

3.12 Sensitivity and resistance

When an antimicrobial drug can kill an organism, the organism is **sensitive** to that drug. When a drug cannot kill an organism, the organism is **resistant** to that drug.

Antiseptics and disinfectants, such as iodine and lysol, can kill *all* kinds of micro-organisms. They can also kill children. But antimicrobial drugs can only kill *some*

SULPHADOXINE 500 mg with PYRIMETHAMINE 25 mg, compound tablets

QUININE HYDROCHLORIDE, for injection, 60 mg in each ml, ampoules of 5 ml (This is a specially dilute solution which makes children's doses easier. The standard BP formulation is 300 mg in each ml)

PYRIMETHAMINE, tablets 25 mg, tin of 1000 tablets $2·66, UNIPAC 1560200

Giardiasis and amoebiasis

METRONIDAZOLE, tablets 200 mg, tin of 1000 tablets $11·26, UNIPAC 1555650

MEPACRINE, tablets 100 mg

Worms

TETRACHLORETHYLENE, capsules of 1 ml or bottle of liquid

BEPHENIUM, granules, sachets of 5 g

PIPERAZINE citrate, mixture 500 mg of piperazine hydrate in 5 ml

PIPERAZINE ADIPATE (or phospate) tablets equal to 500 mg of piperazine hydrate, tin of 1000 tablets $4·02, UNIPAC 1560000

TIABENDAZOLE, tablets 500 mg, bottle of 100 tablets $4·73, UNIPAC 1569575

NICLOSAMIDE, tablets 500 mg

MAGNESIUM SULPHATE, a purge (3.30)

PYRANTEL PAMOATE, mixture 250 mg in 5 ml

NIRIDAZOLE, tablets 500 mg

METRIFONATE, tablets 100 mg

Asthma

EPHEDRINE, tablets 15 mg, bottle of 100 tablets $1·81, UNIPAC 1544900

ADRENALINE, injection, 1 ml ampoules of 0·1 per cent solution, box of 10 ampoules $0·54, UNIPAC 1501000

Pain and fever

PARACETAMOL, tablets of 500 mg

ASPIRIN, soluble tablets 75 mg

ASPIRIN, tablets 300 mg, tin of 1000 tablets $1·28, UNIPAC 1506002

Fits

PHENOBARBITONE, tablets 30 mg, bottle of 100 tablets $0·31, UNIPAC 1559300

PHENOBARBITONE, injection, ampoules of 200 mg in 1 ml

PARALDEHYDE injection, ampoules of 5 ml

Coughs

COUGH MIXTURE, packets or tins of powder for dilution

An antihistamine

PROMETHAZINE mixture, 1 mg in 1 ml, 250 ml bottle $0·78, UNIPAC 1559205

kinds of organisms. When we treat a child we have to try to find out what kind of organism is infecting him. We must then give him a drug which can kill that organism. Sometimes, we can take a specimen from him and examine it in a laboratory. For example, we may find that he has amoebae in his stool. We know that amoebae are sensitive to metronidazole, so this is the drug for him. But we cannot always do this. Often we have to guess, and give the drug which is *probably* right. For example, the organisms that cause pneumonia in an older child are usually sensitive to penicillin. So, when we diagnose pneumonia, we give a child penicillin, even though we cannot find the organisms.

Some kinds of organisms are always sensitive to a drug. For example, the bacteria which cause sore throats (streptococci) are always sensitive to penicillin. Other kinds of organisms are always resistant. TB bacilli, for example, are always resistant to penicillin. There are some antibiotics for killing fungi, but they are very expensive. All viruses are resistant to all antibiotics. So, only treat virus diseases with antibiotics, if there is also secondary bacterial infection.

ANTIBIOTICS DON'T KILL VIRUSES

Sometimes, an organism which used to be sensitive to a drug changes and becomes resistant. This kind of resistance is called **acquired** resistance. It is unfortunate, because it means that a drug which used to work has now become useless. For example, if you use streptomycin for TB without isoniazid, the TB bacilli acquire resistance to streptomycin. If you treat a child this way, he will not be cured. If these resistant organisms infect another person he too will not be helped by streptomycin.

Acquired resistance is common with some drugs and with some organisms, but is uncommon with others. Worms, for example, never become resistant to piperazine or tetrachlorethylene. But some bacteria, especially TB bacilli, easily become resistant to streptomycin. Many pyogenic bacteria have now become resistant to penicillin. Many of the organisms causing diarrhoea used to be sensitive to sulphonamides, but are now resistant to them. So sulphonamides are now almost useless for treating diarrhoea (9.30). Unfortunately, gonococci are becoming resistant to pencillin (26.40).

3.13 Rules for using antibiotics

Bacteria of many kinds can grow in a child's body, and cause septic infections (2.4), such as tonsillitis (18.11), lower respiratory infections (8.21), otitis media (17.9), septic skin infections (11.3), septicaemia (26.24), bacilliary dysentery (9.3), and urinary infections (23.4). We use six antibiotics for septic infections—**sulphadimidine, penicillin, ampicillin, streptomycin, tetracycline,** and **chloramphenicol.** Tetracycline, chloramphenicol and ampicillin can kill more kinds of organisms than the others, so we call them

PROMETHAZINE, tablets 25 mg, UNIPAC 1559200

Poisoning

IPECACUANHA syrup, bottles of 100 ml

Scabies

BENZYL BENZOATE, application, tin, one US quart $3·38, UNIPAC 1520000
GAMMA BENZENE hexachloride, application, tin of 500 ml $3·37, UNIPAC 1551900
SULPHUR, ointment 5 per cent
MONOSULPHIRAM 25 per cent alcoholic solution

Skin Sepsis

GENTIAN VIOLET, crystals (or crystal violet), bottle 25 g $1·23, UNIPAC 1552002
POTASSIUM PERMANGANATE, crystals, or tablets, bottle 500 g $1·76

Ringworm

BENZOIC ACID COMPOUND OINTMENT, half strength

Symptomatic skin treatments

CALAMINE LOTION
PLAIN OINTMENT (emulsifying ointment)
ZINC AND CASTOR OIL OINTMENT

Nutrients

DRIED SKIM MILK, or other supplementary high protein food
GLUCOSE–SALT POWDER, tins
GLUCOSE–SALT POWDER, packets, salts oral rehydration 'Oralyte', packet to make one litre $0·12, UNIPAC 1561100
or the raw materials to make glucose–salt powder (9.21). Excluding common salt (7 parts), which it is assumed will be locally available. These are required in the following proportions:
GLUCOSE (40 parts), bottle 500 g $1·48, UNIPAC 1024300
SODIUM BICARBONATE (5 parts), bottle 1 kg $1·05, UNIPAC 1073800
POTASSIUM CHLORIDE (3 parts), bottle 500 g $0·84, UNIPAC 1066940
DARROW'S SOLUTION, half strength in 2·5 per cent glucose, 500 ml with giving set
GLUCOSE injection 25 per cent, 5 ml vial, box of 10 vials $3·03, UNIPAC 1543500
FERROUS SULPHATE mixture paediatric BPC, 'Children's iron mixture', tins of powder for dilution
FERROUS SULPHATE with folate, 300 mg tablets, bottle 1000 tablets $1·06, UNIPAC 1550010
IRON DEXTRAN INJECTION, 50 mg per ml, ampoules 5 ml
IODIZED OIL, fluid injection B.P.
FOLIC ACID, tablets of 5 mg

broad-spectrum antibiotics. If we use penicillin with streptomycin, or sulphadimidine, the two drugs work together like a broad-spectrum antibiotic. Some of the six drugs can be given together and some cannot. Here are some rules for using antibiotics, for preventing resistance, and for stopping waste.

One. Only use antibiotics if they are necessary. Don't treat colds with antibiotics.

Two. Give antibiotics in the right dose for the right course. Organisms become resistant more easily if the dose is too small, or if treatment is too short. The shortest course with any of these drugs is three days. The longest course is usually two weeks. One day of treatment with any antibiotic is useless.

Three. Never give streptomycin by itself. Always give it with isoniazid for TB, or with pencillin for a septic infection. Buy penicillin and streptomycin separately. Don't buy them ready mixed, because the quantities of each drug may be wrong for children.

Four. Use penicillin alone or with either sulphadimidine or streptomycin,

Five. Use chloramphenicol or tetracycline by themselves, except when the manual tells you to give them with another drug.

Six. The manual gives the best drug for each disease first. So, if possible, use the *first* drug. For example, you can treat otitis media with ampicillin, penicillin, or sulphadimidine. Ampicillin is best.

DON'T GIVE ANTIBIOTICS FOR LESS THAN THREE DAYS. ONE INJECTION OF PROCAINE PENICILLIN IS USELESS BY ITSELF

Broad-spectrum antibiotics can cause diarrhoea or thrush (18.5). They kill the normal organisms (2.2) in a child's gut and mouth. When the normal organisms are dead, the organisms causing diarrhoea or thrush can grow more easily. So stop giving antibiotics. If he has thrush, give him gentian violet. If he has diarrhoea, he will usually recover by himself in a few weeks.

Septic infections

3.14 Sulphadimidine

This is one of a family of drugs called sulphonamides. We can use some drugs in this family, such as sulphadiazine, in the same way as sulphadimidine. Other sulphonamides are different. We have to use them in a different way, so be careful. Sulphaguanidine, for exam-

VITAMIN A, capsules of 200 000 units, bottle of 500 capsules $5·08, UNIPAC 1583000

VITAMIN A, retinyl palmitate, water miscible for intramuscular injection, ampoules of 100 000 units (55 mg)

PHYTOMENADIONE (vitamin K), ampoules for injection 1 mg in 0·5 ml

MULTI-VITAMIN with iron and folate capsules, bottle of 1000 capsules $2·28, UNIPAC 1555810

YEAST TABLETS, 300 mg

Vaccines and antisera

DIPHTHERIA, PERTUSSIS AND TETANUS VACCINE (DPT, vaccine)

POLIOMYELITIS VACCINE, oral, live

MEASLES VACCINE

BCG VACCINE

TETANUS ANTITOXIN 1500 units per ml

TETANUS TOXOID

Diagnostic materials

FLUORESCEIN papers

Other expendable supplies

WATER FOR INJECTION sterile, pyrogen free, 10 ml ampoule $0·06, UNIPAC 1543804

SPIRIT, surgical

IODINE, solution

HYDROGEN PEROXIDE

LYSOL

BENZOIN TINCTURE, B.P.C. (26.52)

COPPER SULPHATE (26.35)

SODIUM THIOSULPHATE (11.14)

CALCIUM HYPOCHLORITE, technical, 4 lb bottle $3·77, UNIPAC 1525000

PARAFFIN, liquid (or cooking oil)

GAUZE, absorbent, non-sterile, 100 m roll, $11·49, UNIPAC 0521900

GAUZE, vaseline, 10 × 10 cm, tin of 12

COTTON WOOL, absorbent, non-sterile, 500 g roll $0·88, UNIPAC 0519600

BANDAGE, gauze,
25 mm × 9 m, roll $0·04, UNIPAC 0512100
50 mm × 9 m, roll $0·12, UNIPAC 0512101
75 mm × 9 m, roll $0·18, UNIPAC 0512102

TAPE, adhesive strapping, zinc oxide, 4·5 metre roll $0·75, UNIPAC 0501000

SUTURE MATERIAL

TUBING PLASTIC, general purpose child care, UNIPAC 0382300

SET, intravenous infusion

PHENOL, bottle 500 g

DDT dusting powder 10 per cent in talc, 2.3 kg bags $2·23, UNIPAC 1540000

INSECTICIDE SPRAY

SOAP

ple, is not absorbed from the gut. It can only work in the gut, and not in other parts of the body. Sulphonamides are useful because a mother can take the tablets or the mixture home with her. She does not have to come to the clinic for injections.

We can use sulphadimidine for many septic infections, especially urinary infections. It is seldom helpful in diarrhoea or dysentery. Most of the bacteria which cause these diseases have become resistant to sulphadimidine. Don't use it for abscesses until they have opened. Don't use it in babies less than one week old because it causes jaundice. If necessary, you can give sulphadimidine to babies less than three months old, but other drugs are better.

Side effects. Sulphadimidine (and the sulphonamides like it) are excreted in the urine. The dose is large—about 2 g a day for a two-year-old child. If he is making little urine, sulphadimidine is not washed through his kidneys. It blocks the small tubes of his kidney so that he cannot pass any urine. He may also have haematuria (23.6). Prevent these side effects. Give a child plenty of fluids, especially water. This is very important in hot weather. When you give a child a sulphonamide, tell his mother that he must have plenty of fluids. Sulphadimidine may also cause a rash (11.25).

SULPHADIMIDINE, OR SULPHADIAZINE, FOR SEPTIC INFECTIONS, 150 mg/kg/day

White 500 mg tablets, or a mixture containing 500 mg in 5 ml.

Give four doses a day.

At each dose give—

- adults, 4–6 tablets (2–3 g) for the first dose, then 2–3 tablets (1–1½ g) for the other doses
- children over 25 kg, 2 tablets, or two teaspoons of mixture (1 g)
- children between 17 and 25 kg, 1½ tablets, or 1½ teaspoons of mixture (0.75 g)
- children between 10 and 17 kg, 1 tablet, or one teaspoon of mixture (0.5 g)
- babies between 5 and 10 kg, ½ tablet or ½ teaspoon of mixture (0.25 g)
- babies under 5 kg, ¼ tablet or ¼ teaspoon of mixture (0.125 g)
- newborn babies. Sulphadimidine is not a good drug for newborn babies

CHILDREN HAVING SULPHONAMIDES MUST DRINK PLENTY OF FLUIDS

3.15 Penicillin

This was the first antibiotic, and it is still the best. The dose of penicillin is measured in milligrams (mg) or in mega-units (M). Mega means million, so there are a million units in a mega-unit. There are several kinds of penicillin.

Supplies for recording and reporting
WEIGHT CHARTS
POLYTHENE BAGS, for weight charts
CONTINUATION CARDS for weight charts

SPECIAL CARE CARDS
CHILDREN'S TALLY SHEETS

NOTE The costs in Tables 3:1 and 3:2 are from UNICEF's 1976 catalogue.

WAYS OF USING THE DOSE FIGURES

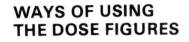

adults are above the wavy line

5ml teaspoon of mixture or syrup

tablet

injection

capsules

powder

tablets or ml or mixture needed for a course of the drug

(48)

★ 26.24 look in the text

The dose figures tell you how much of each drug to give. These doses are the numbers of tablets, or the teaspoons of a mixture, or the 'ml' or 'mg' of a drug for injection. They are only for the sizes of tablet or strengths of mixture shown. Other tablets and other mixtures are different. If, for example the adult dose of procaine penicillin is shown as 2–4 ml, this means that you can give any dose between 2 and 4 ml, it does not mean 24 ml!

Courses are only shown for causal drugs. You can usually give symptomatic drugs for as long as a child has symptoms.

The weights of children are shown rising 2½ kg each year after the first year. This is useful for doses, but it is not exact. The extra ½ kg has been left out. 12½ kg, for example, has been shortened to 12 kg.

If a child comes exactly on a line, use the lower dose.

If a child is very underweight for his age, use his weight not his age. If he is over 35 kg give him the adult dose.

Adults can take tablets, so adult doses are not usually shown for mixtures.

The numbers with a ring round them show the smallest number of tablets or ml of a mixture that a child needs for a course of a causal drug. A mother must take these home with her. They are the amounts of drugs for prepacking (3.4). They allow for one or two tablets to be broken, and a little mixture to be split. Where a course lasts for longer than a month, as with dapsone, only a month's course is shown. Prepack the drugs you use most often.

Fig. 3.11b Using the dose figures on the next few pages.

Benzyl penicillin. This is also called penicillin G, aqueous penicillin, crystalline penicillin, or soluble penicillin. It is destroyed in the gut if we give it by mouth, so we must inject it. After an injection benzyl penicillin goes round a child's body in his blood. For a few hours there is plenty of penicillin to begin killing the bacteria that are infecting him. But he quickly excretes it in his urine and in a few hours it has all gone. *So we must inject benzyl penicillin every six hours* (except in newborn babies, 26.24). So it is a drug for severely ill children who can be given four injections a day.

Procaine penicillin. Because benzyl penicillin leaves the body so quickly, we use procaine penicillin or procaine penicillin aluminium monostearate (PAM). Procaine penicillin goes more slowly into the blood from the place where it is injected. It stays in the body for about a day, so one daily injection is enough.

Procaine penicillin forte (strong) or PPF. This is a mixture of benzyl penicillin and procaine penicillin. The benzyl penicillin goes quickly into the blood and lasts a short time. The procaine penicillin goes slowly into the blood and lasts all day.

Benethamine and benzathine penicillin. Penicillin from these injections goes into the blood very slowly, during four days. This is useful, because a child usually needs one injection only. His mother does not have to bring him to the clinic each day. These penicillins are usually fortified (made stronger). They have some benzyl and procaine penicillin mixed with them. There is 'fortified benethamine penicillin injection BPC' and 'fortified benzathine penicillin injection BPC'. These are usually sold in vials containing about one gram (1 M), which is the adult dose. These penicillins are sometimes called **depot penicillins**. They make a depot or store in a child's buttock which slowly goes into his blood. Use these depot penicillins for infections which are not serious, such as impetigo (11.4), or pyoderma (11.6). Seriously ill children need benzyl penicillin, or procaine penicillin.

Dose. If necessary, we can give penicillin in very large

DRUGS FOR SEPTIC INFECTIONS

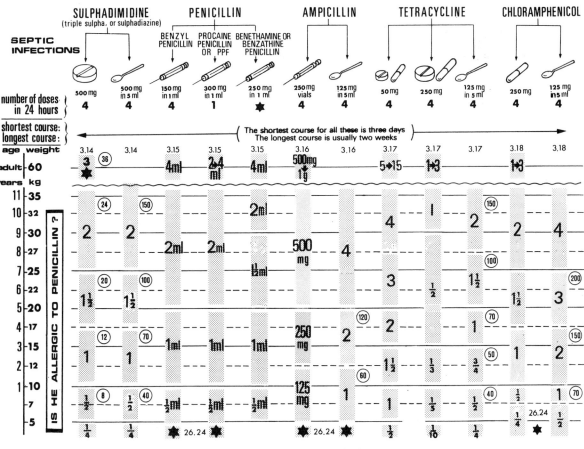

Fig. 3–12 Drugs for septic infections.

doses without causing harm (except in small babies). Most drugs are not like this. Large doses are harmful.

Side effects. All these penicillins have the same side effects. Occasionally a child is allergic to them. Soon after an injection he gets sudden difficulty breathing, wheezing, and shock. He is having an allergic reaction to penicillin and needs adrenaline quickly (3.2). Before you inject penicillin, always ask a child's mother if injections have caused symptoms before.

There is a less serious kind of allergy—penicillin can give a child fever and raised itchy spots (urticaria, 11.24).

A CHILD WHO IS ALLERGIC TO PENICILLIN MUST NEVER HAVE PENICILLIN OR AMPICILLIN AGAIN

Many diseases are NOT cured by penicillin. Penicillin does not cure colds, most kinds of diarrhoea, most urinary infections, sprained ankles, and backache.

PENICILLIN FOR SEPTIC INFECTIONS

A white powder to which water for injection is added to make solutions of these strengths—

benzyl penicillin injection 150 mg in 1 ml (600 mg is one mega-unit).

procaine penicillin injection (PAM) 300 mg in 1 ml (1 g is one mega-unit).

fortified procaine penicillin injection (PPF) 300 mg of procaine penicillin and 60 mg of benzyl penicillin in 1 ml.

fortified benethamine penicillin injection, or *fortified benzathine* penicillin injection. Usually in vials of *about* 1 g (in all) or 1 M. Dissolve this in 4 ml of water, to make a solution of about 250 mg or 0·25 M in 1 ml.

ORDINARY SEPTIC INFECTIONS

Ask his mother if he ever became ill after having an injection (allergic reaction).

EITHER, inject procaine penicillin (PAM, or PPF) *once a day.*

DRUGS FOR TB AND LEPROSY

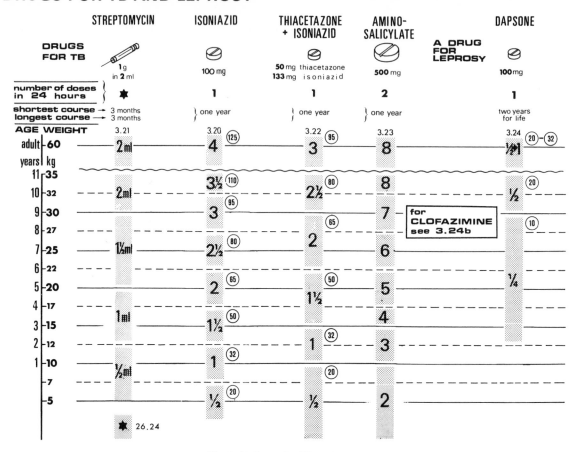

Fig. 3–13 Drugs for TB and leprosy.

At each injection give—
- adults, 2–4 ml (PAM 600–1200 mg or 0·6–1·2 M)
- children over 20 kg, 2 ml (PAM 600 mg or 0·6 M)
- children between 10 and 20 kg, 1 ml (PAM 300 mg, or 0·3 M)
- babies under 10 kg, ½ ml (PAM 150 mg, or 0·15 M).
- newborn babies, go to Section 26.24

OR, inject depot penicillin (benethamine, or benzathine penicillin). Give one injection every three or four days. Often, one injection is enough.

Give—
- adults, 4 ml (about 1 g or 1 M)
- children over 30 kg, 2 ml (0·5 g or 0·5 M)
- children between 20 and 30 kg, 1½ ml (0·4 g or 0·4 M)
- children between 10 and 20 kg, 1 ml (0·25 g or 0·25 M)
- babies under 10 kg, ½ ml (0·12 g or 0·12 M)
- newborn babies, go to Section 26.24

SEVERE INFECTIONS
IF POSSIBLE give benzyl penicillin four times a day.
At each dose give—
- adults, 4 ml (600 mg or 1 M)
- children over 20 kg, 2 ml (300 mg, or 0·5 M)
- children between 10 and 20 kg, 1 ml (150 mg, or 0·25 M)
- babies under 10 kg, ½ ml (75 mg, or 0·125 M)
- newborn babies, go to Section 26.24

OR, but this is not so good, give *twice* the normal dose of procaine penicillin for an ordinary infection. A good way of treating moderately severe infections is to give procaine penicillin each day. On the first day give an extra injection of benzyl penicillin.

DON'T GIVE PENICILLIN FOR LESS THAN THREE DAYS

3.16 Ampicillin

This safe, broad-spectrum (3.13) antibiotic, is very useful for babies. You can give it by mouth as a syrup or capsules, or by injection. It was very expensive, but it is becoming cheaper. Keep it for severe septic infections in

DRUGS FOR MALARIA AMOEBA GIARDIA

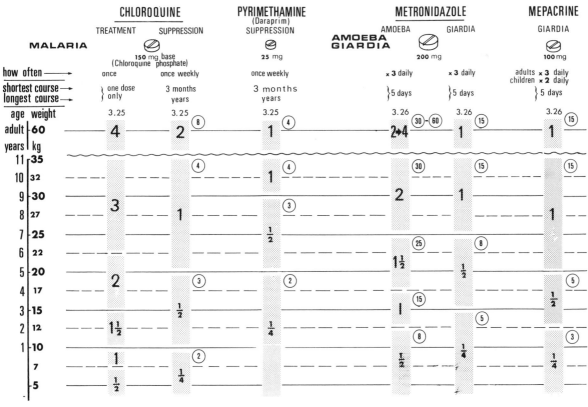

Fig. 3–14 Drugs for malaria, amoebae, and Giardia.

babies, especially septicaemia (26.24). Drugs easily harm babies, but ampicillin is safer than the other broad-spectrum antibiotics. We give you the doses for ampicillin injections, and ampicillin mixture. If you are using ampicillin capsules, give them in the same doses as for chloramphenicol. The doses below are at about 75 mg/kg/day.

Ampicillin is like penicillin, so if a child is allergic to penicillin, don't give him ampicillin.

AMPICILLIN FOR SEPTIC INFECTIONS
50–200 mg/kg/day

BY MOUTH—
A bottle or packet of powder to which water is added to make a syrup with 125 mg of ampicillin in 5 ml.
Give four doses a day.
At each dose give—
- children 20 to 35 kg, four teaspoons (500 mg)
- children 12 to 20 kg, 2 teaspoons (250 mg)
- babies less than 12 kg, 1 teaspoon (125 mg)
- newborn babies, go to 26.24

BY INJECTION—
Vials of 250 mg
Give four doses a day
At each dose give—
- adults, 500–1000 mg (2–4 250 mg vials)
- children between 20 and 35 kg, 500 mg (two 250 mg vials)
- children between 12 and 20 kg, 250 mg (one 250 mg vial)
- babies less than 12 kg, 125 mg ($\frac{1}{2}$ a 250 mg vial)
- newborn babies, go to 26.24

3.17 Tetracycline   3.17

We can give this broad-spectrum (3.13) antibiotic by mouth. It is more expensive than penicillin or the sulphonamides. For many infections it is not so good. We use a kind of tetracycline called **chlortetracycline** as an eye ointment for treating trachoma and conjunctivitis (16.9). Keep this ointment cool, or it will spoil.   3.16

Side effects. Tetracycline is yellow and it colours a child's teeth yellow or brown while they are growing. While he is having the drugs his teeth look normal. You

DRUGS FOR WORMS

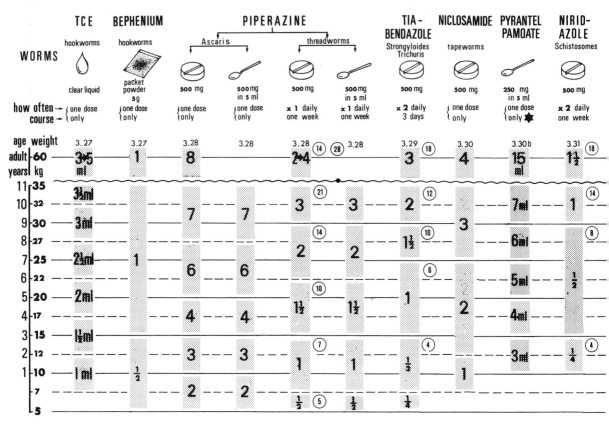

Fig. 3–15 Drugs for worms.

can only see the yellowness months or years later, when his teeth have grown through into his mouth. The yellowness lasts all his life. Prevent it. Don't give a mother tetracycline after the fourth month of pregnancy. If possible, give a child some other antibiotic. Don't give him tetracycline before he is 7 years old, unless his life is in danger. When a child is very sick a *few days* of tetracycline treatment may cure him without harming his teeth.

TETRACYCLINE FOR SEPTIC INFECTIONS, 25 mg/kg/day

Yellow tablets or capsules of 50 mg, or 250 mg, or mixtures with 125 mg in 5 ml.
 Give tetracycline by mouth four times a day
 At each dose give—
  ● adults, one to three 250 mg tablets (250 to 750 mg)
  ● children over 27 kg, four 50 mg tablets (200 mg) or two teaspoonfuls of mixture (250 mg)
  ● children between 20 and 27 kg, three 50 mg tablets (150 mg) or 1½ teaspoons of mixture (190 mg)

  ● children between 15 and 20 kg, two 50 mg tablets (100 mg) or one teaspoon of mixture (125 mg)
  ● children between 10 and 15 kg, 1½ 50 mg tablets (75 mg) or ¾ teaspoon of mixture (90 mg)
  ● babies between 5 and 10 kg, one 50 mg tablet or ½ a teaspoon of mixture (60 mg)
  ● babies less than 5 kg, ½ a 50 mg tablet (25 mg) or ¼ of a teaspoon of mixture (30 mg)
  ● newborn babies, go to Section 26.24

DON'T USE TETRACYCLINE FOR MILDLY ILL CHILDREN

3.18 Chloramphenicol

This is another broad-spectrum (3.13) antibiotic for septic infections. Use it for treating whooping cough in babies (8.17), typhoid, meningitis, osteomyelitis, and severe low respiratory infections.

Side effects. Chloramphenicol sometimes kills pre-

SOME SYMPTOMATIC DRUGS

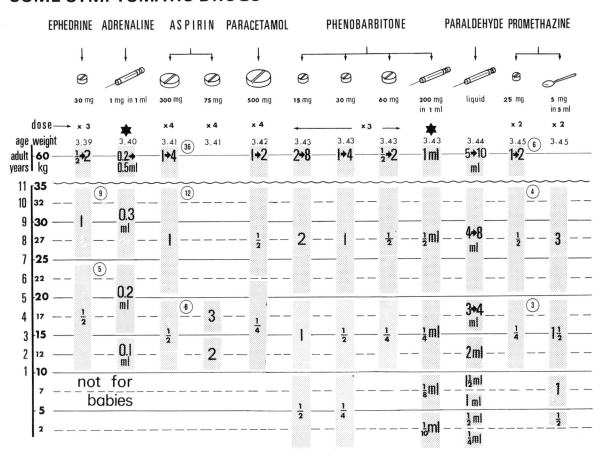

Fig. 3–16 Some symptomatic drugs.

mature babies, so try not to give it to them, or to any baby less than one month old. If you have to give it to a full-term baby, be very careful to give the right dose—too much is dangerous. Give premature babies 25 mg/kg/day. Give full-term babies and babies up to one month 25–50 mg/kg/day. If possible, give them penicillin and streptomycin or ampicillin instead (26.24).

Rarely, chloramphenicol harms the white cells in a child's blood so seriously that he dies. We can risk this if a child is seriously ill, because chloramphenicol is a very good antibiotic, and cheap. But we must not risk harming his white cells *if he is only mildly ill*. So *never* give chloramphenicol to a child with a cold, or a sore throat, or mild diarrhoea. It may kill him, and he does not need it.

CHLORAMPHENICOL, 50–100 mg/kg/day

Capsules, usually 250 mg, or a mixture of 125 mg in 5 ml.

Give chloramphenicol by mouth four times a day.

At each dose give—
- adults, 1–3 capsules (250–750 mg)
- children over 25 kg, two capsules or four teaspoons of mixture (500 mg)
- children between 17 and 25 kg, 1½ capsules, or 3 teaspoons of mixture (375 mg)
- children between 10 and 17 kg, 1 capsule, or 2 teaspoons of mixture (250 mg)
- babies between 7 and 10 kg, ½ a capsule or 1 teaspoonful of mixture (125 mg)
- babies under 7 kg, ¼ of a capsule or ½ a spoonful of mixture (62 mg)
- newborn babies, look in the section above. Also go to Section 26.24

3.18

DON'T USE CHLORAMPHENICOL FOR MILDLY ILL CHILDREN

3.19 Tuberculosis—isoniazid, streptomycin, thiacetazone, aminosalicylate (PAS) and ethambutol

TB bacilli grow slowly and are slowly killed by drugs. So TB is a chronic disease which has to be treated for a long time. Never give streptomycin to children with TB for less than a month. Give the other drugs for not less than one year.

TB bacilli easily become resistant to drugs, especially streptomycin. So a child should always have two TB drugs at the same time and one of them must be isoniazid. If he is having streptomycin he *must* have one of the others also. When he is having isoniazid he should, if possible, have either thiacetazone or aminosalecylate or ethambutol. Unfortunately aminosalcylate is expensive, and difficult to take because the dose is large. In some countries, thiacetazone causes side effects so often that it is not useful. So a child may take isoniazid alone. This is not the best treatment, because bacilli sometimes become resistant to isoniazid. But it is often the only treatment we can give him, and it is very helpful.

**ISONIAZID IS THE BEST TB DRUG
FOR CHILDREN**

3.20 Isoniazid

We usually give isoniazid with some other drug, such as streptomycin, aminosalicylate, or thiacetazone.

Side effects. Rarely, isoniazid causes anaemia and nerve pain. This is much more common in adults.

The doses below and in Fig. 3–13 are at 10 mg/kg/day. If a child is seriously ill you can give double these doses (20 mg/kg/day).

ISONIAZID FOR TB, 10–20 mg/kg/day

White tablets of 100 mg
Give isoniazid by mouth once a day for one year.
At each dose give—
- adults, four 100 mg tablets (400 mg)
- children, ½ a 100 mg tablet for each 5 kg they weigh

3.21 Streptomycin

This is used for treating TB, and for acute septic infections, especially septicaemia in young babies. Bacteria easily become resistant to streptomycin, so **always** give some other antimicrobial drug with it.

Side effects. Too much streptomycin for too long may cause deafness.

STREPTOMYCIN FOR TB AND SEPTIC INFECTIONS, 30–50 mg/kg/day

Vials of a white powder which is dissolved in water for injection so that there is 1 g in 2 ml.

TB. **Give one injection daily for three months (13.6). Also, give isoniazid daily.**

SEPTIC INFECTIONS. **Give one injection a day for 3–7 days with procaine penicillin.**
At each dose give—
- adults, 2 ml (1g)
- children over 30 kg, 2 ml (1 g)
- children between 20 and 30 kg, 1½ ml (750 mg)
- children between 12 and 20 kg, 1 ml (500 mg)
- children between 5 kg and 12 kg, ½ ml (250 mg)
- newborn babies, go to Section 26.24

3.22 Thiacetazone

We always give thiacetazone with isoniazid. So the easiest way to give it is as a compound (mixed) tablet. There are two kinds of compound tablet. They both have the same amount of thiacetazone (50 mg), but one has 100 mg of isoniazid and the other 133 mg. Children need more isoniazid for each kilo than adults, so try to use the 133 mg tablets.

Dose. The dose of thiacetazone is important. Too much causes side effects. So weigh him and give him the right dose.

Side effects. Thiacetazone may cause rashes, vomiting, and vertigo (dizziness). It may also stop a child eating. Side effects are most common in the first four weeks of treatment. If they don't come then they seldom come afterwards.

ISONIAZID AND THIACETAZONE (3–5 mg/kg/day) COMPOUND TABLET FOR TB

A white tablet containing 133 mg (or 100 mg) of isoniazid and 50 mg of thiacetazone.
Give this tablet by mouth once a day for one year.
At each dose give—
- adults, 3 tablets (150 mg of thiacetazone)
- children over 30 kg, 2½ tablets (125 thiacetazone)
- children between 22 and 30 kg, 2 tablets (100 mg of thiacetazone)
- children between 15 and 22 kg, 1½ tablets (75 mg thiacetazone)
- children between 10 and 15 kg, 1 tablet (50 mg thiacetazone)
- babies under 10 kg, ½ a tablet (25 mg of thiacetazone)

3.23 Sodium Aminosalicylate (PAS)

We always give this TB drug with isoniazid, and in addition with either streptomycin or thiacetazone. It is more expensive than isoniazid, and the dose is large, so we don't use it much now.

Side effects. Aminosalicylate may make a child want to vomit. It also causes vomiting and diarrhoea.

SODIUM AMINOSALICYLATE FOR TB, 250 mg/kg/day

White or coloured 500 mg tablets.
   Give aminosalicylate by mouth twice a day for not less than one year.
   At each dose give—

- adults, 8 tablets (4 g)
- children over 32 kg, 8 tablets (4 g)
- children between 27 and 32 kg, 7 tablets (3½ g)
- children between 22 and 27 kg, 6 tablets (3 g)
- children between 17 and 22 kg, 5 tablets (2½ g)
- children between 15 and 17 kg, 4 tablets (2 g)
- children between 10 and 15 kg, 3 tablets (1½ g)
- children under 10 kg, 2 tablets (1 g)

3.23b. Ethambutol for TB

Ethambutol has fewer side effects than PAS or thiacetazone, but it is more expensive. We can use it in two ways. (1) With isoniazid and thiacetazone and *instead* of streptomycin for the first three months TB treatment. This is useful because the child has tablets instead of injections. (2) With isoniazid and *instead* of thiacetazone or PAS for one year's TB treatment.

ETHAMBUTOL FOR TB, 25 mg/kg/day for the first two months, then 15 mg/kg/day

White 400 mg tablets.
   Give one dose each day.
   At each dose give—

First two months
- adults, 4½ tablets (1800 mg)
- children over 35 kg, 3 tablets (1200 mg)
- children between 30 and 35 kg, 2 tablets (800 mg)
- children between 22 and 30 kg, 1½ tablets (600 mg)
- children between 12 and 22 kg, 1 tablet (400 mg)
- children between 5 and 12 kg, ½ tablet (200 mg)

From 2 months onwards
- adults, 2½ tablets (1000 mg)
- children over 35 kg, 1½ tablets (600 mg)
- children between 22 and 35 kg, 1 tablet (400 mg)
- children between 10 and 22 kg, ½ tablet (200 mg)
- children under 10 kg, ¼ tablet (100 mg)

3.24 Dapsone (DDS)

Leprosy (12.4) is a very chronic disease, so children must have dapsone for at least two years. Some leprosy patients have to take it all their lives. The old treatment was to give small doses first. The new treatment is to start with the full dose.

Side effects. These are more common in adults than in children. Occasionally, a child gets a rash, fever, pain in the nerves, anaemia, jaundice, or mental symptoms. He is having a **reaction**, so stop his dapsone, and send him for help. If you cannot do this, stop his dapsone, and wait two weeks. Then start again with a small dose and increase it slowly.

DAPSONE FOR LEPROSY, 0·9–1·4 mg/kg/day

White tablets of 100 mg.
   Give dapsone once a day.
   At each dose give—
- adults, ½–1 tablet (50–100 mg)
- children over 30 kg, ½ tablet (50 mg)
- children between 12 and 30 kg, ¼ tablet (25 mg)

   If the child has tuberculoid leprosy, treat him for at least two years. If he has many bacilli in his skin (lepromatous and some kinds of borderline leprosy), treat him for at least four years after no more AAFB can be found in his skin scrapings. He may need treatment for life.

   Dapsone is a dangerous drug, so teach mothers to keep it locked up, so their children cannot take it.

3.24b Clofazimine

Some leprosy bacilli are now becoming resistant to dapsone. So children with lepromatous leprosy need dapsone *and clofazimine*. Children with tuberculoid leprosy have fewer leprosy bacilli, so they need dapsone only.

Side effects. Clofazimine is red and makes a child's skin red. This looks serious, but the redness goes in a few weeks when treatment stops. Clofazimine also makes the urine red.

CLOFAZIMINE FOR LEPROMATOUS LEPROSY

Red capsules of 100 mg
- Adults one capsule daily with dapsone for six months. Then dapsone only.
- Children of all ages one capsule twice a week for six months with dapsone. Then dapsone only.

EXPLANATION. Tell his mother that his skin and urine will go red. Explain that this will stop when he stops taking the capsules.

Malaria

3.25 Drugs for malaria

We can use malaria drugs in two ways. One, we can treat a sick child who has an acute attack of malaria. We treat him for one day, or for a few days only. Two, we can give a healthy child tablets once a week for many weeks to present him getting malaria. We call this suppression. We use some drugs for **treatment** only, some drugs for **suppression** only, and some drugs for both.

Chloroquine is the most important malaria drug. We treat children with chloroquine tablets or injections, or we suppress their malaria with chloroquine tablets. Unfortunately, the falciparum malaria parasites in some districts (but not yet in Africa) have become resistant to chloroquine, so we cannot use it. Fortunately all malaria parasites are sensitive to quinine. So, where malaria parasites are resistant to chloroquine, we treat sick children with quinine injections, or with sulphadoxine and pyrimethamine compound (mixed) tablets. Most parasites are sensitive to these compound tablets. We *only* use them for malaria parasites which are resistant to chloroquine. If parasites are sensitive to chloroquine, we *always* use it.

Pyrimethamine *alone* is NOT useful for treating an acute attack of malaria. But pyrimethamine alone is useful for suppression – unless parasites are resistant to it. Unfortunately, they often are. If parasites are resistant to pyrimethamine alone, we suppress them with chloroquine.

CHLOROQUINE TABLETS FOR TREATING MALARIA

White tablets, 250 mg of chloroquine phosphate, or 200 mg of chloroquine sulphate, both containing about 150 mg of chloroquine base. Some tablets contain only 100 mg base. If you use these, give more tablets.

Give one dose of chloroquine by mouth like this—
- **adults, 4 tablets (600 mg base)**
- **children over 22 kg, 3 tablets (450 mg base)**
- **children between 15 and 22 kg, 2 tablets (300 mg of base)**
- **children between 10 and 15 kg, 1½ tablets (225 mg of base)**
- **babies between 7 and 10 kg, 1 tablet (150 mg of base)**
- **babies under 7 kg, ½ a tablet (75 mg of base)**

In highly malarious districts where children have some immunity, one dose may be enough. In other districts where children have no immunity, and where one dose seems not to be enough, give chloroquine four times. Give HALF the above dose as a second dose 6 hours after the first dose. Give another half dose on the second and third days also.

Chloroquine is a bitter (bad tasting) tablet. So be sure the child takes it.

Most children with malaria can take chloroquine by mouth. But a child cannot take chloroquine if he is vomiting, having fits or is unconscious. These are signs of cerebral malaria (10.7). So he must have *chloroquine or quinine by injection NOW*. Too much chloroquine by injection is very dangerous, so *give him the right dose for his weight.* You MUST know his weight. Give chloroquine by SUBCUTANEOUS injection: ONLY when it is absolutely necessary. DON'T give it intramuscularly or intravenously, because it is absorbed too quickly and is very dangerous. The dose is 4mg/kg and there are usually 200 mg in a 5 ml ampoule. One whole ampoule is the adult dose. A child needs 1 ml for each 10 kg he weighs, so 1 ml is the dose for a 1 year old child. A second dose within 24 hours is very dangerous. So, make sure that someone else has not already given him a chloroquine injection. If you inject chloroquine, and send him for help, write the time of the injection in your letter.

CHLOROQUINE BY INJECTION FOR CEREBRAL MALARIA, 4 mg/kg/dose

An ampoule of 200 mg in 5 ml.
Weigh the child and find the dose from Figure 3–17.
Give one SUBCUTANEOUS injection only (3.5), and don't give another dose until the following day. Only give it then if he is still vomiting, unconscious, or having fits.

Treatment with sulphadoxine with pyrimethamine. This is a mixture of 500 mg of sulphadoxine and 25 mg of pyrimethamine. It is useful for treating malaria parasites which are resistant to chloroquine. Unfortunately, it cannot be injected. So if a child with chloroquine resistant malaria is vomiting, and cannot take tablets by mouth, he must have quinine. (Note. There are no dose figures for sulphadoxine with pyrimethamine or metrifonate. If you want them draw them on the empty table at the end of the book.)

SULPHADOXINE WITH PYRIMETHAMINE FOR CHLOROQUINE RESISTANT MALARIA

White 525 mg tablets, or syrup.
Give one dose only.
Give—
- **adults, 2 tablets**
- **children between 27 to 35 kg, 1½ tablets**
- **children between 20 and 27 kg, one tablet**
- **children between 10 and 20 kg, ½ a tablet**
- **children less than 10 kg, ¼ of a tablet.**

ONLY USE SULPHADOXINE WITH PYRIMETHAMINE FOR MALARIA WHICH IS RESISTANT TO CHLOROQUINE

Treatment with quinine. Quinine is a very good drug for treating malaria, especially cerebral malaria. It is very useful in countries where malaria parasites have become resistant to chloroquine. *If possible, give it intravenously.*

QUININE BY INJECTION FOR SEVERE MALARIA 10mg/kg/dose

Ampoules of 5 ml containing 60 mg in each ml. Check the strength of the ampoule. Some ampoules contain 300 mg in each ml.

If the child is severely ill and is having a drip, add the quinine to the fluid in the bottle. *This is the best way to give quinine.* **Always give quinine by drip, if possible.**

OR dilute the dose with 10–20 ml of sterile saline or water for injection. Give it *slowly* **INTRAVENOUSLY during ten minutes. If necessary, give another dose 8 hours later. Don't let quinine get outside the vein or it may cause a painful ulcer.**

OR, give one INTRAMUSCULAR dose deep into the child's buttock. This is the least good way to give quinine, because it may harm the muscle.

Give one dose—
- **adults 5–10 ml (300–600 mg)**
- **children over 27 kg, 5 ml**
- **children between 21 and 27 kg, 4 ml**
- **children below 21 kg, see Figure 3–17**

If the child is not much improved six hours later, give him one more dose only. As soon as possible give him chloroquine by mouth.

INJECTIONS OF CHLOROQUINE AND QUININE

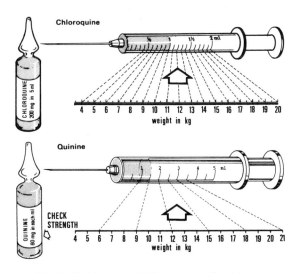

Fig. 3–17 Injections of chloroquine and quinine.

Suppression with chloroquine, or sulphadoxine with pyrimethamine, or pyrimethamine alone. This is useful in young children who live in malarious districts. It is especially useful if they are malnourished or chronically ill. We seldom suppress malaria in all the children coming to a clinic. But we can suppress it in some of them. Suppressing malaria may help an underweight child to climb back onto the road to health. It can also help a child with TB to recover. The most useful age for suppressing malaria is between three months and five years. Give him chloroquine, or pyrimethamine alone, or sulphadoxine with pyrimethamine *once a week*. If you cannot give the drug every week, give it every two or three weeks. Suppression should last several months at least. Suppression for a few weeks only is not helpful.

SUPPRESSING MALARIA WITH CHLOROQUINE

White tablets containing about 150 mg of chloroquine base.
Each week give—
- **adults, two tablets (300 mg base)**
- **children over 35 kg, 1½ tablets (225 mg)**
- **children between 20 and 35 kg, 1 tablet (150 mg base)**
- **children between 10 and 20 kg, ½ a tablet (75 mg base)**
- **babies under 10 kg, ¼ of a tablet (37 mg base)**

SUPPRESSING MALARIA WITH PYRIMETHAMINE ALONE

White 25 mg tablets
Each week give—
- **adults, 1–2 tablets (25–50 mg)**
- **children over 30 kg, ½–1 tablet (12–25 mg)**
- **children between 20 and 30 kg, ½ a tablet (12 mg)**
- **children between 10 and 20 kg, ¼–½ tablet (6–12 mg)**
- **babies under 10 kg, ¼ tablet (6 mg)**

SUPPRESSING MALARIA WITH SULPHADOXINE WITH PYRIMETHAMINE

Give the same doses as for treatment. Give a dose every one or two weeks.

Don't give sulphadoxine with pyrimethamine for more than six months.

EXPLANATION. **Too much pyrimethamine is dangerous. So tell the child's mother to keep the tablets safe where he cannot take them and eat them.**

Amoeba and Giardia

3.26 Metronidazole and mepacrine

Several kinds of diarrhoea need special drugs. Treat

amoebic dysentery (9.4), with metronidazole or tetracycline. Treat giardiasis (9.6) with smaller doses of metronidazole or with mepacrine. Metronidazole is the best drug, but it is expensive. You can also use metronidazole to treat skin ulcers (11.7), Vincent's stomatitis (18.7), and cancrum oris (18.8).

Side effects. Metronidazole sometimes causes vomiting. Mepacrine sometimes makes a child's skin yellow. This yellowness is not jaundice and does not make the sclera of his eyes yellow. It lasts several weeks.

METRONIDAZOLE FOR AMOEBIC DYSENTERY, 12–60 mg/kg/day

White 200 mg tablets
  Give metronidazole three times a day for five days.
  At each dose give—
  ● adults, 2–4 tablets (400–800 mg)
  ● children over 25 kg, two tablets (400 mg)
  ● children between 17 and 25 kg, 1½ tablets (300 mg)
  ● children between 12 and 17 kg, 1 tablet (200 mg)
  ● children less than 12 kg, ½ a tablet (100 mg)

METRONIDAZOLE FOR GIARDIASIS

Give metronidazole three times a day for five days
  At each dose give—
    ● adults, 1 tablet (200 mg)
    ● children over 25 kg, 1 tablet (200 mg)
    ● children between 15 and 25 kg, ½ tablet (100 mg)
    ● children under 15 kg, ¼ of a tablet (50 mg)

MEPACRINE FOR GIARDIASIS

Yellow 100 mg tablets
  Give adults one tablet three times a day for five days.
  Give children mepacrine twice a day for five days.
  At each dose give—
    ● children over 20 kg, one tablet (100 mg)
    ● children between 12 and 20 kg, ½ a tablet (50 mg)
    ● children under 12 kg, ¼ of a tablet (25 mg)

Worms

3.26b Drugs for worms

There are many drugs for worms. They are called **antihelminthics**. Some drugs, such as tetrachlorethylene, kill one kind of worm only. Other drugs, such as pyrantel pamoate, and tiabendazole kill several kinds of worm. Drugs like this are called **broad-spectrum antihelminthics.** Some drugs are cheap (tetrachlorethylene, piperazine). Other drugs are expensive (tiabenazole, pyrantel pamoate). Find out what kind of worm your patient has and how large his worm load is (21.1). Choose the best drug for him from Table 3:1b. Give him

a broad-spectrum antihelminthic if he has several kinds of worms, or if you do not know what worms he has.

3.27 TCE (tetrachlorethylene) and bephenium

Use these drugs for treating hookworm infections (22.5). Bephenium also kills *Ascaris*. This is useful because many children have hookworms and *Ascaris*. TCE is very much cheaper than bephenium. This is important because there may be many infected children. TCE easily evaporates (goes into the air), so put the cap tightly on the bottle. Keep it in a dark bottle, because it becomes dangerous if sunlight shines on it. If possible keep it in a refrigerator.

Side effects. Occasionally, TCE causes abdominal pain and headache. Don't give it to a very anaemic child with a haemoglobin of less than 5 g/dl. Never give more than 4 ml. This is the largest safe dose, and is a little less than a teaspoonful. Measure the dose carefully. Use a small syringe, or count the drops (20 drops in one ml).

DON'T GIVE TCE IF A CHILD'S HAEMOGLOBIN IS LESS THAN 5 g/dl

TCE FOR HOOKWORMS, 0·1 ml/kg

A clear liquid with a strong smell.
  Give one dose by mouth. Two days later give a second dose.
  At each dose give—
    ● adults, 3–5 ml (one teaspoonful)
    ● children, ½ ml for every 5 kg they weigh. Maximum dose 4 ml.

BEPHENIUM FOR HOOKWORMS AND ASCARIS

  Packets containing 5 g
  Give one dose only by mouth—
    ● adults, one whole packet (5 g)
    ● children over 15 kg, one whole packet (5 g)
    ● children under 15 kg, half a packet (2½ g)

IF A CHILD HAS *ASCARIS* AND HOOKWORMS, TREAT HIS *ASCARIS* FIRST, OR GIVE HIM TCE AND PIPERAZINE TOGETHER

3.28 Piperazine for *Ascaris* and threadworms

One large dose of piperazine paralyses *Ascaris* worms (stops them moving 21.3). They can no longer swim in the gut and they come out of a child in his stools. Treat threadworms (*Enterobius* 21.5) with a smaller dose of piperazine once a day for a week.

Table 3:1b   Drugs for worms

	Tetrachlorethylene	Bephenium	Piperazine	Tiabendazole	Niclosamide	Pyrantel pamoate
Ascaris		++	+++	+		+++
Hookworms	++	+++		+		+++
Strongyloides				+++		
Trichuris		+		+		
Treadworms			++	++	+	+++
Tapeworms					+++	

The plusses show how good each drug is for treating each worm.

We can use several kinds of piperazine (adipate, citrate, or phosphate) in the same way. The sizes of the tablets and the strength of the syrups differ. Some tablets are 300 mg, others are 500 mg.

Side effects. Piperazine sometimes makes a small child weak for a few days. This is not serious and soon goes. Occasionally, it causes vomiting.

**PIPERAZINE FOR *ASCARIS*,
120 mg/kg/dose**

Tablets containing 500 mg of piperazine hydrate, or a mixture with 500 mg of piperazine hydrate in 5 ml.
  Give one dose only—
  ● adults, 8 tablets (4 g)
  ● children over 27 kg, 7 tablets or 7 teaspoons (3½ g)
  ● children between 20 and 27 kg, 6 tablets or 6 teaspoons (3 g)
  ● children between 15 and 20 kg, 4 tablets or 4 teaspoons (2 g)
  ● children between 10 and 15 kg, 3 tablets or 3 teaspoons (1½ g)
  ● babies under 10 kg, 2 tablets or 2 teaspoons (1 g)

**PIPERAZINE FOR THREADWORMS,
40 mg/kg/day**

Give one dose daily for a week
  At each dose give—
  ● adults, 2–4 tablets (1–2 g)
  ● children over 30 kg, 3 tablets or 3 teaspoons (1½ g)
  ● children between 22 and 30 kg, 2 tablets or 2 teaspoons (1 g)
  ● children between 15 and 22 kg, 1½ tablets or 1½ teaspoons (750 mg)
  ● children between 7 and 15 kg, one tablet or one teaspoon (500 mg)
  ● children under 7 kg, ½ a tablet or ½ a teaspoon (250 mg)

3.29 Tiabendazole

This is useful for hookworms, *Ascaris*, threadworms, *Strongyloides*, and *Trichuris*. For hookworms, *Ascaris* and threadworms we have other drugs. So use tiabendazole for *Strongyloides* and *Trichuris*, and for children who have several kinds of worm.

TIABENDAZOLE FOR SEVERAL KINDS OF WORMS, 50 mg/kg/day

White 500 mg tablets
  Give the tablets by mouth twice a day for three days.
  Ask the child to chew (bite) them.
  At each dose give—
  ● adults, 3 tablets (1½ g)
  ● children over 30 kg, 2 tablets (1 g)
  ● children between 25 and 30 kg, 1½ tablets (750 mg)
  ● children between 15 and 25 kg, 1 tablet (500 mg)
  ● children between 7 and 15 kg, ½ tablet (250 mg)
  ● children under 7 kg, ¼ tablet (125 mg)

3.30 Niclosamide for tapeworms

Use this for any of the tapeworms in Section 21.4. Niclosamide kills tapeworms, but it does not kill the ova inside them. The ova of *T. solium* may hatch into larvae and spread through the child. Give the child a purge (bowel-opening medicine) two hours after you have given niclosamide for *T. solium*. This will quickly remove the ova from his gut and prevent them spreading. This is not necessary with other tapeworms. Magnesium sulphate is a good purge. The adult dose is 2–12 g in a glass of water. Give a child 4 g or one teaspoonful.

NICLOSAMIDE FOR TAPEWORMS

White 500 mg tablets
  For *Taenia* give one dose only. For children break the tablets into powder, and mix it with water.

At each dose give—
- adults, 4 tablets (2 g)
- children over 25 kg, 3 tablets (1·5 g)
- children between 12 and 25 kg, 2 tablets (1 g)
- children under 12 kg, 1 tablet (500 mg)

If the child has a *T. solium* infection, give him a purge two hours later.

For *H. nana* give one dose as above. Then give half this dose daily for six days.

3.30b Pyrantel pamoate for worms

This is a useful broad-spectrum antihelminthic drug. It is the best drug for threadworms.

PYRANTEL PAMOATE 11mg/kg/dose

A mixture with 250 mg of base in five ml
 Give one dose only
 Give—
- adults, 15 ml (750 mg)
- children above 30 kg, 7 ml (350 mg)
- children between 25 and 30 kg, 6 ml (300 mg)
- children between 20 and 25 kg, 5 ml (250 mg)
- children between 15 and 20 kg, 4 ml (200 mg)
- children between 10 and 15 kg, 3 ml (150 mg)

Don't give it to children under 10 kg.

For threadworms, give another dose two weeks later. For hookworms (*Necator*) give one dose each day for three days.

3.31 Niridazole for schistosomiasis

Use this to treat infections with *Schistosoma haematobium* or *Schistosoma mansoni*. Niridazole sometimes colours the urine brown. It may cause mental symptoms, vomiting, and diarrhoea.

NIRIDAZOLE FOR SCHISTOSOMIASIS, 25 mg/kg/day

White 500 mg tablets
 Give niridazole by mouth twice a day for a week
 At each dose give —
- adults, 1½ tablets (750 mg)
- children over 30 kg, 1 tablet (500 mg)
- children between 15 and 30 kg, ½ tablet (250 mg)
- children under 15 kg, ¼ tablet (125 mg)

3.31b Metrifonate for *Schistosoma haematobium*

This is a useful drug for treating children with *Schistosoma haematobium* infections. It is not useful for treat-

ing other kinds of schistosome. It is easier to give than niridazole. A child only needs three doses of metrifonate. With niridazole he needs two doses a day for a week. Don't give metrifonate to children if they are ill with some other disease, such as malaria or diarrhoea.

Side effects. Occasionally children have abdominal pain and feel they want to vomit. Sometimes they feel weak and have a headache.

METRIFONATE, 7·5 mg/kg/dose

White 100 mg tablets
 Give one dose. Wait two weeks and give a second dose. Wait two weeks and give a third dose.
 At each dose give—
- adults, 5 tablets (500 mg)
- children over 25 kg, 2 tablets (200 mg)
- children between 17 and 25 kg, 1½ tablets (150 mg)
- children between 10 and 17 kg, 1 tablet (100 mg)
- children between 5 and 10 kg, ½ tablet (50 mg)

Nutrients

3.33 Iron

Haemoglobin in the red cells contains iron. If a child lacks iron, he cannot make enough haemoglobin, so his blood becomes anaemic (22.1). We can give older children and mothers ferrous (iron) sulphate tablets. Younger children need children's iron mixture (Ferrous sulphate mixture, paediatric, BPC). Iron mixture does not keep well. It slowly goes brown during a few weeks. It is not harmful when it is brown but the iron is less well absorbed. The mixture should be freshly made. Iron by mouth is cheap, but is absorbed slowly. So we have to give it for a long time — at least three months.

**GIVE IRON FOR AT LEAST
THREE MONTHS**

IRON SULFATE TABLETS FOR ANAEMIA

Green 200 mg tablets
 Give adults and children over 20 kg one tablet twice a day. Don't give these tablets to smaller children.

'CHILDREN'S IRON MIXTURE' FOR ANAEMIA

A pale green mixture
 Give this once a day in a drink of water. Give—
- children over 10 kg, two teaspoons (10 ml)
- children under 10 kg, one teaspoon (5 ml)

Iron medicine or tablets may make a child vomit. This is less likely if he has food or a sugary drink with iron medicine.

46

EXPLANATION. **Too much iron is dangerous. Tell the child's mother to keep iron tablets or medicine in a locked cupboard, where he cannot find them and poison himself (14.6). Explain that his iron medicine may make his stools black.**

Iron dextran injection. Iron treatment by mouth takes a long time and a mother may not give her child his iron medicine. So iron injections are useful. Inject iron deep into the muscle. If you do not inject iron dextran deeply enough, the iron may stain the skin of a light skinned child. The dose of iron depends on the child's weight and how anaemic he is. So we need to know his weight and his haemoglobin.

IRON DEXTRAN INJECTION FOR ANAEMIA

Ampoules of 2 or 5 ml, a dark brown fluid containing 50 mg of iron in each ml.

Haemoglobin above 6 g/dl. **The child's weight in kg multiplied by 2/3 is the number of ml of iron dextran he needs. For example, an 18 kg child needs 12 ml of iron dextran.**

Haemoglobin below 6 g/dl. **His weight in kg is the number of ml of iron dextran he needs.**

Give iron dextran by deep intramuscular injection. Give up to 5 ml into each buttock. If he needs more than 10 ml (5 ml each side), give the rest at his next visits. When he has had the iron he needs, don't give any more iron injections for nine months.

3.34 Iodides

Our bodies need small quantities of iodine. Usually, we get enough iodine from our drinking-water, but in some districts there is not enough iodine in the water. Iodine deficiency causes goitre (19.6), and iodine embryopathy (24.14b). We can prevent both these diseases. We can add a little iodine to all the salt that people eat. If this is not possible, we can inject iodized oil.

IODIZED OIL FOR ENDEMIC GOITRE AND IODINE EMBRYOPATHY

Injection abscesses happen more easily with oily injections, so sterilize the syringes carefully. If possible, use sterile disposable syringes made of plastic (not polystyrene, because this oil dissolves polystyrene). Clean the skin with iodine.
  Don't treat adults over 45
  Give one injection every three years

At each dose give—
  ● **adults under 45 years, 1–2 ml**
  ● **children over 20 kg, 1 ml**
  ● **children between 10 and 20 kg, $\frac{1}{2}$ ml**
  ● **children under 10 kg, $\frac{1}{3}$ ml**
  If there are nodules (lumps) in the patient's goitre, only inject 0·2 ml.

3.35 Vitamin A

3.35
3.30b

Lack of vitamin A causes serious eye lesions which may make a child blind. Vitamin A is supplied as yellow capsules of 100 000 units and as an injection (retinyl palmitate, water miscible). For prevention and treatment, go to Section 16.15.

3.36 Compound vitamin tablets

3.36

There are several kinds of mixed vitamin tablet. They all contain some of the B vitamins and may contain other vitamins also. Each country needs to use the best one for its common deficiencies. Give these tablets to malnourished children only. The dose is not important and large doses are only wasted. Give children less than two years old one tablet three times a day, and older children two tablets. One week of treatment is usually enough.

3.33

3.37 Folic acid

3.37

This is one of the B vitamins and is found in leaves, meat, and liver. The body needs it to make haemoglobin. Lack of it causes anaemia (22.1). Two weeks is the normal course, but a child with sickle cell anaemia may need it for years.

3.31
3.34

FOLIC ACID FOR ANAEMIA
White 5 mg tablets

ADULTS AND CHILDREN. **One tablet (5 mg) a day. If you cannot give children a tablet each day, give them a tablet each week.**

EXPLANATION. **Tell the child's mother that he must eat plenty of dark green leaves.**

3.38 Vitamin K

3.38
3.31b

We use this for preventing and treating haemorrhagic disease of the new born (26.33). Vitamin K is supplied in ampoules containing 0·5 ml of a milky solution in which there is 1 mg of vitamin K. This is the dose for a newborn child. Give one injection to all newborn children who weigh less than 2 kg. Don't give more than one mg, even if the child goes on bleeding. Don't use an ampoule if the fluid in it looks oily. Don't use it if the top part of the fluid looks different from the bottom part.

SYMPTOMATIC DRUGS

Asthma

3.39 Ephedrine

When a child has asthma (8.13) the muscles of his smaller bronchi contract and the mucosa inside them swells. Air has difficulty going in and out of his lungs. Ephedrine and adrenaline make his bronchial muscles relax. They reduce the swelling of his mucosa, and so help him to breathe. Babies have very little muscle in their bronchi, so these drugs don't help them. Don't give children ephedrine, or adrenaline, until they are a year old.

DON'T GIVE EPHEDRINE TABLETS OR ADRENALINE TO A BABY LESS THAN A YEAR OLD

EPHEDRINE FOR ASTHMA 3 mg/kg/day

White 30 mg tablets
  Give ephedrine by mouth three times a day
  At each dose give—
  ● adults, ½–2 tablets (15–60 mg)
  ● children over 25 kg, 1 tablet (30 mg)
  ● children between 10 and 25 kg, ½ a tablet (15 mg)
  ● don't give ephedrine to babies weighing less than 10 kg.

3.40 Adrenaline

Give a child with a severe asthmatic attack an adrenaline injection. But don't give too much, and don't give it too often. Adrenaline is also useful for a child who has severe allergic reaction to penicillin or tetanus antitoxin (3.2).

ADRENALINE INJECTION FOR ASTHMA, OR A SENSITIVITY REACTION 0·01 mg/kg/dose

Ampoules of 0·5 ml, or 1 ml
  Count the child's pulse and give him one injection subcutaneously. If possible, measure it with a 1 ml Microstat syringe (3–8).
  ● adults, 0·2–0·5 ml
  ● children between 25 and 35 kg, 0·3 ml
  ● children between 15 and 25 kg, 0·2 ml
  ● children between 10 and 15 kg, 0·1 ml
  ● don't give adrenaline to babies under 10 kg

Count his pulse again. Don't give a second dose until 30 mins later. If necessary, give a third dose two hours after that. Never give more than three doses. If his pulse goes up by more than 30 beats per minute after one dose of adrenaline, don't give another dose.

Pain

3.41 Acetylsalicylic acid ('Aspirin')

Aspirin helps to stop pain. Aspirin also makes a child sweat, and lowers his temperature (10.1), so it is a useful symptomatic drug for fever. Many of the medicines that people buy for treating pain, contain aspirin. But they are always more expensive than ordinary aspirin.

Side effects. Too much aspirin can cause fast deep breathing, then very weak breathing and coma. Don't give aspirin to children who are dehydrated, or passing very little urine, or who have asthma—it may start an attack. Don't give it to children under 10 kg.

Most aspirin tablets contain 300 mg. There is also a small soluble (easily dissolved) children's tablet which only contains 75 mg of aspirin (aspirin soluble tablets, paediatric BPC). You can use both kinds of tablet. Find out which tablet you have, because one contains four times as much aspirin as the other.

ASPIRIN FOR PAIN AND FEVER 65 mg/kg/day

White 300 mg tablets
  Give aspirin by mouth four times a day
  At each dose give—
  ● adults, 1–4 tablets (300–1200 mg)
  ● children over 20 kg, one tablet (300 mg)
  ● children between 10 and 20 kg, ½ a tablet (150 mg)
  Don't give these tablets to children under 10 kg

SOLUBLE ASPIRIN ('CHILD'S ASPIRIN') FOR PAIN AND FEVER

White tablets containing 75 mg of aspirin
  Give soluble aspirin by mouth four times a day
  At each dose give—
  ● children between 15 and 20 kg, 3 tablets (225mg)
  ● children between 10 and 15 kg, 2 tablets (150 mg)
  Don't give these tablets to children under 10 kg.

3.42 Paracetamol (acetaminophen)

This is a newer drug for treating pain and fever. Paracetamol is safer for young children than aspirin, so always use it if possible.

PARACETAMOL FOR PAIN AND FEVER

White 500 mg tablets

Give paracetamol by mouth four times a day
At each dose give—
- adults, 1–2 tablets (500 mg–1 g)
- children over 22 kg, $\frac{1}{2}$ tablet (250 mg)
- children between 10 and 22 kg, $\frac{1}{4}$ tablet (125 mg)

Fits

3.43 Phenobarbitone

Small doses (3 mg/kg/day) of phenobarbitone tablets by mouth *prevent* fits. Larger doses (6 mg/kg/day) prevent fits *and* make a child sleepy. You can also give phenobarbitone by injection to *treat* fits. Too much (an overdose) causes coma (14.8) and death. So teach mothers to keep the tablets where children cannot find them. Phenobarbitone is sold in tablets of several different sizes, so check the size of tablet you are giving.

The doses of tablets are at 3 mg/kg/day. If necessary, for treating the spasms of tetanus (18.16), you can give twice the dose—but not more. Phenobarbitone works for a long time—12 hours or more. Don't give more until the phenobarbitone you have already given has had time to start working.

PHENOBARBITONE TABLETS TO PREVENT FITS OR THE SPASMS OF TETANUS, 3–6 mg/kg/day

White 30 mg tablets. For other sizes of tablets see Figure 3–16.

Look at the size of the tablet.
Give phenobarbitone by mouth three times a day
At each dose give—
- adults, 1–4 30 mg tablets (30–120 mg)
- children over 20 kg, one 30 mg tablet (30 mg)
- children between 10 and 20 kg, $\frac{1}{2}$ a 30 mg tablet (15 mg)
- babies under 10 kg, $\frac{1}{4}$ of a 30 mg tablet (7 mg)

The doses below of phenobarbitone for injection are at 4 mg/kg/dose. If necessary, you can give twice this dose.

PHENOBARBITONE INJECTION TO TREAT FITS 3–10 mg/kg/dose

Ampoules of 1 ml containing 200 mg of phenobarbitone
Measure carefully, if possible use a Microstat 1 ml syringe.
Give one intramuscular injection—
- adults 1 ml (200 mg)
- children over 20 kg, $\frac{1}{2}$ ml (100 mg)
- children between 10 and 20 kg, $\frac{1}{4}$ ml (50 mg)
- babies between 5 and 10 kg, 1/8 ml (25 mg)
- babies under 5 kg, 1/10 ml (20 mg)

If, after the above dose, the child has not stopped having fits after 15 minutes, give him *ONE* more dose only. If you

have already given him a double dose, don't give him any more.

3.44 Paraldehyde   **3.44**

This is a safe drug for stopping fits, or the spasms of tetanus. It is a thick oily liquid with a strong smell. Paraldehyde dissolves rubber, and some kinds of plastic. So, use either a glass syringe, or a kind of plastic (nylon) which will not be harmed by paraldehyde.

3.41
3.39

Side effects. Paraldehyde sometimes causes a painful sterile injection abscess (3.6).

3.43

PARALDEHYDE FOR FITS OR THE SPASMS OF TETANUS, 0·1–0·2 ml/kg/dose

Liquid in ampoules containing 2, 5, or 10 ml.

FOR FITS
Give one dose by deep intramuscular injection
- adults, 5–10 ml
- children over 20 kg, 4–8 ml
- children between 15 and 20 kg, 3–4 ml
- children between 10 and 15 kg, 2 ml
- children between 7 and 10 kg, $1\frac{1}{2}$ ml
- babies between 5 and 7 kg, 1 ml
- babies between 2 and 5 kg, $\frac{1}{2}$ ml
- very small babies under 2 kg, $\frac{1}{4}$ ml

If the child has not stopped having fits after 15 minutes give him ONE more dose only.

FOR THE SPASMS OF TETANUS

Two or even three times the above dose may be needed every four hours to stop the spasms.
If you give paraldehyde into the rectum, give three times (0·6 ml/kg) the intramuscular dose, in ten times its volume of saline. Give it through a plastic tube or rubber catheter.

3.40

An antihistamine

3.45 Promethazine   **3.45**

A substance called histamine is formed in some lesions and helps to cause inflammation and itching (2.4). An antihistamine (against histamine) drug helps some kinds of inflammation, which are not caused by infection. Promethazine is an antihistamine, and helps urticaria (11.24), and angioneurotic oedema (19.7). Promethazine also makes a child sleepy. It is useful symptomatic treatment for a dry cough or an itchy rash which keeps a child awake at night. It helps to prevent vomiting. It may prevent a child vomiting when he goes on a bus (travel sickness, 25.8). Even so, antihistamines are not very useful and health workers often give them when they are not helpful. Antihistamine tablets do *not*

3.42

help asthma, and there is no need for antihistamine injections.

PROMETHAZINE HYDROCHLORIDE, 1 mg/kg/dose

White 25 mg tablets, or an elixir (mixture) with 5 mg in 5 ml. Give promethazine twice a day.
At each dose give—
- **adult, 1–2 tablets (25–50 mg)**
- **children over 20 kg, $\frac{1}{2}$ a tablet or 3 teaspoons (15 mg)**
- **children between 10 and 20 kg, $\frac{1}{4}$ of a tablet or $1\frac{1}{2}$ teaspoons (7 mg)**

If necessary, you can give twice these doses.

Cough mixture

3.46 A placebo

Most coughs are useful because they remove pus or mucus which might block a child's respiratory system. The best way to treat a serious cough is to treat the disease which is causing it. Serious coughs are usually caused by septic respiratory infections, and need an antibiotic. Mild coughs are usually caused by viruses, and do not need an antibiotic. But a child's mother always wants some treatment, so you need a cough mixture to give him. 'Children's cough mixture' does not cure a cough. It is a placebo to give a child while you observe him to make sure he has no serious infection.

If necessary, you can make this cough mixture from 1 per cent ammonium chloride, a few drops of peppermint water and some colour.

CHILDREN'S COUGH MIXTURE

Put 100 ml into the bottle that the child's mother has brought with her. The dose for children of all ages is 5 ml, or one teaspoon four times a day.

Poisoning

3.47 Syrup of ipecacuanha

This drug causes vomiting and is useful in some kinds of poisoning, see Section 14.6. Keep some syrup of ipecacuanha in your clinic. Don't use extract of ipecacuanha. It is too strong. You will not want ipecacuanha often, but it may save a child's life.

SYRUP OF IPECACUANHA FOR POISONING

Give the child 15 ml of syrup of ipecacuanha, and then a cup of water. Most children vomit in 15 minutes. If he has not vomited in 15 minutes, give him another dose.

Drugs for the skin

3.48 Ointments, lotions, and skin antiseptics

The best way to treat some skin diseases, such as severe skin sepsis, is to give a child drugs by mouth, or by injection. We can treat other diseases by putting drugs onto his skin. We can put them into thick ointments or into liquid lotions.

We can treat scabies (11.10) with lotions made with **25 per cent benzyl benzoate**, or **1 per cent gammebenzine hexachloride**, which is much cheaper, because we can dilute it more. We can also treat scabies with **5 per cent sulphur ointment in vaseline**, or with monosulphiram.

You can treat ringworm (11.13) with benzoic acid compound (mixed) ointment (Whitfield's ointment). You can treat septic infections (11.3) on the outside of the skin, such as impetigo, or pyoderma, with **gentian violet** (crystal violet). This kills pyogenic bacteria. You can also use gentian violet to treat thrush (18.5). Dissolve half a teaspoonful of gentian violet crystals in two cupfuls of water. This will make a 0·5% solution which you can paint on the skin. It will make his skin dark blue and also colour his clothes.

We can help septic skin infections by washing the skin in **potassium permanganate solution**, which is an antiseptic. Dissolve a pinch (1 g) of crystals in a litre of water. This makes a dark red solution containing one part of permanganate in a thousand parts of water.

Hypochlorite is a good antiseptic and disinfectant. Make hypochlorite solution by adding 1 teaspoonful of calcium hypochlorite (3:1) to a litre of water. You can also use dilute hypochlorite solution BPC ('Milton') containing 1 per cent of chlorine. Even this is too strong to use on the skin, so dilute it with at least one part of water before you use it. A cheaper way of using hypochlorite is to buy strong hypochlorite solution BPC ('Choros', 'Deosan', 'Jik' etc.) containing 8–18 per cent of chlorine. These solutions are usually used for bleaching (whitening) clothes. Dilute them with at least 30 times as much water before you use them for the skin. We can also use hypochlorite solutions for disinfecting babies' feeding bottles (N 8.11) or plastic tubes for nasogastric drips (9.24). Very dilute hypochlorite solutions soon become useless, so make a fresh solution each time you need it.

Explain to mothers that permanganate and hypochlorite solutions are for the skin, and are NOT to be taken by mouth.

Saline is a dilute solution of salt in water. You can use it for cleaning septic skin lesions. You can also use it for cleaning lesions in the mouth and nose and eyes. Put *half* a level teaspoonful of salt in a cupful of water. More salt will not help.

As usual, the best treatment is curative, but symptomatic treatment is sometimes useful also. If a lesion is dry, cracked, and scaly, an oily medicine helps. If it is very itchy, **calamine lotion** may help. **Zinc and castor oil ointment** is useful for treating nappy rash (26.43).

EQUIPMENT FOR DIAGNOSIS

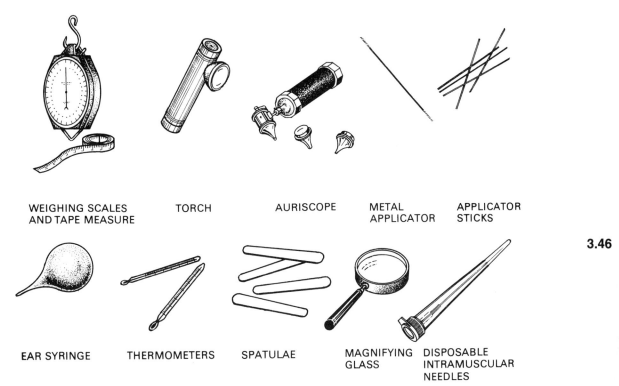

WEIGHING SCALES AND TAPE MEASURE   TORCH   AURISCOPE   METAL APPLICATOR   APPLICATOR STICKS

3.46

EAR SYRINGE   THERMOMETERS   SPATULAE   MAGNIFYING GLASS   DISPOSABLE INTRAMUSCULAR NEEDLES

Fig. 3–18 Equipment for diagnosis.

3.49 Some other expendable supplies

The clinic needs other supplies also. It needs **fluorescein paper** (16.7) for diagnosis. It needs **sterile water** to dissolve the dry drugs in ampoules. You need **iodine** as a skin antiseptic. **Hydrogen peroxide** is useful for sore mouths (18.8). You need lysol for disinfection, and liquid paraffin (or cooking oil) to lubricate (make oily) nasogastric tubes (9.24). Dry gauze is for cuts. Vaseline gauze is for burns (14.3). Cotton wool, bandages, and adhesive tape are for dressings. You need 'plastic tubing, general purpose' for making scalp vein sets (9.27), for nasogastric drips (9.24), for feeding children who are too weak to eat, for feeding newborn babies (26.18), and for feeding malnourished children (7.11). You can boil this tube to sterilize it. You can soften it in a match flame so that you can squeeze it tight round a needle. Larger tube, such as the tube from used drip sets, is useful for older children. For sterilizing this tube, see Section 9.24. You need phenol (carbolic acid) for Pandy's test (15.3). Insecticide (insect killing 'medicine') helps to keep flies out of the clinic. You need soap to wash your hands after the examination of every child. The clinic also needs weight charts, continuation cards (6.2), and plastic bags for weight charts.

EQUIPMENT

3.50 'The important 20'

Most clinics already have some equipment, such as bowls, basins, and trays. But many of them do not have all the things which they need to examine and treat children. The extra equipment for this has been listed in Table 3:2. You can easily carry the weighing scale (5–3) on a bicycle, and hold a clinic in another village. The measuring tape is for measuring the arm circumference (N 1.5) to diagnose malnutrition. There is an electric torch, a rectal and an oral thermometer, and 20 wooden spatulae. There is an auriscope and some applicator sticks. The rubber bulb can suck and blow. You can easily sterilize this, so you can use it for ears (17–6) and noses, and for newborn babies. There is a pressure cooker (6–9) for sterilizing, and a kerosine pressure stove to heat it with. There are three sizes of syringe (3.5), and two sizes of ordinary needle. There are some sterile disposable needles for lumbar puncture. There are also some curved needles, a needle holder, and tissue forceps, so that you can stitch (14–4). There is a measuring scoop for making glucose saline. Lastly there is a jug, a funnel, and some bottles and spoons for liquid medicines.

Table 3:2 Equipment for the clinic

For Diagnosis

SCALE, Salter Model 235, 0 to 25 kg in half kg graduations to match the weight chart, ECHO.

TAPE MEASURE, fibre glass, graduated in cm, each $0·15, UNIPAC 0567000, one only.

FLASHLIGHT, prefocused, two cells, right-angled plastic, each $1·06, UNIPAC 0630000, one only (18–1).

AURISCOPE, set, electric with spatulae, spare battery and bulb, each $23·55, UNIPAC 0660000, one only (17–2).

APPLICATOR, metal ear and nose, double ended, each $0·21, UNIPAC 07030000, five (17–4).

APPLICATOR STICKS, wooden, one packet (17–4).

MAGNIFYING GLASS, one only.

SYRINGE, ear and ulcer, 90 ml, conical tip, rubber, each $0·52, UNIPAC 0364000, one only (17–6).

THERMOMETER, clinical, rectal, Celsius, 35 to 42°C, each $0·25, UNIPAC 0482500, one only (10–1).

THERMOMETER, clinical, oral, Celsius, 35 to 42°C, each $0·25, UNIPAC 0481500, one only (10–1).

DEPRESSOR, tongue, wooden, child size, box of 500 $2·09, UNIPAC 0621000, one box only (18–1).

For treatment, and records

PRESSURE COOKER, seven litres, aluminium, each $13·43, UNIPAC 2039505, one only (6–9).

STOVE, kerosine, single burner, pressure type, each $12·40, UNIPAC 0170000, one only.

LAMP, alcohol, brass, 150 ml, each $2·42, UNIPAC 0955100, one only (17–4).

SYRINGE, hypodermic, 5 ml, glass, Luer adaptor, five (3–20), or autoclavable plastic equivalent.

SYRINGE, hypodermic, glass, Luer adaptor, 2 ml, each $0·25, UNIPAC 0783500, thirty (3–8), or autoclavable plastic equivalent.

SYRINGE, microstat, glass, 1 ml, Luer adaptor, each $1·13, UNIPAC 0786500, three (3–8, 13–2), or autoclavable plastic equivalent.

RING, rubber, red, for Microstat syringes, four, $0·04, UNIPAC 034990

NEEDLES, hypodermic, $0·7 \times 38$ mm, regular bevel, Luer adaptor, box of twelve $0·33, UNIPAC 0750000, ten boxes (3–8).

NEEDLES, hypodermic, $0·45 \times 10$ mm, Luer adaptor, UNIPAC 0751502 box of 12, $0·58, three boxes.

NEEDLES, $0·9 \times 40$ mm, short bevel, Luer adaptor,

EQUIPMENT FOR TREATMENT

TREATMENT

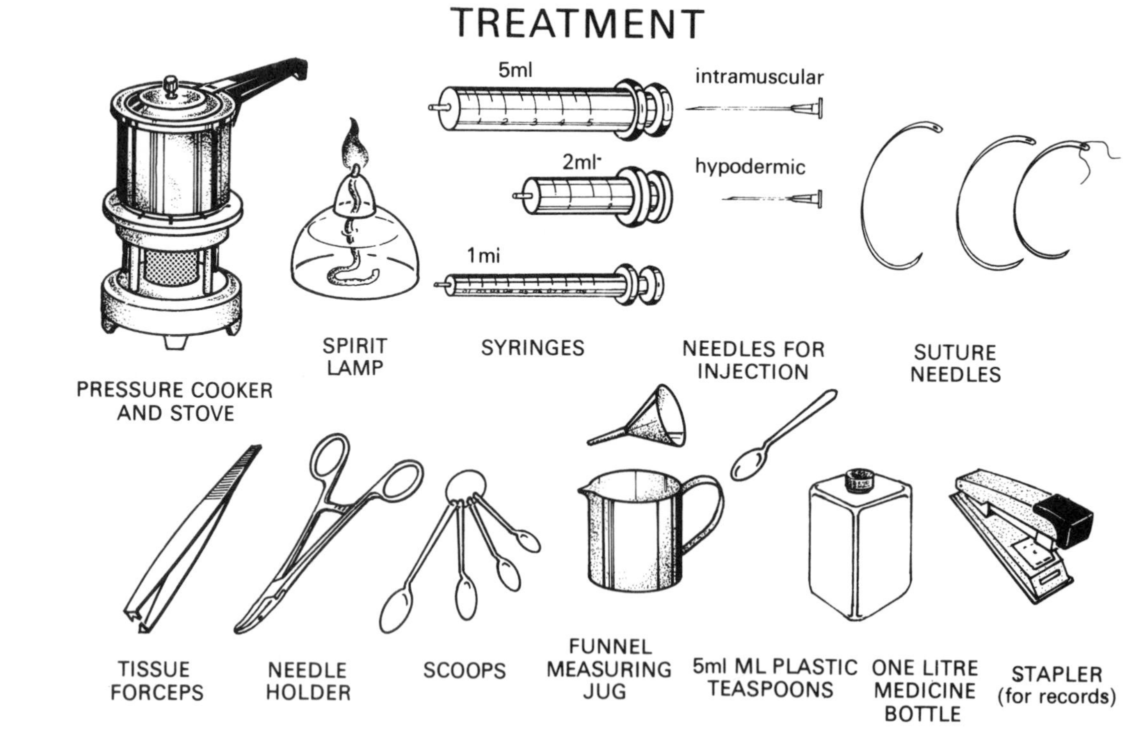

Fig. 3–19 Equipment for treatment.

sterile, disposable in individual plastic wrapping, twenty (15–2).

NEEDLES, suture surgeons, ⅜ inch circle, cutting No 12, packets $0·52, UNIPAC 0759332, two (14–4).

FORCEPS, tissue 150 mm, stainless steel spring type, 1 × 2 teeth, each $0·83, UNIPAC 0737000, one only (14–5).

HOLDER, needle, curved Metzenbaum, stainless steel, each $1·91, UNIPAC 0742985, one only (14–4).

SCOOPS, measuring, for preparing glucose-salt solution, TALC, one set only (9–10b).

MEASURE, 1,000 ml. with handle graduated, stainless steel, each $1·54, UNIPAC 0261000, one only.

FUNNEL, lab 75 mm diam, polypropylene, each $0·14, UNIPAC 0945900, one only (3–7).

BOTTLE, plastic, one litre, square form, three (3–7).

TEASPOONS, plastic, 5 ml, twenty (3–1).

STAPLING MACHINE, and staples, each $4·31, UNIPAC 2680002, one only.

Twenty of these pieces of equipment are so important that *all* clinics should have them. They are in bold type and are called the 'Important 20'. They form part of the quality score (6.8).

YOU CANNOT GIVE GOOD CHILD CARE WITHOUT THE RIGHT EQUIPMENT

---

4 Caring for a healthy child

4.1 'Bloke is not ill, so why should I take him to the clinic?'—the well child

Many mothers think that we can only help a sick child. They do not understand that we can also prevent a healthy child becoming ill. We can do this in three ways.

One. We can give a child special 'medicines' called **vaccines,** which prevent him getting some diseases. We call this **immunization**.

Two. We can look carefully at a child's growth curve on his weight chart (7–1). His growth curve tells us if he is growing, or if he is malnourished. We call this **monitoring his growth** (watching it). A child who is growing is usually healthy. So, if we monitor his growth we monitor his health (N 1.2).

Three. We can teach a child's mother how to look after him. This is **health education** (2.11). It is one of the most useful ways to help mothers and their children.

We can also help children in another way. Some mothers do not know the difference between a healthy child and a mildly sick child. They may think that a child is healthy when he is not. Chronic disease comes so slowly that a mother may not see that her child is slowly becoming sick. Other children in her village may be sick in the same way as he is. She can easily think that he is normal. Most of the children in her village may be underweight, and have worms, anaemia, impetigo, chronic malaria, mild vitamin A deficiency, or scabies. Mothers may not know that we can prevent and treat all these diseases. So every mother should bring her child to see us every two months during his first year. She should bring him at least every three months during his second year. She should do this even if she thinks he is healthy and has no symptoms. He may be mildly sick and need treatment. Mothers soon learn to bring their healthy children to us when they know what we can do.

**HEALTHY CHILDREN SHOULD
COME TO A CLINIC**

Immunization

4.2 Immunity and antibodies

A child only gets whooping cough once. He does not get whooping cough again because he is immune to it. He becomes immune by making **antibodies**. Antibodies are special proteins in his blood. Antibodies 'fight' the

HEALTHY CHILDREN SHOULD COME TO THE CLINIC

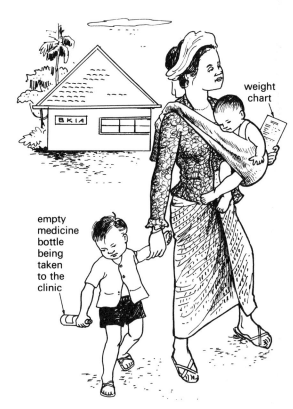

weight chart

empty medicine bottle being taken to the clinic

Fig. 4–1 Healthy children should come to the clinic.

organisms that cause disease, or the toxins (poisons) that organisms make. Antibodies fix onto an organism and kill it. They can also fix onto toxins and stop them causing harm. The antibodies which fight toxins are called **antitoxins**. So an antitoxin is a special kind of antibody. A different kind of antibody fights each organism or toxin. For example, measles antibodies only fight the measles virus. They cannot fight malaria. Antitoxins against tetanus are not helpful in diphtheria. The white cells in the blood are also important for immunity, but we only describe antibodies here.

While a child is ill with measles, his body begins to make the special antibody against the measles virus. He goes on making measles antibody for the rest of his life. He becomes immune, and never has measles again. When a child makes his own antibodies, he has an **active immunity**. He can become actively immune in two ways. He can become ill with the disease itself, or we can give him a vaccine. We grow the harmful organisms in a factory and kill them (dead vaccines), or make them weak (live vaccines). Because the organisms in a vaccine are weak or dead they cause no harm. When we give a child a vaccine, he makes antibodies against the dead or harmless organisms of the vaccine. He has no symptoms, or only mild symptoms, such as a mild fever. The antibodies which he makes can fight the harmful organisms of that disease, and so prevent him becoming ill. When disease makes a child immune he has a **natural active immunity**. When we give him a vaccine to make him immune he has an **artificial active immunity**.

Active – the child makes his own antibodies. Slow to come Slow to go

Natural. The child makes his natural active immunity himself, after he has had the disease.

Artificial. The child makes his artificial active immunity himself, after we have given him a vaccine.

Immunity

Passive – the child is given antibodies. Quick to come Quick to go

Natural. His mother gives him antibodies while he is in her uterus – natural passive immunity.

Artificial. Health workers inject him with antibodies – artificial passive immunity.

BACTERIA, TOXINS AND ANTIBODIES

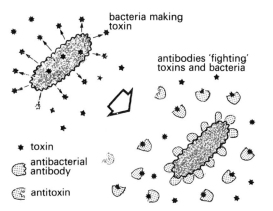

* toxin
antibacterial antibody
antitoxin

4.1
4.2

Fig. 4–2 Bacteria, toxins, and antibodies.

Active immunity is the best kind. But a child does not become immune until two weeks or more after we give him a vaccine. He may need immunity much sooner than this. If necessary, we can make him immune immediately. We can give him antibodies from another person, or from an animal. When we give a child antibodies we give him a **passive immunity**.

There are two kinds of passive immunity. A child's mother can give him a **natural passive immunity** while he is in her uterus. If she is immune to tetanus, for example, she has tetanus antitoxins (anti-tetanus antibodies) in her blood. Some of these antitoxins go from her blood into her child's blood before he is born. He is born with tetanus antitoxins in his blood. He is immune to tetanus. But these antibodies are slowly destroyed. They can only protect him for a few months after birth. But they last long enough to protect him from tetanus of the newborn. Natural passive immunity also explains why children do not usually have measles or malaria, until they are about three months old. By this age, most of the antibodies they were given at birth have gone.

We can give a child an **artificial passive immunity**. We can inject antibodies into him. These antibodies come from an immune person or animal. For example, we can inject tetanus antitoxin into an injured child who might have tetanus bacteria in his wound (18.16). The antitoxin makes him immune immediately, before he has had time to make his own antitoxin. The antibodies which we inject are soon destroyed. So an artificial passive immunity lasts a short time—usually about two weeks.

4.3 Vaccines

Live and dead vaccines. Live vaccines contain live organisms. But we make these organisms weak so that they cause no harm. The live vaccines are BCG (TB vaccine), polio vaccine, and measles vaccine. The organ-

4.3

ACTIVE IMMUNITY

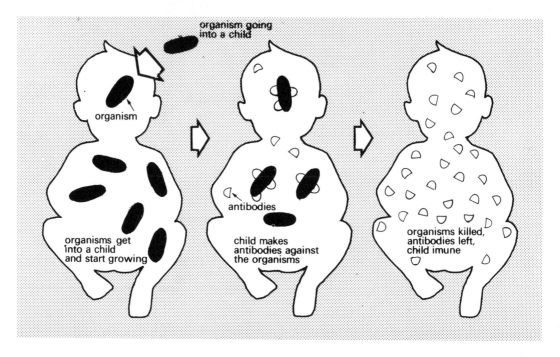

organism going into a child

organism

organisms get into a child and start growing

antibodies

child makes antibodies against the organisms

organisms killed, antibodies left, child imune

Fig. 4–3 Active immunity.

isms in these live vaccines infect a child, grow in him, and cause him to make antibodies against them.

Dead vaccines contain dead organisms or toxoids. **Toxoids** are harmless substances which are made from the toxins (poisons) of bacteria. The vaccine against whooping cough (pertusis) contains dead bacteria. Vaccines against diphtheria and tetanus contain toxoids. These dead bacteria and toxoids are mixed together to make DPT vaccine (Diphtheria, Pertusis, Tetanus). DPT is a vaccine against all three of these diseases. Sometimes, we give tetanus toxoid by itself (18.16).

There is an important difference between live and dead vaccines. The living organisms in live vaccines easily die if you do not store and use them carefully. Dead vaccines spoil less easily. If the organisms in a live vaccine have died they cannot infect a child and cause him to make antibodies. They are not harmful but they are useless. Live vaccines die if you do not keep them in a refrigerator, or if strong light (especially sunlight) falls on them.

Vaccines quickly become useless if you leave them outside a refrigerator for too long. The temperature of a refrigerator should be between 2°C and 0°C. But, if you open the door of a refrigerator often, it will probably be between 15°C and 20°C. The temperature is usually low in the morning and higher in the evening. The temperature of its freezing part should be below 0°C. In a warm room (37°C) BCG vaccine dies in two weeks, DPT in four days, polio in one day, and measles in one hour. If warmth has spoiled a vaccine, cold will not make it work again. Live vaccines also die if spirit or some other antiseptic touches them. *When you give live vaccines, use syringes which you have sterilized by heat*, **not** *by an antiseptic.*

Live vaccines	Dead vaccines	
BCG (against TB)	Diphtheria	
Polio	Whooping cough	DPT vaccine
Measles	Tetanus	
	Tetanus toxoid	

LIVE VACCINES EASILY DIE

Freeze drying. Because live vaccines die so easily, they are usually freeze dried, so that they stay alive longer. Liquid live vaccine is put into an ampoule, and then frozen into ice. The water vapour in the ampoule is then sucked off. This makes the organisms dry, and the ampoule looks almost empty. You must pour a special fluid called a **diluent** into an ampoule of freeze dried vaccine before you use it.

VACCINES AND ANTITOXINS

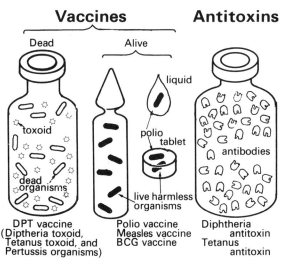

Fig. 4-4 Vaccines and antitoxins.

MAKING A FREEZE DRIED VACCINE READY FOR USE

Keep the diluent in the refrigerator, so that it will be cool when you want to use it.

Make a scratch with an ampoule file on the neck of the ampoule of cold diluent. Make another scratch on the neck of the ampoule of vaccine. Wrap a piece of plastic film round the neck of the ampoule. This prevents vaccine being blown away when air goes suddenly into the empty ampoule. Bend the neck away from the scratch. Open the vaccine and the diluent.

Fill a sterile 5 ml syringe with the diluent using a sterile 0·7 × 38 mm needle.

Add it to the vaccine. Draw it in and out of the syringe several times until the vaccine is dissolved.

Keep the vaccine cold with ice or a cold pack until you want to use it.

The cold chain. Vaccines are like ice cream. They must be cold from the time they are made until the time you use them, or they spoil. Ice creams melt and vaccines become useless if they become warm on their journey from a factory to a child. So vaccines must travel down a 'cold chain' from one refrigerator to another. When vaccines are in a bus, a train or a plane, they must be in a thermos flask with ice, or cold packs, or in special cold boxes. Cold packs are special bags that hold 'cold' and help to keep vaccines cool. Vaccines must not wait and get warm at a bus stop, a railway station, or an airport or in your clinic. This is difficult. It is one reason why many children are not immunized, or are given useless spoiled vaccine.

Shelf life. If a vaccine is carefully stored at the right temperature it should work for about two years. This is its **shelf life**—the time it can stay on the shelves of a refrigerator. If it becomes warm, its life is much shorter. If you look on a box of vaccine you will see a date printed. This is the **expiry date**. It shows the end of the shelf life and it is the date when a properly stored vaccine expires or becomes useless. Don't use vaccines after the expiry date.

KEEP VACCINES COLD

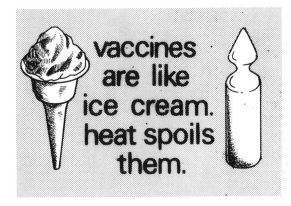

Fig. 4-5 Keep vaccines cold.

If vaccines are dead, they don't work, and they waste the time of the workers who give them. They waste money and transport. They don't protect children. Mothers become angry if their children have diseases which they were immunized against. They stop believing what health workers say.

***
**VACCINES MUST BE REFRIGERATED—
ALWAYS KEEP VACCINES BELOW 8°C**
***

4.4 An immunization timetable

You must give vaccines the right number of times at the right age. If a child needs more than one dose, he must wait for the right time between each dose.

The right age. We must immunize children *before* the usual age when they have the disease. So we must start immunizing them early in their first year. Very young children are not good at making antibodies. So we must not immunize children too early. There is a 'best' age to give every vaccine. For example, you can give **BCG** at birth or at any time afterwards, but 3 months is the best age.

You waste **measles** vaccine if you give it to a child less than about nine months old. He still has antibodies from his mother. These antibodies prevent infection by the harmless virus in the vaccine. So, he does not become immune. You may waste vaccine if you give it to children over one year old. By this age, some children have already had measles. So we have a very short time to immunize children against measles—between nine months and one year. If an older child has not had measles, immunize him.

Give **polio** vaccine at any age after three months. Try to complete the course before a child is a year old. Polio often paralyses children while they are learning to walk. So they should be immune before this time.

Give a baby his first **DPT** at three months. Some workers give the first DPT at one month because whooping cough often kills young babies (8.17).

Table 4:1 Immunization Timetable

Vaccine	Age
DPT 1st dose BCG 1st dose Polio 1st dose	3 months or older
DPT 2nd dose Polio 2nd dose	6 months. Two or three months after the first dose
DPT 3rd dose Polio 3rd dose Measles	9 months (DPT and polio can be given later, but measles should be given at 9 months)
DT BCG	When the child goes to school

The right number of doses. We give a child **BCG** twice—once when he is three months old and again when he goes to school. One injection of **measles** vaccine is enough.

A child needs three doses of live **polio** vaccine. There are three kinds of dangerous polio virus which may cause disease. So there are three kinds of weak polio virus in the vaccine. A child must be infected by all three of them. So he needs three doses with at least a month between doses.

Dead vaccines are not so good as live vaccines. They don't cause a child to make antibodies so easily. So we give dead vaccines, like **DPT**, three times. One injection of DPT gives very little immunity. Two injections give more but not enough.

A child needs a fourth dose of diphtheria and tetanus toxoids when he goes to school. He is past the dangerous age for whooping cough, so he does not need whooping cough (pertussis) vaccine. Also the pertussis part of DPT vaccine causes more side effects in older children. So he needs DT, not DPT vaccine. This increases his immunity to diphtheria and tetanus.

Extra doses of vaccine are usually not helpful, except for tetanus toxoid and DT. If a mother wants an injection for her child, give him an extra dose of one of these vaccines.

The right time between doses. If the doses of a vaccine are too close together, the child will not get a strong immunity. There should be at least six weeks between each dose of polio vaccine. There should also be at least four weeks between the first two doses of DPT vaccine. If the time between doses is shorter than six weeks or longer than four months, his immunity will be less. The time between the second and third doses is less important.

You can give vaccines one at a time, or several together. Some children come to the clinic very seldom. When a child comes, try to give him all the vaccines he needs. If necessary, give him BCG into his right arm, and a drop of polio vaccine into his mouth. Inject DPT vaccine into his thigh.

You can immunize mildly ill children. If a child is severely ill, don't immunize him. But if a child is only mildly ill, you can immunize him. This is useful, because some mothers only come to a clinic when their children are ill. We must not lose this chance to immunize them.

'He has missed the right time for his second or third dose.' This is not serious. If he has only had one dose of DPT or polio vaccine, give him two more doses. Leave six weeks between them.

Your immunization timetable may be different. The times we say are in the immunization timetable in Table 4:1. But diseases behave differently in different countries. So the immunization you give and the ages at which you give them may be different. Measles, for example, is such a mild disease in some countries that immunization against it is not necessary. Each country usually has its own special immunization timetable. Follow the timetable for your country.

FOLLOW THE IMMUNIZATION TIMETABLE FOR YOUR COUNTRY

4.6 BCG immunization

This live vaccine prevents TB—See Section 13.4. It is usually freeze dried. In most countries BCG is given in the *right* arm. In some countries it is given in the left arm. Do whatever is right for *your* country.

BCG VACCINE

STORAGE. **Keep the vaccine between 4°C and 8°C. Keep the liquid vaccine away from sunlight.**

AGE. **If possible immunize him at birth and give him a smaller dose (0·05 ml). If you don't immunize him at birth, 3 months is the usual age.**

IMMUNIZATION. **Sterilize a 1 ml 'Microstat' syringe, a 0·7 mm hypodermic needle and some 10 × 0·45 mm hypodermic needles. USE THE SYRINGE FOR BCG ONLY.**

THE RIGHT PLACE FOR BCG VACCINE

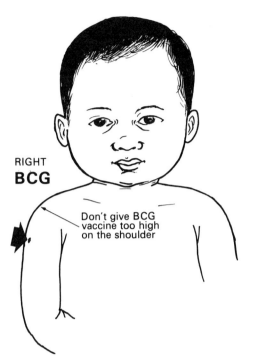

RIGHT
BCG

Don't give BCG vaccine too high on the shoulder

Fig. 4–6 The right place for BCG vaccine.

Add diluent to the freeze dried vaccine—see Section 4.3.

Fit a thin 0·45 × 10 mm hypodermic needle (3–8), so that the bevel on the needle faces the graduations. This makes the vaccine easier to measure.

Fill the syringe from the ampoule of liquid vaccine.

Hold the syringe upwards and remove any air in it.

Pass the end of the needle through the flame of a spirit lamp so that it becomes a dull red. If you flame the needle each time, you need not use a different needle for each child.

Stretch the skin over the child's *right* upper arm (deltoid region) with your thumb and first finger. Throw away a few drops of vaccine from the needle. This cools the needle and removes the heated vaccine.

Push the needle with its bevel facing upwards *into the skin*—not into the tissue underneath it. Keep the needle as flat as possible. Inject 0·1 ml of vaccine. This should make a small raised swelling in the skin at least 5 mm across. If the child is newborn, inject 0·05 ml.

Flame the needle before you use it for another child.

PUTTING A NEW RING IN A MICROSTAT SYRINGE. Sometimes the red rubber ring becomes worn, so that the syringe leaks. Take off the old ring with a knife. Fit a new one. This will be easier if you wet it.

EXPLANATION. **Tell the child's mother why you are immunizing him. Explain what is going to happen at the place of the immunization. Ask her if she has any questions.**

The swelling made by a BCG immunization goes away in about half an hour. Two or three weeks later a small red slightly tender swelling comes, and grows for about another week. Then this becomes a small abscess which ulcerates and crusts. The crust goes and leaves a small red swollen scar. The scar becomes smaller, pale, and sunken, and stays for many years. Always immunize children with BCG on their right upper arms. A scar there will show that a child has had BCG (13:2). But it does not mean he is immune, because even dead vaccine causes an ulcer and a scar. Dead vaccine makes a skin lesion, but it does not protect the child.

KEEP SUNLIGHT AWAY FROM VACCINES

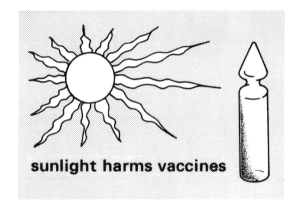

sunlight harms vaccines

Fig. 4–8 Keep sunlight from vaccines.

4.6

Side effect—'Eni's ulcer has lasted three months, and there are lumps (BCG lymphadenitis) under his arm.' This sometimes happens but it is not serious. BCG organisms normally spread to the lymph nodes. If they cause abnormally severe ulceration, put isoniazid powder on the lesions. Treat them as ordinary ulcers. *Don't* open any enlarged nodes. Tell his mother he will have a strong immunity to TB. BCG lymphadenitis is more common in newborn babies. So we immunize them with a smaller dose of vaccine.

4.8 Measles vaccine

4.8

Measles vaccine is expensive, live, and easily killed. Antiseptics in a syringe kill it, so only use a syringe sterilized by heat. Any chemicals in the water used to dilute the vaccine can also kill it, so always use the diluent made specially for it.

MEASLES VACCINE

STORAGE. **Keep it in the freezing part of the refrigerator. It must never be at more than +8°C. But the ampoules of diluent crack in the freezer, so keep them in the ordinary part of the refrigerator.**

AGE. **Immunize the child between 9 months and 1 year. 9 months is the best time.**

IMMUNIZATION. **Add** *COLD* **diluent to the freeze dried vaccine (4.3). Use the liquid vaccine within one hour.**
   Clean the skin of the child's thigh or buttock with spirit.
   Inject 0·5 ml subcutaneously.
   Don't let the vaccine stay in the syringe more than half an hour before you use it.

EXPLANATION. **Tell his mother that he may get a fever in eight or nine days. This will go by itself. Occasionally a child gets a mild measles rash.**

DON'T WASTE MEASLES VACCINE ON CHILDREN WHO HAVE ALREADY HAD MEASLES

4.8b Polio vaccine

Polio vaccine contains three kinds of live harmless polio virus. Sometimes it is a tablet, sometimes a liquid.

POLIO VACCINE

STORAGE. **Keep the vaccine in the freezing part of the refrigerator. Thawing it (making it liquid) weakens it. So only take it from the freezer when you need it. Take out one bottle at a time. Keep the bottle you are using cool with ice.**

AGE. **Immunize the child three times—at 3 months, 6 months, and 9 months. Don't immunize him if he is 'ill' or if he has diarrhoea, because the vaccine is less likely to protect him.**

IMMUNIZATION. **Put three drops of liquid into the child's mouth, or give him a tablet. Make sure he swallows it.**

EXPLANATION. **Explain why you are immunizing him. Tell her when to bring him for his next dose. Has she any questions?**

Dead vaccines

4.9 DPT, DT vaccine and Tetanus toxoid

DPT protects a child against diphtheria, pertussis (whooping cough) and tetanus. DT protects against diphtheria and tetanus. Tetanus toxoid protects against tetanus alone. They are all turbid fluids, and are usually in 5 ml bottles with rubber caps.

DPT VACCINE

STORAGE. **Keep DPT, DT and Tetanus toxoid in a refrigerator at 2–8°C.** *Don't* **freeze them solid in the freezing part of the refrigerator. This destroys them.**

CHECK. **Shake the vaccine. Leave it for five minutes. If the liquid is clear, the vaccine is useless. Send it back to the stores.**

AGE. **Immunize a child with DPT at three months, six months, and nine months. Give him a dose of DT when he goes to school.**

IMMUNIZATION. **Clean the outer side of his arm, buttock, or thigh with spirit.**
   Fill a sterile syringe and needle with vaccine.
   Inject 0·5 ml subcutaneously.

EXPLANATION. **Tell his mother why you are immunizing him. Has she any questions? Explain that he may have a mild fever, which 'shows that the vaccine is working'. The fever starts within 12 hours, and stops within 24 hours of the injection. Give her some paracetamol for it. Tell her when to bring her child for his next dose.**

DON'T FREEZE DPT

4.10 Immunization in the clinic

You should be able to give all the immunizations from your own table every working day of the week. But this may be difficult because you may not have enough equipment. Sometimes ampoules of vaccine are so big that you need many children to use up all the vaccine. So you may have to give each vaccine only once a week or less often. If you do this, be sure to tell mothers which are the 'immunization days'.

RULES FOR IMMUNIZATION

Every child MUST have a sterile needle for himself only. Every child should have a sterile syringe for himself (3.5, 6.13). If possible, sterilize a pressure cooker full of 2 ml plastic syringes before the clinic starts.
   Don't immunize children for diseases they have already had.
   Immunize malnourished children, they are in special danger.
   Keep a thermometer in your refrigerator. Read it every morning and evening and keep a record of the temperature.
   Put polio and measles vaccine in the freezing compartment of the refrigerator.
   Put DPT vaccine, DT vaccine, BCG vaccine, tetanus toxoid, and measles diluent in the outer part of the refrigerator. *Don't* **let DPT freeze solid.**
   Pack the vaccines loosely, so that cold air can go between the packets.
   Don't put vaccines in the door of the refrigerator. They warm up each time you open the door.

Keep several plastic (not glass) bottles of water in the refrigerator. They will keep the vaccine cold for longer if the refrigerator fails.

Don't use vaccines after the end of their shelf life—throw them away. Rotate (turn round) your supply of vaccines. Use your oldest vaccines first, before they expire. When you put new vaccine into a refrigerator, put it at the back behind the old vaccine.

Keep vaccines cold in a refrigerator or cold box, until you want to use them.

Never let strong sunlight fall on a live vaccine, especially measles vaccine or BCG, or the vaccine will die. If you are immunizing outside a building, shade the vaccine with a piece of paper, or a large leaf.

Don't keep open ampoules of live vaccine from one day to another. If you take vaccine out of a refrigerator to use in a clinic, don't put it back.

Read the paper that comes with the vaccine. You may need to use vaccines from different makers in different ways.

Never give any live vaccine with a syringe that has been 'sterilized' in an antiseptic. Always sterilize your syringes by heat for live vaccines.

Don't add 'water for injection' to vaccines. This sometimes contains antiseptics which kill live vaccines.

Remember, the times at which vaccines become useless in a warm room (37°C) are—BCG two weeks, DPT four days, polio one day, measles one hour.

KEEP THE REFRIGERATOR DOOR SHUT. INJECT VACCINES WHILE THEY ARE STILL COLD. DON'T GIVE CHILDREN VACCINES WHICH DON'T WORK

Treating children without symptoms

4.11 Four diseases

These diseases are so common in some districts that every child needs prevention or treatment for them. If they are common in your district, prevent or treat them like this—

Malaria (10.7). Prevent malaria from harming a child by giving him chloroquine or sulphadoxine with pyrimethamine, or pyrimethamine alone for suppression (3.25). When you give these drugs, put a large dot in one of the 'Malaria pill' boxes on his weight chart.

Worms. Sometimes there are very many children with either *Ascaris*, or hookworms. If so, treat them all every six months without looking at their stools. If hookworms are common (22.5), give TCE (tetrachlorethylene, 3.27). If *Ascaris* is common, give piperazine (3.28).

Vitamin A deficiency (16.13). In districts where this is common give children vitamin A every six months.

Start when they are six months old. Under one year give them 100 000 units (one capsule). Over one year give them 200 000 units (two capsules). There are no special boxes for vitamin A printed on the card. So write 'A' in a circle opposite the month when you give him a capsule.

Iodine deficiency (19.6). If many children and adults have goitres, give every child an injection of iodized oil every three years. Give him the right dose of iodized oil (3.34) with a carefully sterilized needle. Record this injection. Write 'I' in a circle on his weight chart.

USING THE WEIGHT CHART TO RECORD MALARIA SUPPRESSION AND VITAMIN A

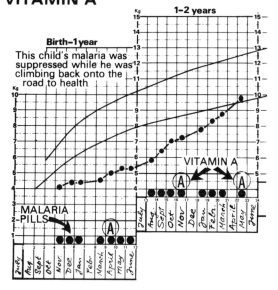

4.8b
4.10

4.11

Fig. 4–9 **Using the weight chart to record malaria suppression and vitamin A.**

4.12 Caring for a healthy child on his first visit

4.12

When mothers understand what a clinic can do, they will bring their healthy children to you. Immunize these children and chart their weights. Examine them, because they may have abnormal signs which their mothers have not seen, or which they think are normal. A complete examination takes a long time, and you may have many children to see. What should you ask for and look for? *This depends on what diseases are common in your district, and on what you can do for them.* You will need to do different things on a child's first visit and on his later visits. Don't do the same things for every child. Do the things each child needs most.

4.9

Spend a little time getting to know the child's mother. Weigh him, and fill in a weight chart for him. If he is below the road to health, go to Section 7.13.

HISTORY

BIRTH. **Was this normal? (This may help to explain problems he has later, 24.12.) Was he born too early? What did he weigh? Did he cry quickly?**

PAST ILLNESSES. **What illnesses has he had? Were there any complications? Did he recover completely from them? (If he has not had measles or whooping cough, he needs immunization.)**

NUTRITION HISTORY. **Make sure his mother is following the rules of good nutrition (7.2, 7.13).**

Rule one. **Is she breast-feeding him until he is eighteen months or two years old? Explain that this is very important.**

If he is bottle-fed, find out if this is necessary, because bottle-fed children are in danger (26.15). If she has any breast milk, he must go on sucking. If she has no breast milk, explain how she can make artificial feeding safer. Try to persuade her to use a cup and spoon or a jug instead of a bottle. Explain that he must eat plenty of porridge with protein food, so that he can stop his bottle as soon as possible.

Rule two. **If he is four months old, or more, has he started to have porridge?**

Rule three. **Is she adding protein food to his porridge?**

Rule four. **How often does she feed him? Be sure she knows that a child needs to eat at least four times a day?**

Rule five. **Is he having some protective food every day?**

MILESTONES. **Check that he is passing them. Here are some of them: 6 weeks—smiles; 9 months—sits without help; 18 months—walks; 21 months—speaks single words; 36 months—speaks short sentences. If he is not passing his milestones, go to Section 24.16.**

BROTHERS AND SISTERS. **How many are there? What ages are they? Are any of them sick? Have any of them died? What diseases did they die from? Has anyone in the family got a chronic cough which might be TB? Fill in the 'brothers and sisters box' on his weight chart (6–1). If several of his brothers and sisters have died, he may need to go in the special care register (6.3).**

EXAMINATION.
Take off all his clothes.
Are his skin and scalp normal?
Is he well nourished (7.13)?
Is he anaemic (22.1)?
Has he got a BCG immunization scar?
If lack of vitamin A is a common problem in your district (16.13), has he any signs of it?
Has he any ear discharge?
Are his mouth and teeth normal?

IMMUNIZATION, ETC. **Have all her children been immunized? How many doses of vaccine have they had? What does she know about the immunization programme? If necessary start to immunize him. Give him malaria tablets, or vitamin A, if they might be useful.**

FAMILY PLANNING. **Talk to his mother about this. Does she know about it? Would she like to use it?**

EXPLANATION. **Tell her that you are pleased to see her. Praise her for something. Has she any questions? Explain what the clinic tries to do. Explain the immunization programme. Explain the weight chart to her. If she is breaking the rules of good nutrition, explain how she could follow them. Explain any problems you have found, and ask her if she has any questions. There will be too much to say on her first visit, so say what is most important. Leave the rest until later. Tell her when you would like to see her again.**

HEALTH EDUCATION. **Teach mothers to recognize healthy children. Healthy children have rising growth curves. They are always running about and playing. Between their first and fifth birthday their arm circumference is greater than 14 cm. They are not anaemic and have red lips and conjunctivae. They have no signs of disease, such as coughs, diarrhoea, skin lesions, or discharge from the nose. They pass their milestones and have been immunized.**

EXAMINE ALL CHILDREN FOR PEM, ANAEMIA, VITAMIN A DEFICIENCY, AND BCG SCARS

4.13 Caring for a healthy child on his later visits

If there are several workers in the clinic, be sure that each mother always sees the same worker. This will help you to know your own patients, and understand their special problems. This is continuity of care (5.2)—care by the same person.

Do a short monthly check, and a longer check every three or six months. If a child comes up after a few days or a week, don't weigh him again. Don't weigh a healthy child more often than once a month.

Sometimes a mother has lost her child's weight chart and you do not know what immunizations she has had. If you always give a child his first dose of polio and DPT with his BCG, you can easily find out. If a child has a BCG scar, he needs his second or third doses of polio and DPT. If he has no scar, he needs BCG and his first DPT and polio.

MONTHLY CHECK
Tell the child's mother that you are pleased to see her. Has she any questions?
Weigh him and fill in his weight chart. If he has grown

since his last visit, he is probably healthy. If his curve is flat, go to Section 7.13.

Look at his weight chart to see what is written about any problems he may have. Ask about these. Has he any new problems? Is he having special care (6.3)?

Give him any immunizations, vitamin A, or malaria pills that might be useful.

Can you help his mother with family planning?

Ask her something about his feeding.

Make sure that she has learnt something useful. Praise her about something.

SIX MONTHLY CHECK

Do all the things in the monthly check, and these things:

Check that she is following the rules for good nutrition.

Check that the child is passing his milestones.

Don't forget to ask about family planning.

Take off his clothes. Examine his nutrition (7.13), and look for anaemia. If vitamin A deficiency is common in the district, look for signs of it. Look for ear discharge and examine his mouth, teeth, skin, and scalp.

4.14 'When should he come to the clinic again?'

If the clinic is not busy there will be plenty of time to see healthy children. But if there are many sick children you cannot see healthy children often. Some healthy children come to the clinic every week, which is too often. Tell the mothers of these children that once a month is enough.

DECIDING WHEN TO SEE A CHILD AGAIN

Before a mother leaves the clinic, tell her when you would like to see her child again. Explain carefully, so that she comes back on the right day. Tell her also that if she is worried about something she can come back any time.

A healthy child should come at least every two months

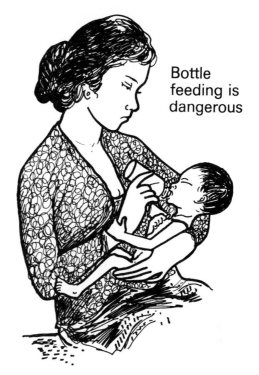

Bottle feeding is dangerous

4.14

Fig. 4–10 Bottle-fed babies are in danger.

during his first year. He should come about every three months during his second year. There is no need to examine him on every visit, but you should weigh him.

A child who is not gaining weight should come to the clinic at least every month.

4.13

Keep a special care register. Ask the mothers of the children in the register to bring them every week, if necessary.

Bottle-fed children should come more often than breast-fed children.

5 Caring for a sick child

5.1 Ten steps

We must follow ten steps when we care for a sick child. Although we cannot follow all of them with every child, we need to follow most of them, with most children.

First, we must weigh a child and put his weight on his road to health chart (6.2). So **weighing** is the first step. Next, we ask his mother about his symptoms. We call this taking a **history**, and it is the second step. Then we examine him. The **examination** is the third step. We may need to look for signs of disease in his blood, stools, or urine. We call this doing **special tests**, and it is the fourth step in caring for a sick chlid.

Now we can decide what disease he has, so **diagnosis** is the fifth step. Then we decide what to do for him. For example, we might have diagnosed that he has pneumonia, and is very ill. We must decide if we are going to treat him ourselves, or if he must go to hospital. We call this **management** and it is the sixth step. Some children need **treatment** with a drug, or in some other way, so this is the seventh step.

THE TEN STEPS IN CARING FOR A SICK CHILD

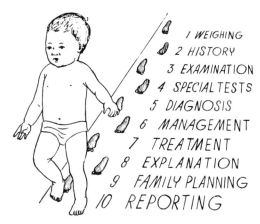

1 WEIGHING
2 HISTORY
3 EXAMINATION
4 SPECIAL TESTS
5 DIAGNOSIS
6 MANAGEMENT
7 TREATMENT
8 EXPLANATION
9 FAMILY PLANNING
10 REPORTING

Fig. 5–1 The ten steps in caring for a sick child.

Next, we explain to his mother why he is ill, We must tell her how we are going to manage and treat him. So **explanation and education** is the eighth step. All mothers need to know about family planning. So when a mother brings us her child, we should talk to her about it. The ninth step is thus **family planning**.

So many children may come to our clinic that we easily forget what we have done for each of them. So we must write this down, or record it. The government wants a report about the work of our clinic. So the tenth and last step is **recording and reporting** (6.1).

All these steps are for a sick child on his **first visit**. But we usually need to see him again, so that we can be sure that he is recovering. These other visits for the same illness are called **follow-up visits** (5.28).

The next few pages tell you how to examine a child completely. This takes about 20 minutes, so we call it examining him as a **long case**. We don't have enough time to examine every child like this. We have to examine most children as **short cases** (5.27).

5.2 Making the clinic ready for integrated care

Try to make everything in the clinic easy for the child, his mother, and for yourself. Figure 5–2 shows how you can do this. But each clinic is different and you will have to choose the way that is best for your clinic.

Make sure that all waiting mothers have somewhere to sit. This must be far enough away, so that they cannot hear what you say to the mother you are seeing. Always ask a mother to sit down before you talk to her. You cannot examine a child across a table, so put her chair beside or in front of your chair. Don't let her sit at the other side of your table. Young children can be examined on their mother's knees, but it is useful to have a couch also. Put the couch on your left side. Leave enough space for a mother to go around to the other side to hold her child. You will want the couch for maternity care and family planning, so put a curtain or screen round it. You cannot examine a child in the dark, so make sure you have plenty of light.

DON'T PUT A DESK BETWEEN YOURSELF AND YOUR PATIENTS

Put a bowl of water, soap, and a towel near you, to wash your hands after each child. Get a table with a shelf underneath it. Keep on the shelf all the things you need often, so that you don't have to go and fetch them. If there is not enough room on the table, find a place near by, where you can reach them easily. You will want bowls and trays, a torch, an auriscope, an ear syringe, a thermometer in a jar of lysol, spatulae, a magnifying glass, applicator sticks, cotton wool, and a bucket with a lid for dirty dressings. You may also need a children's tally (6.4), and some continuation cards (6.2).

In some clinics another worker gives out drugs, but it is useful to have some drugs prepacked on your table (3.4). You will also need some sterile syringes and needles, and some bottles of mixtures.

Put the equipment and records for family planning and antenatal care on your table also. After you have cared for a child, you should care for his mother. One health worker should give a mother and her child all the care they need, and so get to know them. This is **integrated care**—several kinds of care together.

Each time a child comes to the clinic the same person

MAKE YOUR CLINIC EASY TO WORK IN

5.1

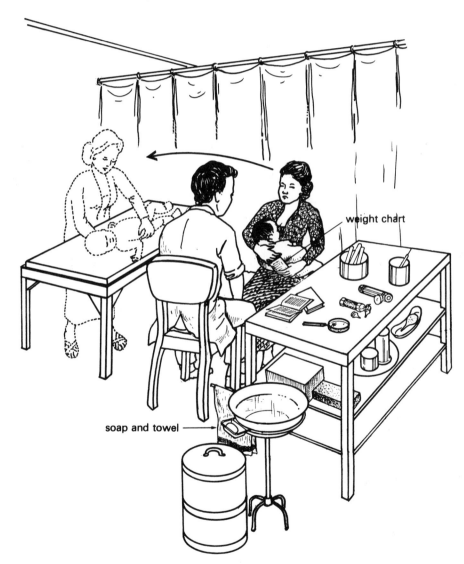

5.2

soap and towel

weight chart

Fig. 5–2 Make your clinic easy to work in.

65

must see him. This is **continuity of care**—care by the same person.

**CONTINUITY OF CARE MEANS
CARE BY THE SAME PERSON**

CARING FOR A CHILD AS A LONG CASE

5.3 First step—weighing

Usually, you should weigh a child first before you do anything else. If he is very ill, you can weigh him later. One dot on his chart will tell you if he is on the road to health. If he has several weight dots on his chart, you can see if he is growing or losing weight. This is much more useful (N 1.3). If the clinic is busy, ask a helper, such as a clerk, or one of the mothers, to weigh children. Write down a child's weight on his continuation card and put a dot on his weight chart. Some clinics measure length as well as weight. This is not necessary, because it does not help in management.

**IF POSSIBLE, TEACH SOMEONE ELSE
TO WEIGH CHILDREN**

Second Step—History

5.4 The ten parts of the history

There are so many questions to ask that we divide the history into ten parts. The first part is the introduction (beginning) when we start to make friends with a child's mother. The next parts are about him, and the last three are about his family.

**TAKING A HISTORY IS
ASKING QUESTIONS AND
LISTENING TO THE ANSWERS**

5.5 The introduction—making friends with his mother

The mother of a sick child may be worried, and perhaps frightened. Be kind to her. She will only give you a good history if she feels that she can talk to you easily. If you cannot speak her language, try to learn a few words of

WEIGHING A CHILD IS THE FIRST STEP

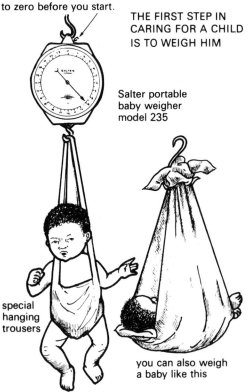

this is the zero adjustment knob.
Be careful to set the scale
to zero before you start.

THE FIRST STEP IN
CARING FOR A CHILD
IS TO WEIGH HIM

Salter portable
baby weigher
model 235

special
hanging
trousers

you can also weigh
a baby like this

Fig. 5–3 Weighing a child is the first step.

Table 5:1   The ten parts of a history

1 **Introduction**—making friends with the child's mother.

The child's history

2 What is his **presenting** (most important) **symptom** (PS)?
   How much of it is there (quantity)?
   What is it like (quality)?
   What has been happening to it (time)?

3 What **other important symptoms** have there been?

4 What **other treatment** has he had?

5 Was his **birth** normal? What diseases has he had before? What diseases has he been immunized against? This is his **past history** (PH).

6 Is he passing his **milestones**?

7 What does he eat? This is his **nutrition history** (NH).

The family history (FH)

8 What has happened to his **brothers and sisters**?

9 **What kind of family** has he got?

10 **What kind of house, water and latrine** do they have?

it, so that you can greet her. Use her name when you talk to her. Listen carefully to what she says. She may be frightened and not talk much at first. She may have waited a long time. She may be trying very hard not to go home and give her child local medicine. Put yourself in her place. Think of yourself as the mother of a sick child. He may have been crying all night. She may have come a long way. Ask her where she lives, or look at the address on his weight chart.

USE A MOTHER'S NAME

Find out if the child is a boy or a girl. Do not say 'she' for a boy, or 'he' for a girl. If he is old enough, ask for his name and use it, and let him answer some questions himself. Say a few kind words to him as soon as you see him. Try to make friends with him. Lend him a toy that you can easily wash. Try not to look straight at him or frighten him.

Find out if the person who brings him to the clinic is the person who usually looks after him. His grandmother, or a servant may have brought him. Sometimes, a servant knows more about a child than his mother does.

Ask about his age and birthday. Fill in his weight chart. If you cannot find his age, you may have to use a 'local events calendar' (N 1.6e).

Ask one question at a time. If his mother starts to answer another question, let her say what she wants to say first. Then ask your question again in another way. If you want to get a good history, go on asking each question until she answers it.

ASK ONE QUESTION AT A TIME.
MAKE SURE THAT YOUR QUESTION
IS UNDERSTOOD AND ANSWERED

The child's history

5.6 What are his present symptoms?

Let the child's mother tell you what is wrong with him in her own way. He will probably have one or two presenting symptoms, such as diarrhoea and 'hotness of the body' (fever). Let her tell you about any other symptoms he may have had by asking 'Anything else?'. She may not know that something is important, or she may be so worried about it that she is too frightened to tell you. If you are using this book, look up these presenting symptoms in the index. They will tell you which 'Caring for . . .' section to go to.

Find out *three things* about each presenting symptom.

How much of the symptom has there been? (Quantity). For example, if a child has had diarrhoea, how many stools has he had each day? Ask if there is a lot or a little stool each time. If he has had fits, ask how many fits he has had.

What have the symptoms been like? How severe are they (Quality)? If a child has had diarrhoea, ask what his stools look like. Has there been blood or mucus in them? If he has a cough, does he whoop?

Pains are difficult to diagnose in children. If a child is old enough to tell you, find out as much as possible about his pain. Ask him to point with one finger to where it is worst.

What is happening to the symptoms (Time)? This is very important. Ask how long a child has had symptoms. *How often he has had symptoms?* Go back to the beginning of his illness. Ask when he was last completely well. Ask if his symptoms came slowly or suddenly.

Symptoms such as cough, diarrhoea, or skin sepsis are probably not serious if they only last a few days. But if a child has had them most days for many weeks or months, they are serious. They help to cause malnutrition.

5.3
5.4

HOW LONG HAS HE HAD SYMPTOMS?
HOW OFTEN DOES HE HAVE THEM?
HOW SEVERE ARE THEY?

5.5

Many people cannot remember when things happened. Things which happened to them a short time ago are often more important than things which happened a long time ago. They make their history too short or too long. A month of trouble may seem like a week, and a year of trouble like a month. Six months may seem like 'always'. Often, a mother will time her child's illness by something which happened, such as a harvest.

Ask if a child's symptoms are getting better or worse. This is useful, because there is less need to do anything about a symptom which is getting better. Symptoms which have lasted a long time in a 'well' child are probably not serious.

SYMPTOMS WHICH ARE GETTING WORSE
ARE MORE DANGEROUS THAN SYMPTOMS
WHICH ARE GETTING BETTER

5.6

Ask if the child has had his symptoms before, and has recovered from them. If his mother tells you he has had a cough for 3 days, she may mean that a month ago he coughed for 3 days, but then recovered. Asking if he has had a cough before may help you to get the right answer.

5.7 What other important symptoms have there been?

5.7

For each presenting symptom there are some other symptoms which are important to ask about. For example, if a child has diarrhoea, ask if he has also been vomiting. This will help you to decide how to rehydrate him (9.20). The 'Caring for . . .' sections tell you what other symptoms to ask about. Remember to record the important symptoms he did *not* have, as well as those which he did have. This may be useful later.

5.8 What treatment has he already had?

Many children have already been treated before they come to you. A mother might have treated her child herself. She might have taken him to a traditional healer, or she might have bought medicine for him in the market. She might also have taken him to another clinic or doctor. Ask what treatment he has already had before you give him any more. He may already have been given an injection of chloroquine. If you give him another one too soon afterwards, you may kill him (3.25).

5.9 What is his past history?

Was his **birth** normal? If he was born too small (26.22), he may stay small for a long time afterwards. Has he had any other illnesses? Has anything been written about his **past illnesses** on his weight chart? Measles, for example, may harm a child's lungs so that he coughs for a long time. Has he had any injections or been to hospital? The hospital doctor should have recorded what happened to him on his weight chart. What **immunizations** has he had?

5.10 Is he passing his milestones normally?

Some children are late passing their milestones (24.10). They may have a brain disease, or chronic infection, or malnutrition. Ask his mother what he can do. Can he sit, walk, or talk?

WHAT OTHER TREATMENT HAS HE HAD?

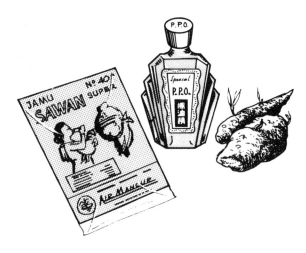

Fig. 5–4 What other treatment has he had?

5.11 Eating—his nutrition history

This is important in two ways.

Is he eating normally now? If he is hungry, he is probably 'well'. 'Not eating' and especially 'not sucking' (26.20), is a sign that he is 'ill'.

A hungry child is 'well'.

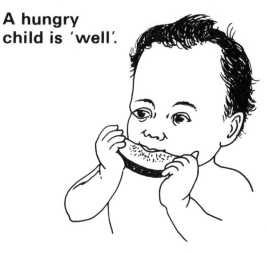

Fig. 5–5 If a child is eating normally, he is probably 'well'.

NOT EATING IS A SIGN OF AN 'ILL' CHILD

What foods does she usually give him? Might he be malnourished? Is he breast-fed? If breast-feeding has stopped, why did it stop? Is he bottle-fed? When did he start eating porridge? What did he eat yesterday? How often is he fed? Decide if he is getting enough of the right foods. Is his mother breaking any of the five rules of good nutrition? (7.2).

Here are two very important questions that you will often need to ask.

CAN HE DRINK?—Dehydration (9.20) CAN HE EAT NORMALLY?—Malnutrition (7.11)

The family history

5.12 What has happened to his brothers and sisters?

He may catch their diseases, so ask if any other children, or any adults in the family are ill. Some illnesses, such as scabies, are usually shared by the whole family (11.10).

Ask where he comes in his family. Fill in the 'family box' on his weight chart for his brothers and sisters. Find out how many of them are alive. Don't ask about deaths immediately. First ask a mother how many pregnancies she has had. Then ask how many of her children are still alive. From this you can find out how many have died. This is the best way to find this out, because mothers may not like to say how many of their children have died.

Sometimes, more than one child in a family dies of the same disease. If several of a child's brothers and sisters have died, he may die also. Put him in the special care register (6.3).

ASK ABOUT A CHILD'S BROTHERS AND SISTERS

5.13 What kind of family is it?

Anything that we find out about a child's home and family may help us to manage him better. There are two useful things to know.

Is the family rich or poor? This tells us if they can pay for treatment and transport, and if they can feed their children properly. We want to know how much land a family has, or what job the child's father does. If his mother works away from home, who looks after the children?

How strong (stable) is the family? Sometimes we want to know if a child's parents are divorced, or if his mother is living with his father. Perhaps his grandmother is caring for him?

Is his mother alone, or is she part of a large family? How much help has she? How much work does she have to do?

You can learn much about a child's family as you take his history. Does his mother look clean and well dressed? If his clothes are clean, she probably looks after him carefully. Does she understand what you say easily, or not so easily? If she is not good at understanding, you must do step eight—the explanation—very carefully.

5.14 What kind of house, water, and latrine do they have?

The kind of house a family has depends mostly on how rich they are. It is not as important as how much water they have or what kind of latrine they have. In many districts only about one family in a hundred has enough safe water. A mother who has to fetch water from a long way cannot fetch very much. Her children have many skin infections, because she cannot wash them often.

**THE BEST WAY TO LEARN ABOUT
A CHILD'S HOME IS TO VISIT IT**

Third Step—the examination

5.15 Is he 'well' or is he 'ill'?

Look at a child while you are taking his history. Decide if he is 'well' or 'ill'. This may be difficult, and you may have to change your mind later. But *start to think about it as soon as you see a child*. When you have seen many children you will be able to do this very quickly. Look carefully at the children waiting in the clinic. If you see any that are seriously ill, examine them first and don't

keep them waiting. All clinic staff, including cleaners should watch for them and make sure they are seen quickly. Remember to thank the cleaner who brings you a sick child.

Several signs which tell us how 'well' or 'ill' a child is depend on his brain. As he becomes more ill his brain stops working normally. He goes through the stages shown by the letters A to F in Table 5:2. Finding out which stage he is at is easier if he is awake.

Stage A Well. A child is well if he looks happy and is interested in what is going on around him. He sleeps normally. He is well if he plays, and eats, or sucks strongly from the breast.

Stage B Tired. At some times in the day even a healthy child becomes hungry and tired. At these times he is quiet and still in his mother's arms, or becomes irritable and restless. An irritable child becomes angry and cries easily. A restless child moves around more than normal and will not sit still. When a healthy child

BEGIN LOOKING CAREFULLY AT A CHILD WHEN HE IS FIRST BROUGHT IN TO SEE YOU

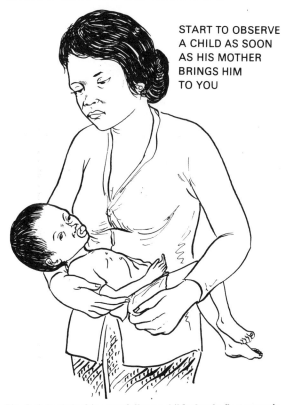

START TO OBSERVE A CHILD AS SOON AS HIS MOTHER BRINGS HIM TO YOU

Fig. 5–6 Begin looking carefully at a child when he first comes in to see you.

5.8

5.13

5.9

5.10

5.14

5.12

5.15

5.11

has sucked, eaten, or slept, he is happy and active again, and goes back to Stage A.

Stage C   *Mildly or moderately ill.* A healthy child is only irritable, restless, or quiet at *some times in a day.* He is irritable for about the same amount of time each day. Each child is different, but his mother will know what is normal for him. If he is irritable at unusual times, or all the time, he may be becoming ill. An ill child cries and his mother cannot comfort him. Or he may be abnormally quiet and will not leave his mother's arms. He wakes and cries in the night. He holds a breast or teat, but does not suck. An older child will not eat. If he has just learnt to walk or talk, he stops doing these things. He does not run about and play. 'He has stopped running around and playing' is one of the earliest signs that a child is 'ill'. A child who sits quietly and does not run about is **apathetic**. As he gets worse, he becomes **drowsy** (abnormally sleepy), weak, and 'floppy' (hypotonic). When he is carried, his arms and legs hang loosely from his body like the child in Figure 5–7.

LEARN TO RECOGNIZE THE 'ILL' CHILD

The 'ill' child.

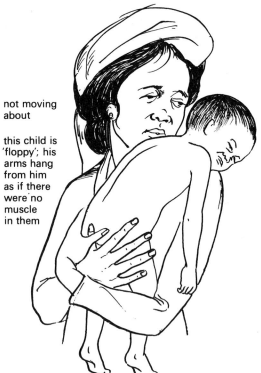

not moving about

this child is 'floppy'; his arms hang from him as if there were no muscle in them

Fig. 5–7 Learn to recognize the 'ill' child.

Table 5:2   Is he 'well' or is he 'ill'?

NORMAL

A WELL   Happy, smiling, playing, running about, sucking from the breast, or eating. Active and interested in what is going on around him. Cries and fights strongly when he is awakened and examined. Sleeps well.

B TIRED   Sleepy, cross, irritable, and restless, or quiet—*at the usual times.*

ABNORMAL

C MILDLY OR MODERATELY ILL   Cries and will not be comforted. Irritable and restless, or abnormally inactive and quiet—at unusual times, or all the time. Drowsy. Wakes up and cries at night. Weak and 'floppy'. Unhappy when he is examined, but not strong enough to fight.

D SEVERELY ILL   Looks very 'ill'. Keeps his eyes half open. Seems to be asleep, but can be only half woken up. Talks nonsense—delirium.
Any of these signs also show he is severely ill—

Hypothermia (cold, 10.4)	Stridor (noisy breathing 8.9)
Shock (cold, pale, sweating, 14.2)	Sunken eyes (dehydration, 9.18)
Cyanosis (blue, 8.2)	Fits (15.1)

E VERY SEVERELY ILL   Coma, looks as if he is asleep, but cannot be woken up.

F   DEAD

Stage D   *Severely ill.* As a child becomes more ill, he becomes even more sleepy and waking him is difficult. An older child may be half asleep and talk nonsense. This is **delirium**, and is common in any severe fever. When a severely ill child is awake, his eyes do not seem to see anything, even if they are open.

Stage E Very severely ill. When he becomes very ill, he cannot be awakened. This is called **coma** (unconsciousness), and is very serious (14.8).

Stage F Dead. Death is the last stage.

The last stage is death.

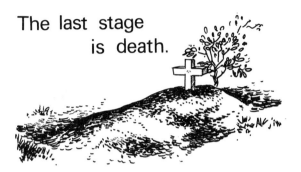

Fig. 5–8 Most deaths can be prevented.

BEGIN TO DECIDE IF A CHILD IS 'WELL' OR 'ILL' AS SOON AS YOU SEE HIM

A child may have something wrong with a part of his body, such as a skin lesion, sore eyes, or a cut foot. Local lesions like this are usually not serious. They do not harm the rest of him and he stays 'well'. If something is wrong with the whole of a child, he is 'ill'. We can treat a child's local lesion, and need not worry much about the rest of him. But if a child is ill, we must take a complete history, examine his whole body, and manage him carefully.

AN 'ILL' CHILD NEEDS A CAREFUL HISTORY AND EXAMINATION

5.16 Examining a child

We examine adults lying flat on a couch. This may frighten a child, so examine him on his mother's knees. Let him suck from the breast if he wants to. You can examine most children sitting or standing.

We usually examine an adult from his head downwards. We look at his face and his head first, then at his hands and arms, and so on down his body. When you examine a child, start with the parts that do not make him fight. Examining his throat and ears may make him kick and cry, so that he has to be held. Examine these last. Crying and fighting do not spoil an examination if they happen at the end.

EXAMINE THE DIFFICULT PARTS OF A CHILD LAST

If he fights hold him in a blanket.

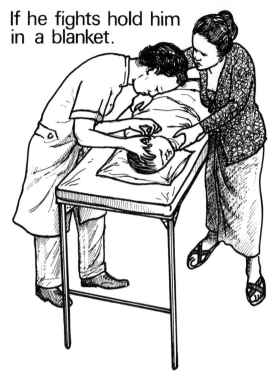

Fig. 5–9 If a child fights, he must be held while you examine him.

Some abnormalities, such as dehydration (9.17), cause signs in several parts of a child's body. Don't look for all these signs at the same time. Look for a dry mouth last, when you examine his throat.

You can see the signs in a child's face when he is dressed. But you cannot see signs in the rest of his body if it is covered with clothes. Take them all off before you finish examining him. Don't only pull them up or down. Some health workers like to undress children during the examination. Other workers ask mothers to take their children's clothes off (except for nappies) while they are waiting in the queue. Mothers soon know that a worker will only see children if they are undressed. Mothers start to undress their children when they see that their turn is next. Do whatever you find best, *but all children must be undressed at some time.* Don't forget to look under a baby's nappy, and remember that signs can also be hidden under his hat or his shoes.

EXAMINE CHILDREN UNDRESSED

A nappy can hide a rash (26.43), an obstructed hernia, or disease in a child's foreskin (23.11). Abnormal urine may stain his nappy red with blood, or dark because he has jaundice. If his nappy is dirty, leave it on until the end of the examination. If he passes urine or stools

5.16

71

ALL THESE THINGS CAN HIDE THE SIGNS YOU READ TO MAKE A DIAGNOSIS

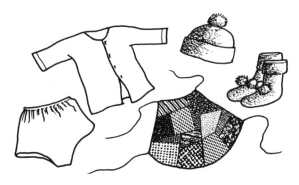

Fig. 5–10 All these things can hide the signs you need to make a diagnosis.

during the examination, notice if these are normal or not.

5.17 Before he is undressed

If a child is sleeping, examine as much of him as you can while he sleeps. Don't wake him up until you have to. You may be able to examine his eyes and his ears while he sleeps.

Breathing. Look at the way he breathes. Fast breathing helps you to diagnose pneumonia (8.9). Is he breathing noisily (stridor)? Does he move his nose as he breathes? Is he breathing through an open mouth because his nose is blocked? If he might have pneumonia, count his breathing before you wake him (8.9).

COUNT HIS RESPIRATIONS BEFORE YOU WAKE HIM UP

Signs in his face, head, and neck. Look carefully at his face while you are taking his history. You may see the sunken eyes of dehydration (9.18), the pale lips of anaemia (22.1), the yellow colour of jaundice (22.10), the 'old man's face' of marasmus (7.9), the misery and thin pale hair of kwashiorkor (7.10), or perhaps the face of Down's syndrome (24.13). Is there a discharge from the child's nose (25.11)? or his ears (17.14)? Look at his face whenever you touch some part of him. His face will show you if you are hurting him.

Look for anaemia. Pull down one of his lower eyelids or his lower lip (22.1). Look at his hair. Is it pale, thin, and weak because of malnutrition (7.10)? If he is less than a year old, feel his fontanelle (15–9). Feel for large tender tonsilar lymph nodes under both angles of his jaws (18–3), and in his neck. Use *both* hands.

Meningeal signs (15.6). You can look for these while a child has his clothes on.

Now that you have learned all that you can with his clothes on, take them off.

TRY TO UNDRESS HIM WITHOUT MAKING HIM CRY

5.18 After a child is undressed

Nutrition (7.13). Is he well or badly nourished? The best way to find out is to look at the growth curve on his weight chart. But looking at him is helpful also. Has he got enough fat underneath his skin to give him the smooth round look of a healthy child? Are his muscles wasted? Look at his legs and arms, shoulders, and buttocks. Their round shape is made by muscle. They are flat in malnutrition. Does he have oedema of his legs? Measure his arm circumference (7.1). If it is less than 14 cm between his first and 5 birthday, he is malnourished.

Skin (11.2). Look for lesions in his skin. Has he got a rash? Pick up a fold of skin at the side of his abdomen, and see if it is normally elastic (9–8).

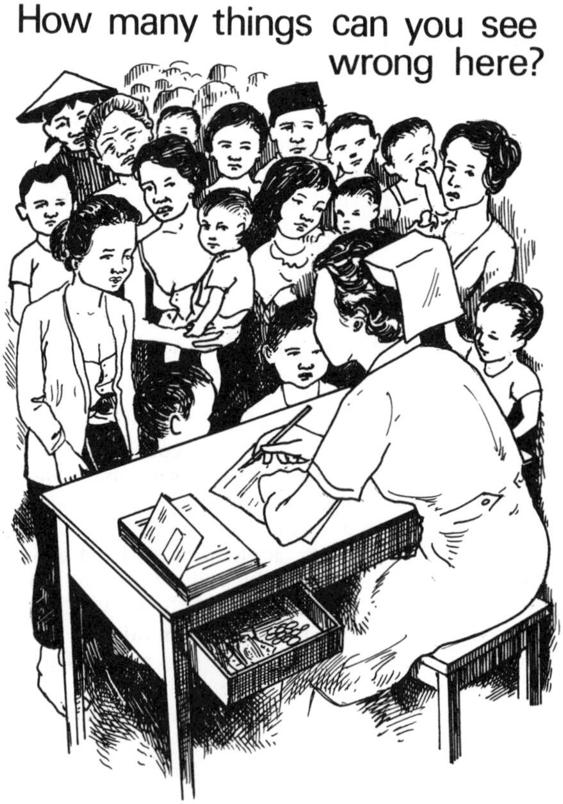

How many things can you see wrong here?

Fig. 5–11 List all the things you can find wrong here, then look for the answer in Section 5.29.

Chest. Look for insuction (8.9). If necessary, test for it as shown in Figure 8–7.

Mouth (18.2) and ears (17.3). Leave these to the end, but don't forget them.

You may need to examine many other parts of him. For example, has he been passing his milestones normally (24.10)? Can he do the things which he should do for his age?

When the examination is finished, wash your hands, or they may carry harmful organisms to the next child.

AFTER THE EXAMINATION WASH YOUR HANDS

Some signs, such as stridor (8.10) are easy to recognize the first time. Other signs, such as a swollen fontanelle (15–9) are difficult. Often, you cannot be sure if something is normal or abnormal. Look for signs in many normal children. In this way you learn all the different ways a healthy child can look or feel. You can then tell more easily if something is abnormal or not.

LEARN TO DIAGNOSE WHAT IS ABNORMAL BY EXAMINING MANY NORMAL CHILDREN

5.19 Fourth step—Special tests

Special tests are very helpful for diagnosis. The haemoglobin (13.5), for example, helps us to diagnose anaemia. Occasionally we can send a child to a hospital to have his chest X-rayed. Most special tests are done in a laboratory. Every health centre should have a small laboratory to examine a child's blood, urine, CSF, and stools. We can do these tests easily and quickly while a child and his mother wait for the answer. They should not have to come back on another day.

Here are some of the tests that a health centre laboratory can do. They are all described in the laboratory book (1.4).

Blood. Haemoglobin (L 7.1), haematocrit (L 7.2), thin blood film (L 7.11), sickle cells (L 7.24), total white cell count (L 7.29), and thick blood film (L 7.31).

Urine. Protein and sugar (L 8.3), acetone (L 8.7), isoniazid and aminosalicylate (L 8.9), dapsone (L 8.10), pus cells (8.11), centrifuged deposit (L 8.13), and ova of *S.haematobium* (L 8.15).

CSF. Cells (L 9.9), Pandy's test (L 9.10), stained film (L 9.11), and protein (L 9.13).

Stools. Saline smear (L 10.2a), 'Cellophane thick smear' (L 10.2b), 'Sellotape swab' for threadworms (L 10.4), and lactose (L 10.12).

Some other specimens. Sputum for AAFB (L 11.1), pus for bacteria by Gram's method (11.5), skin scraping for leprosy (L 11.11b) or fungi (L 11.15).

5.18

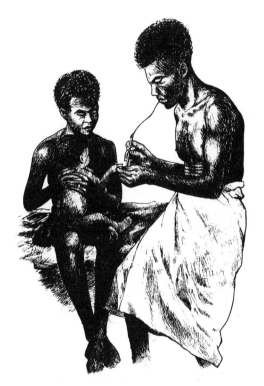

5.17

5.19

Fig. 5–12 Taking blood for haemoglobin in the laboratory.

5.20 Fifth step—Diagnosis

5.20

Diagnosing a child means deciding what diseases he has. We find which disease pattern ('picture') of symptoms, signs, and special tests is most like the symptoms and signs which he has. When you diagnose a child use as many signs and symptoms as you can. For example, if you think a child might have meningitis, look for *all* the meningeal signs (15.6). If you think he may have TB, ask about *all* the symptoms in Table 13:1.

USE AS MANY SIGNS AND SYMPTOMS AS YOU CAN TO MAKE THE DIAGNOSIS

Some signs, symptoms, or special tests are much more useful for diagnosis than others. A few of them are caused by one disease only. This means that if we find that sign, we can be sure a child has that disease. For example, if a child whoops, he must have whooping cough. If his skin lesions are anaesthetic (without feeling, 12.3) he must have leprosy. Signs like this are **diagnostic** of a disease. Anaesthesia in a skin lesion is diagnostic of leprosy. Koplik's spots are diagnostic of measles (10.6). Many special tests are diagnostic. For example, if an anaemic child has many hookworm ova in his stool, he must have hookworm anaemia.

Often, a disease does not cause *all* the signs you read about here. For example, you will not see Koplik's spots in all children with measles. Some children with whooping cough don't whoop. Often you will have to make a diagnosis from *some* signs only.

If you are not sure about a sign, it is probably negative. For example, if you are not sure if there is pus on the tonsil, there is probably no pus there.

A sign which is not there (a negative sign) is as important as a sign which is there (a positive sign). For example, if there is no protein in the urine, the child has *not* got the nephrotic syndrome. This disease always causes protein in the urine.

Some diagnoses have several parts. Each part is necessary. For example, 'diarrhoea' by itself is not enough for a diagnosis (9.31). We also want to know if a child with diarrhoea is dehydrated, and if he has hyperpyrexia. We want to know if he is malnourished and, if there is some special cause for his diarrhoea.

Try to make all a child's signs and symptoms fit one disease before you decide that he has several diseases. For example, cough, fever, and red eyes can all be caused by measles.

Some children have more than one disease. So you may need to make more than one diagnosis. For example, many children are mildly malnourished, and have scabies and hookworms. Okeke at the end of the book is a child like this.

There is a list of diagnoses towards the end of each 'Caring for . . .' section. The most common disease is first, and the rarest last.

The right diagnosis is important, because without it we cannot manage and treat a child in the right way. So always try to make a diagnosis. Use a 'D' for diagnosis for recording it. If, for example, a child has pyoderma, write D = pyoderma.

Sometimes, diagnosis is difficult. For example, a child has a mild cough. You are sure that he has not got whooping cough, and moderately sure that he has not got TB. He might have a chronic upper respiratory infection or 'URI' (8.6), but you are not sure. If you are not sure of a diagnosis, put a question mark beside it. Write 'D = ? URI' on his card.

IF YOU CANNOT MAKE A DIAGNOSIS, DO NOT BE AFRAID TO SAY SO

Sixth step—Management

5.21 The ten ways of managing a child

Usually, you know what to do with a child. Sometimes, however, a child is too ill to treat at home. You are worried about him, and not able to make a diagnosis. What can you *do* with him? This is only another way of asking yourself—How can I *manage* him? There are many ways you could manage him. Here are ten ways. Often, you will need to manage a child in more than one way at the same time. Read them carefully, but don't learn them by heart.

One. The most common way of managing a child is to tell his mother to bring him to the clinic next month. If he needs any immunizations, give them to him. Manage all healthy children like this (4.12) and children with only mild symptoms.

Two. If he is only mildly ill, you might give him symptomatic treatment and send him home. Explain to his mother that he is not seriously ill. Tell her to bring him back after one, two, or three days. Tell her to come sooner if he becomes worse, or if he has any new symptoms. So you **observe** him. If his illness becomes serious, you will know before it is too late to treat him. To observe a child like this is one of the most useful ways of managing him. He might need to come back every day, or every two or three days, until you are sure he is well. Sometimes, you need to observe a child's growth curve by weighing him each week for several weeks.

TO OBSERVE A CHILD MEANS TO WATCH HIM CAREFULLY

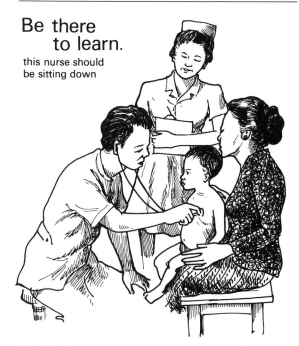

Be there to learn.

this nurse should be sitting down

Fig. 5–13 Never lose any chance of learning about how to care for children.

Three. If a child has an easily treated disease like *Ascaris* infection, you can treat him and send him home.

Four. You can send him home and visit him to see if he is getting better. Seeing his home might be very helpful.

Five. He might be sent to a laboratory for a special test that you cannot do.

Six. The child can be sent for an X-ray.

Seven. If the health centre has beds, he and his mother might stay in it for a few days.

Eight. You might ask someone who knows more about children to see him. If this person is also working in the clinic, this is easy. If he is far away and expensive, it is difficult. If you ask someone else to see a child, try to be there yourself at the same time. This helps you to learn.

Nine. If you see a sick child in a sub-centre, you might send him to the main health centre. Or you might send him to hospital. This is easy if the hospital is near and transport is cheap. It is difficult if the hospital is far away and the family is poor. *If you could treat him, but you have not got the right drugs, you will have to send him for help.*

Ten. A seriously ill or injured child might need to go to hospital very quickly as an emergency.

Which of these ways is best for the child? Deciding is often difficult. We all go on learning how to choose the best way all our lives. What you decide to do depends on how you answer the **ten management questions** in Table 5:3.

Table 5:3   The ten management questions

A How sure am I about the diagnosis?

B How ill is the child now?

C How far away does he live? Can he easily come back and see me?

D If he is not treated, will he recover or get worse quickly or slowly?

E Can I treat him myself?

If you can treat him there is no need to ask some of the next questions.

F Does he need to be treated either by a doctor, or in hospital?

G How near are we to a doctor or a hospital?

H How much will transport and treatment cost his family?

I How much money has the family got? They may have no money and have to pay with rice or chickens or something else.

J What does the family want to do?

Here are examples of how two children, Agus and Yanto, might be managed. We do not need all the ten management questions.

AGUS

A 'How sure am I of Agus's diagnosis?'

I don't know what his diagnosis is. He is two-and-a-half years old, and is on the road to health. He has had fever for three days, and a mild cough, but I can find no signs of any disease. He has not got a moving nose, stridor, or dyspnoea. His respiratory rate is 36, so he has not got a lower respiratory infection (8.21). His throat, ears, and eyes are normal and he has no neck stiffness. He went to town three weeks ago, and he has not yet had measles. There are no malaria parasites in his blood slide. He may have almost any disease that causes fever.

B 'How ill is he?'

He has a fever of 39·5°C. He is not eating. He wants to be carried all the time, and is very irritable. He is an 'ill child' (5.15).

C 'How far away does he live?'

He lives in the next village, and can easily come to the clinic.

HOW MUCH IS TRANSPORT AND TREATMENT GOING TO COST THE FAMILY?

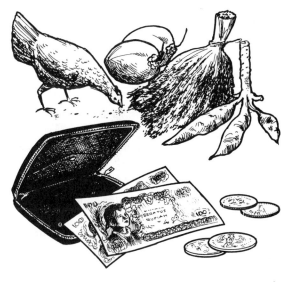

Fig. 5–14 How much is transport and treatment going to cost the child's family?

5.21

D *'If he is not treated, will he recover or get worse quickly or slowly?'*

I don't know.

E *'Can I treat him myself?'*

I can give him symptomatic treatment for his fever. He has probably got a virus infection for which there is no causal treatment.

The second way of managing a child is the best one—Agus needs observing. So, treat his fever with aspirin, wet cloths, and fluids (10.3). Ask his mother to bring him back every day until he is well. Tell her that you will see her quickly each time and she need not wait. Agus has probably got some mild virus infection and will be well in a few days. If he has a serious disease you will be able to diagnose it before it is too late. You may find that tomorrow he will have a measles rash and diagnosis will be easy.

OBSERVING A CHILD IS ONE OF THE THE MOST USEFUL WAYS OF MANAGING HIM

YANTO

A *'How sure am I about Yanto's diagnosis?'*

I am not sure of the diagnosis. He is 18 months and weighs 13 kg. He has had three fits, and I think that he has neck stiffness. He may have meningitis, but I am not sure. He needs a lumbar puncture, but I cannot do one.

B *'How ill is he now?'*

He seems to be seriously ill.

D *'If he is not treated, will he recover or get worse quickly or slowly?'*

If he has got meningitis, he may get worse and die very quickly.

E *'Can I treat him myself.'*

No.

F *'Could he be treated either by a doctor or in a hospital?'*

Yes, he must have a lumbar puncture, and he probably needs hospital treatment now.

G *'How far are we from a hospital?'*

Our nearest hospital is about ten kilometres away, so it is quite near.

H *'How much are transport and treatment going to cost?'*

The hospital is free, but transport is expensive.

I *'Has the family got enough money or can they borrow it?'*

The family are poor but Yanto's mother tells me she can borrow enough money.

J *'What does his mother want to do?'*

At first she did not want to go to hospital, but now that I have explained how seriously ill he is, she will go.

The tenth way of managing a child is the best one. Yanto should be sent to a hospital as an emergency. He needs a lumbar puncture to find out if he has meningitis. If he has meningitis, he will be treated. If he has not got meningitis, he can come home. The family will have spent their money well.

Yanto will need a letter to take to the hospital. This is how to write it.

'PLEASE SEE THIS CHILD'— WRITING A HOSPITAL LETTER

Whenever you send a child to hospital, or to see someone else, send a letter with him. Be sure to write all these ten things on it.

The name and address of your clinic so they can send the answer to you.

The date.

The child's name and age.

The most important parts of his history.

The most important signs.

Any special tests you have done.

What you think the diagnosis is.

Any treatment you have given him.

Anything else which you think might be useful. Write anything important you know which a hospital may not easily find out. For example, his brother may have epilepsy, or the family may be very poor.

'Thank you' and your name, and who you are.

Tell his mother to take his weight chart to the hospital, and to bring it back afterwards.

WHENEVER YOU SEND A CHILD FOR HELP, SEND A LETTER WITH HIM

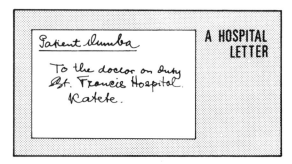

Fig. 5–15 Whenever you send a child for help, send a letter with him.

After the child has been seen at a hospital, the hospital should send a letter back to you. This is impossible if you have not given your name and address clearly. Try to visit the child in hospital, and find out what has happened to him. Ask the child's mother to bring him to see you after he has come out of hospital.

5.23 Seventh step—Treatment

If you have made a diagnosis, treatment is usually easy. Find the right page in this book and see what drug or other treatment he needs. The most serious diffficulty is not having the right drug. For many illnesses, such as colds, there are no drugs which help much. Fortunately, most of these children get better without drugs.

Sometimes you have to do things to a child. You may have to give him a scalp vein drip (9.27) or take a foreign body out of his ear (17.13) or do a lumbar puncture (15.3). Any of these things can be difficult. If you cannot do something after two tries—STOP. Send the child to someone else.

If possible, explain how she can prevent her children getting this disease again. Explain the weight chart, and how to feed the child better. Tell her when you would like to see her child again. If the child's father is there also, talk to him too. Say that you are very pleased that he came.

In a busy clinic, there is little time for teaching, but try to teach each mother something.

**TEACH EVERY MOTHER SOMETHING.
MAKE SURE A MOTHER KNOWS WHEN TO
COME AGAIN**

5.25 Ninth step—family planning

Family planning is important for a mother and her family, for the country and for the world. We must help mothers to use it. Whenever you have time, talk to mothers about family planning. Does a mother know

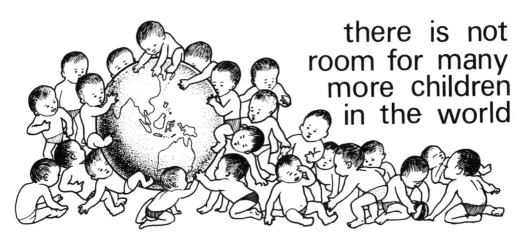

there is not room for many more children in the world

Fig. 5–16 Family planning is a very important step in caring for children.

5.24 Eighth step—Explanation and education

First decide how you are going to manage and treat a child. Then explain this to his mother.

Has she any questions? Give her time to think. Try to answer them? Ask her why she thinks he became ill, and then tell her why you think he became ill. Tell her what treatment you are going to give him, and when he will be well again. This is very important with diseases that take a long time to treat, such as TB (13.6), leprosy (12.4), and iron deficiency anaemia (22.4). If she should help in treatment, show her what to do. Ask her to do it while you watch.

**HAVE YOU ANY QUESTIONS YOU
WOULD LIKE TO ASK?**

---

about it? Has she already had enough children? Look at the 'brothers and sisters box' on her child's weight chart. Is she having difficulty with family planning? Explain how bad it is for children to come too close together. The best **birth interval** (time between births) is three years. It should never be less than 18 months (N 9.17a).

Mothers know that many children die. They want large families so that some children will grow up. If a mother sees that you can help her children when they are sick, she may not want so many. Don't waste this chance of talking to her about family planning, but wait until you have finished caring for her child. Try to help her the same day, so that she need not come to the clinic again. This is integrated MCH care (5.2).

Record on a child's weight chart what his parents are doing about family planning. There is a space for this on the top of the chart (7–1). There is only room for a few words, but this is enough. For example, you might write 'mother interested', or 'wants loop', or 'father unwilling', or 'on the pill'.

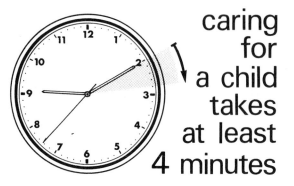

caring for a child takes at least 4 minutes

Fig. 5–17 You cannot care for a child in less than four minutes.

5.26 Tenth step—Recording and reporting

This is in the next chapter. You might only have the time and paper to record a little. However, always try to record a child's symptoms and how long they have lasted.

When you have finished caring for a child, ask his mother what you can do for her. Perhaps she needs antenatal care? Perhaps his brothers and sisters need help?

WHAT CAN WE DO FOR HIS MOTHER?

CARING FOR A CHILD AS A SHORT CASE

5.27 Short cases

In a busy clinic there is not enough time to examine every child as a long case. Fortunately, most children are not very ill. Many diagnoses are not difficult, so you can diagnose and treat most children quickly. These children are the short cases.

How long we spend with each child depends on how ill he is. It depends on how difficult he is to diagnose, and on how many other children are waiting. We cannot ask every mother every question, or examine every child for everything. We have to choose which are the most important questions to ask, and the most important signs to look for. With a few difficult 'ill', children we need to go through all the ten parts of the history. We must examine them all over, to make a complete record like Okeke's at the end of the book. This takes a long time, so these are the long cases. We need to spend much less time on most of the other children. These are the short cases with easy diagnoses. We need only ask their mothers a few questions and look for the most important signs. The 'Caring for . . .' sections for each presenting

symptom will help you to know which these are. Here are some of the more important things you should do. If you always do these things you will be giving good care.

CARING FOR A CHILD AS A SHORT CASE

HISTORY. **What is his presenting symptom, and how long has he had it?**

What other symptoms has he got? How long has he had them?

What treatment has he had?

Is he feeding or sucking well?

Look at his weight chart.

Is he 'well' or 'ill'?

EXAMINATION. **Look at him undressed.**

Examine his mouth and eyes (anaemia, stomatitis, xerophthalmia).

If he has fever, always examine his throat and ears. if he has a cough, watch him breathing. If necessary, count his respirations.

If he has diarrhoea, look for signs of dehydration.

DIAGNOSIS. **Make a diagnosis and record it.**

EXPLANATION. **Always give his mother some explanation about why he is ill and how she can help him.**

Don't let short cases get too short. You cannot care for a child in less than about four minutes. So don't try to see more than 15 children in an hour, or about 45 in a morning.

CARING FOR A CHILD TAKES AT LEAST FOUR MINUTES

When you start to care for children, see as many of them as you can as long cases. Even after you have worked in a clinic for many years, always see some children as long cases. In this way you will get better at caring for children. If you never see any sick children as long cases, you will never learn any more about them.

ALWAYS SEE SOME CHILDREN AS LONG CASES

FOLLOW UP CASES

5.28 All sick children need following up

You must see again, or 'follow up' all sick children. If you don't follow up a child, you will never know if he recovered or not. The first time you see a sick child, go through all the ten steps. The next time you see him, *show that you remember him and his mother*. Ask her how he is. Ask a few questions, and look for a few signs. Look at the last record on his chart. Is he recovering? Is his mother giving him his treatment in the right way? Perhaps she stopped giving him his drugs when he seemed a little better? If there are several workers, be sure that children come back to the worker who saw them before. Like this you can each get to know your patients. This is continuity of care.

SICK CHILDREN NEED TO BE FOLLOWED UP

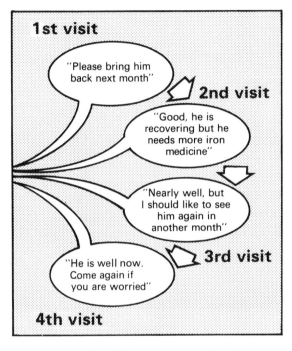

Fig. 5–18 Sick children need to be followed up.

NEVER FORGET TO ASK—HOW IS HE?

Now turn to the end of the book. Look on the back of the tear-out dose tables. You will find an example of how one child was cared for.

TELL HER WHEN TO RETURN

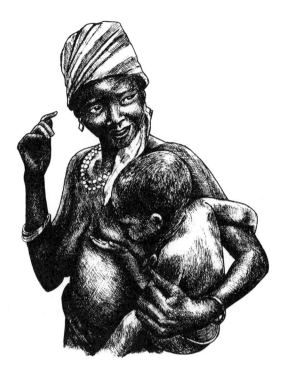

5.26

Fig. 5–19 Tell her when to return.

5.29 Some of the things which are wrong in Figure 5–11

5.29

There are too many mothers crowding round the table, There is too much noise. The nurse cannot talk to a mother about family planning without all the other mothers hearing what she says.

There is no chair for a mother to sit on while the nurse is examining her child.

5.27

There is no equipment for examining children and there are no prepacked drugs.

There is a table between the nurse and the mothers (5.2).

This nurse spends much of her time taking money from the mothers and putting it in the drawer of her table!

Now wash your hands

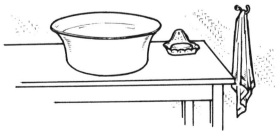

5.28

6 Working in a clinic

6.1 Records and reports

This chapter describes three important parts of our work—recording, reporting, and sterilizing.

To *record* something means to write it down. We make records for a child, so that when he comes again, we can read what we have done. We don't need to ask his mother, or try to remember. We also need records so that we can evaluate our clinic. This means finding out how well it is working.

To *report* something means to tell it to someone else. Reports from each clinic go to the district, then to the

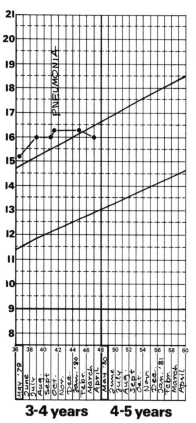

Road to Health Chart

Clinic	Child's no.
TANETE RIAJA	0007

Child's name	
AMIRUDDIN NURNI	Boy/~~Girl~~

Mother's name	Registration No.
SWARNI NAJAMUDIN	87410

Father's name	Registration No.
LATIF AMIRUDDIN	23961

Date first seen	Birthday-birthweight
JAN/1/	MAY 14 '76 / 3.2 kg

Where the family live: address
RT 1, RW2, DESA TANETE RIAJA

BROTHERS AND SISTERS		
Year of birth	Boy/Girl	Remarks
Junawarni	girl	died 3/12
Damari	girl	died 13/12
Wahayuddin	boy	
Amiruddin	boy	
Mupayani	boy	

ANTI-TUBERCULOSIS IMMUNISATION (BCG)

Date of BCG immunisation ....
..........July '76

POLIOMYELITIS IMMUNISATION

Date of first immunisation ....Aug. '76
Date of second immunisation ....Nov. '76
Date of third immunisation ....Febr. '77

WHOOPING COUGH, TETANUS & DIPHTHERIA IMMUNISATION

Date of first immunisation ....Aug. '76
Date of second immunisation ....Nov. '76
Date of third immunisation ....Feb. '77

MEASLES IMMUNISATION

Date of immunisation ....Feb. '77

OTHER IMMUNISATIONS

....
....

SENSITIVE TO PENICILLIN

SS

Fig. 6–1 The outside of the weight chart.

80

province, and then to the ministry of health. This tells the ministry how its clinics are working. Sometimes the reports go to the district health committee.

Recording and reporting uses time. We could use this time for helping more children. So we must make only the most useful records and reports. We must not spend too much time on them. Caring for mothers and children comes first. Recording and reporting comes second. Record and report things which can help make decisions. If something is not going to help make decisions, don't record it. So, when you use the records described here, try to stop using the ones you are using already. If you keep twice as many records as you need, you waste time.

**ONLY RECORD THINGS WHICH HELP
TO MAKE DECISIONS**

A child's own records

6.2 The weight chart

A child's weight chart (N 1.3) is printed on strong card. His mother keeps it in a plastic bag. Each time she comes to a clinic or hospital, she should bring it with her. If you

teach mothers carefully, they soon learn to bring their weight charts. If clinics keep children's records, mothers have to wait a long time while a clerk looks for them. But, if mothers keep them, there is no waiting, and fewer charts are lost. If a mother keeps her child's weight chart, it is always ready for you to see, when you visit him at home. This is why home-based (home-kept) records are used in many countries. The only record for each child that the clinic keeps is the special care register. This is for the few children who need special help.

The inside of the weight chart is shown in Figure 7–1. Outside the chart there are spaces for the child's name, his address and his clinic number. There are also spaces for the names of his father and his mother. There are spaces to record his immunizations, and important things about his brothers and sisters. There is little space to write on a child's weight chart. He needs another card **6.1** also for his history and follow up. This card is his **continuation card** (6–2). It goes into the same plastic bag as his weight chart. If you do not have this card, use a piece of paper, and fix it to his chart with a staple. **6.2**

TEACH MOTHERS TO BRING WEIGHT CHARTS

The clinic's records

6.3 The special care register   6.3

Some children especially need our help. These children are at 'special risk'. They are more likely to become more ill or die. These children are seriously underweight, or backward (24.10), or have TB (13.7), or leprosy (12.5). These children are not seriously ill, but their diagnosis is difficult and they need observing (5.21). They are the small babies (26.22), the twins, and the babies whose birth was difficult. Or their mothers have difficulty breast-feeding (26.21). They are the last children in large families, the children of very poor families, the children without fathers or mothers, and the children whose brothers and sisters have died. Some children need special care for several of these reasons.

We must be sure who these children are, and where they live. So we must record them in a special care register. If their mothers do not bring them to see us, we must visit them at home. We can make the special care register in a note book, with a page for each child. Or we can use a card and keep it in a file. This card has spaces for a child's address, his reason for being on the register, and the date. Underneath there is space to write his history, examination and diagnosis. There is also space to record what we found at each home visit, and when he came to the clinic. On the right of the card there are spaces to record when he should come up again. We can look at these spaces, and we can quickly find out which children have not come to the clinic. We must visit these children at home. You can keep all the special cards of each kind together. For example, you can keep the cards

THE CONTINUATION CARD
FOR THE WEIGHT CHART

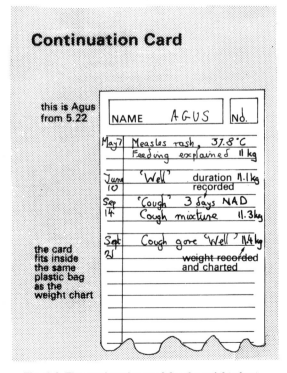

Fig. 6–2 The continuation card for the weight chart.

for all the malnourished children together, or the cards for all the children from each village.

Some clinics care for very many underweight children, or children who are last in large families, or very poor.

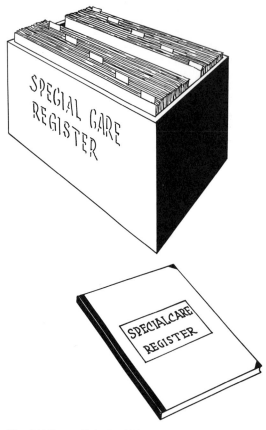

Fig. 6–3 Every clinic should have a special care register.

All of them could go on the register. But a register is useless if it has so many children that we cannot give them all special care. So choose the children whom you can help most, and register them. Don't put acutely ill children in the special care register. See them every day. They either recover quickly or die.

REGISTER THE CHILDREN WHOM YOU CAN HELP MOST

6.4 The children's tally

An easy way to record the work of a clinic is to keep a tally like that in Figure 6–4. When you use a tally like this put a stroke through one of the 'O's each time you record a child. The tally in Figure 6–4 records children under one year and children between one year and five years. The tally records new attendances, and children who have attended before this year. The tally also records children who have not attended since last year. The tally records some diseases, such as kwashiorkor and severe anaemia, and also immunizations. You may want to record other diseases, so there are spaces for these diseases on the tally. The worker who used Figure 6–4 recorded children with hookworms. When there are several workers in a clinic, each worker needs his own tally sheet. At the end of the month add all the tally sheets together to make the clinic's report.

The tally records the percentage of children who have gained weight since they last came to the clinic. This is

A CHILDRENS TALLY SHEET

CHILDREN'S TALLY SHEET

Worker K. Zulu Clinic Matero Date 7 Nov.

	New attendances	Old attendances (This year)	Old attendances (Last year)
Under One year	Total 16	Total 30	
One to Five years	Total 8	Total 25	

Total new attendances 24   Total repeat attendances 80

DISEASES/COMPLICATIONS	Totals
Gaining weight	60 B
Kwashiorkor	8
Marasmus	5
Severe anaemia	12
Measles	27
Scabies	31
Hookworm	7
Other children sent for help	18

IMMUNIZATIONS

BCG

DPT	1st Dose Total 15	2nd Dose Total 13	3rd Dose Total 12
Polio	1st Dose Total 15	2nd Dose Total 20	3rd Dose Total 10
Measles			
Tetanus toxoid (for mother)	1st Dose Total 11	2nd Dose Total 13	Booster Total 10

Health education lessons — Given; topic(s) danger signs in diarrhoea / Not given; reasons

Malaria suppression — Given to all / Not given; / Given to some children only

Fig. 6–4 The children's tally.

82

very useful. All children should gain weight. So the percentage should be 100 per cent. A falling percentage is an early sign that food is becoming short in a district.

When you send in your report at the end of the month remember to report anything special or unusual. This might be an epidemic (many cases) of some disease, or a disease which you had not seen before. It might be more deaths than usual in the village, or something else.

6.6 How to make records

Writing takes time, so make every word tell you as much as possible. **Medical shorthand** (a quick way of writing) makes recording quicker. But if we want to read other worker's records, we must all use the same shorthand. Table 6:1 shows some of the shorthand we can use.

When you make a child's records, write down his symptoms and how long he has had them. Record his diagnosis also. There is an example of how you should make a record at the end of the story of Okeke at the end of the book.

Reporting

6.7 Are we reaching our objectives?

In Section 1.2 we set ourselves two objectives, *quality*, and *coverage*. How can we measure if we are reaching them? We can make scores. There are many ways of making scores, and *the scores you use may be different.* We will describe three scores. **The quality score** measures how good the work of a clinic is. The **patients per worker per day** measures output. It tells us how much work each worker does. The **average yearly visits per child under five** tells us how often an average child in our community comes to our clinic each year. It shows how much care we are giving children. It tells us something about **coverage**—how well our clinic is covering the community.

These scores make us look at our work in a new way. For example, a quality score of only 10 per cent makes us ask how we could increase it. If an average child comes to the clinic less than once a year, this is too little. These scores are useful, but they are not perfect. For example, the average yearly visits score does not tell us if we are seeing a few children often, or many children once. The quality score only tells us a few things about the quality of our clinic.

Sometimes, we must change the way a score is made, so that it measures something different. So each score has a date. The scores here are for 1979, but after a few years they might have to be changed.

6.8 The quality score (1979)

This book describes the things we can do in a clinic. The quality score measures *some* of them.

Integrated care. Every clinic should care for well and sick children on every day from Monday to Saturday. *On the same day* the clinic should give antenatal care, and help with family planning. This is integrated care.

Table 6:1 Medical Shorthand

PS	Presenting symptoms	C	Child
OT	Other treatment	FP	Family planning
PH	Past history	AN	Antenatal
FH	Family history	PN	Postnatal
NH	Nutrition history	NAD	Nothing abnormal discovered (found)
OE	On examination		
IV	Intravenously	0	Absent or negative
IM	Intramuscularly	✓	Examined and found normal
SC	Subcutaneously	×	Number of times present, for example × 6 = six times
PEM	Protein energy malnutrition		
URI	Upper respiratory infection	↑	Increased
		↓	Reduced
Ⓕ	Supplementary food	→	Unchanged
DSM	Dried skim milk	Ⓡ	Right
EBM	Expressed breast-milk	Ⓛ	Left
SSW	Salt and sugar water	D	Diagnosis
GS	Glucose–salt solution	♀	Female, girl
Ⓐ	Vitamin A	♂	Male, boy
Ⓘ	Iodized oil injection	5/52	Five weeks
PP	Procaine penicillin	5/12	Five months
PPF	Procaine penicillin forte	TCA	To come again to be followed up
W	Weight		
Hb	Haemoglobin	Ⓢ	Special care
BS	Blood slide	✓ (boxed)	Clinic visit
AFB	TB bacilli (13:1)	▢	Should have come to the clinic but did not
HW	Hookworm	⟋✓	Home visit, family in
SS	Sickle cell anaemia	⟋◯	Home visit, family out
A	Adult	℞	Treatment

Mothers are busy and many mothers walk a long way to the clinic. Each time a mother comes to the clinic she may lose a day's work and a day's pay. So she should *not* have to bring a well child on one day, and a sick child on another day. She should not have to come for family planning, or antenatal care on a third day. Integrated care has 15 points. Unless a mother can get *all* these kinds of care on one day, there is no score for it.

If there is integrated care on one day, score one point; two days, score 2 points; three days, score 5 points; four days, score 10 points; five days, score 12 points; six days score 15 points.

Highest score—15 points

Monitoring growth with weight charts. Do you give all children weight charts, so that you can monitor their growth? Mothers should keep these charts in plastic bags. Score 10 points if you have weight charts *and* plastic bags in stock. Score 0 if you have no weight charts in stock. Score 5 if you keep them in the clinic and don't give them to mothers.

Highest score—10 points

Health education, Has the clinic got a health education plan listing the behaviour changes needed by the community? Are these lessons written out for each change (2.12, N 10.2)? For each written lesson with visual aids, and questions for evaluation, score one point. If there are no visual aids or evaluation questions, there is no score. You must write out lessons again when they become old. So don't score for lessons which are more than two years old.

Highest score (10 lessons)—10 points

Special care register. Have you got a register (6.3)? If you have, score one point for each child who has been visited *during the last month*. If nothing has been written on his card about what was found, there is no score. Divide the number of points by the number of health workers in the clinic who see sick children.
Highest score (15 children visited per worker)—15 points.

Drugs and expendable supplies. You must have the necessary supplies. Start with 30 points. Take away one point for any of the 'Important 50' supplies which you do not have. The 'Important 50' are the supplies in bold type in Table 3:1. If you don't need a drug, because you don't have the disease for it in your district, score that point.

Lowest score—0; highest score—30 points.

Equipment. The important pieces of equipment are in bold type in Table 3:2. Score one point for each piece you have. If something, such as an auriscope, is not working, there is no score. You must have at least 15 spatulae, 10 syringes, 30 needles of all sizes, and ten 5 ml measuring spoons before you score the point for them.

Lowest score—0; highest score—20.

Add up your score. If no doctor works at the clinic, or if he visits it less than two days a week, this is your score. But, if a doctor works in it more than two days a week, subtract five points for each of the things that have *not* been done on the children from the clinic during the last six months.
Measuring the haemoglobin
Examining the stools for ova
Tube feeding
Lumbar puncture
Examining the sputum for AAFB
Final quality score . . . per cent (highest score—100)
The lowest score is 0. There is no minus score. Above 70 per cent is a good score, above 90 per cent is a very good score.

6.9 Patients per worker per day (1974)

This measures the average number of patients that a health worker sees every day.

Count the number of patients of all kinds who came to your clinic during a month. This is the number of *patients seen*. If some patients had more than one kind of care at the same time, such as antenatal care and family planning, they count as one patient seen.

Count the number of workers who examine or treat patients in the clinic every working day, such as midwives, and doctors. There are about 25 working days in the month, so multiply the number of workers by 25. This gives the number of *worker days* at the clinic during the month.

Divide the patients seen during the month, by the worker days. This tells you the average number of patients each worker sees each day. For example, say there are three workers in the clinic. The number of 'worker days' will be $3 \times 25 = 75$. Say 3000 patients were seen at the clinic during the month. The patients per worker per day will be 3000 divided by 75 = 40.

Above 20 is a good score. If you think that 20 is too many, remember how many sick children there are, and how few health workers!

6.10 Average yearly visits per child under five (1978)

How much care do we give to the average child in our community? First, we must find out how many children live in the area (part of the town or district) in which we work.

You can find your clinic area in several ways. Here is one way. Take a map. Mark each clinic on it which gives child care. Join each clinic to the clinics nearest to it by lines. Make a mark half way along each line. Join up these marks. This makes a line around each clinic. If a line cuts across a village or street, move the line. Move it so that the whole of a village or street is in the same clinic area. Find out the number of people there are in the area round your clinic. Ask the headman of each village or street in your area. Add them together.

About one sixth of the people in your area are children under the age of five. So, divide the number of people in your area by six. This is the number of children your clinic has to care for. Look at your children's tally to find out how many children under five you saw last month. Multiply this number by twelve to tell you how many children you see each year. Divide the number of visits by the number of children. This tells you the average number of visits each child makes.

For example, let us say there are 18 000 people in your districts. There will be 18 000 divided by 6, equals 3000 children under the age of five. If you saw 100 children during the month, you would see 1200 during the year. So the chances of each child being seen once during the year are 1200 divided by 3000. This equals 0·4 which is a little less than half. This means that the average child has less than half a clinic visit each year.

A healthy child should come to the clinic at least every two months when he is under one year old (6 visits). He should come every three months during his second year (4 visits). If he is sick, he should also come after he is two years old. But, to make calculation easier, we will not count these later visits. So each child should make 6 + 4, or *at least ten visits* during the first five years of his life. This is an average of at least two visits a year. Unfortunately, few clinics see children as often as this.

Above 2 visits per child per year is a good score.

Above 4 is a very good score.

So your score of less than half a visit a year is low.

A CHILD SHOULD COME TO A CLINIC TEN TIMES BEFORE HE IS TWO

6.12 'But the scores for our clinic are so low'

Perhaps the quality score for your clinic is 0. *Don't worry.* Your beginning score does not matter. Chart your scores, and try to make them better. Try to make your score curves rise a little every month, like a child's growth curve. Some points are easy to get. If you give integrated care every day of the week, you get fifteen points for your quality score immediately. If few children come, try to make your care as good as possible. Mothers will bring their children when they know you can help them.

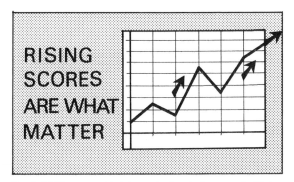

Fig. 6–6 Where we get to is important, not where we start from.

Sterilizing

6.13 Using a pressure cooker

Sterilizing something means killing all the organisms on it. We can prevent infection in a clinic. We can sterilize everything that goes into a child's body. We must sterilize syringes, needles, forceps, and spatulae. We can boil a few needles and syringes each time we use them. But this uses much fuel, because water must be boiling all the time while a clinic is working. Sterilizing in the hot steam of a pressure cooker is better.

When we heat water, it gets hotter until it boils at 100°C. If the water is in an open pan, it cannot become hotter than 100°C. If we heat it more, it boils faster, and

it makes more steam. But, if we boil water in a strong pan **6.9** with a lid fixed on, steam cannot come out. So it becomes much hotter. Steam in the pan tries to come out. It presses against the lid—it is under pressure. We measure pressure as the number of kilos pressing on every square centimetre of the inside of the pan and the lid. We write this as kg/cm². The usual pressure for sterilizing is one kilo pressing on every square centimetre—1 kg/cm². Steam at this pressure is about 120°C. It kills organisms much faster than does steam or boiling water at only 100°C.

Organisms do not die immediately, even at 120°C. So the length of time we sterilize equipment is important. Steam at 1 kg/cm² kills almost all organisms in *15 minutes*. Most harmful organisms die in *five minutes* at this pressure.

The pressure cooker in Figure 6–9 has a pan and a lid. **6.12** Between them is a thick rubber ring called a **gasket** to keep in the steam. Steam kills organisms quicker than hot air, or a mixture of hot air and steam. So there is a **vent** (hole) to let out the air before you start sterilizing. When the air has gone, you can sterilize the equipment in pure steam. The vent is closed by a metal weight. When the vent is closed steam can only come out when it has reached more than 1 kg/cm². There is also a small piece of metal called the **safety valve**. This melts **6.10** (becomes liquid) if the cooker becomes too hot and the pressure becomes dangerously high. Melting lets out the steam and stops the cooker bursting. You need a new safety valve before you can use the cooker again.

Inside the cooker there is a metal plate called the **trivet** (shelf). This keeps equipment out of the water while you sterilize it. The trivet has a rim (edge) on one side. Always use it with its rim *down*. UNICEF pressure cookers have a bowl to put equipment in.

NEVER LET A PRESSURE COOKER BOIL DRY

USING A PRESSURE COOKER TO STERILIZE SYRINGES, FIGURE 6–9

(1) Put the trivet into the cooker, with its rim downward. Put about two cupfuls of water into it.

Put the equipment into the bowl and put the bowl into the cooker.

(2) Put the lid on the pan like this. Place the arrow on the **6.13** **edge of the lid opposite the line on the handle of the pan. Move the handle of the lid to the left, until the handles are together and the cooker is closed.**

(3) Heat the cooker strongly. In a few minutes steam will come out of the vent. Wait until steam is coming strongly—about one minute. During this time it will blow away air from inside the cooker.

Put the weight on top of the vent. Leave the cooker for two or three minutes with the heat high. During this time the pressure will rise to 1 kg/cm².

(4) A *loud* hissing noise shows that the pressure inside the pan has reached 1 kg/cm², so turn the stove low.

Start timing. Keep just a little heat during the 5 or 15 minutes of sterilization. A small hissing noise may come from the weight. This is normal.

(5) At the end of 5 or 15 minutes, take the cooker off the stove. Don't touch the weight. First cool the cooker. Don't take off the weight until the cooker is cool. Cover the cooker with a wet cloth, or put it under a tap, or put it into a bucket of water. The steam in the cooker will become water again. Lift up the weight a little after about half a minute. If there is a hissing noise, there is still some steam inside, and the cooker is not cool enough.

When there is no steam in the cooker, take off the weight and open the lid.

(6) A pressure cooker is easy to use, but *there must always be some water in it to make the steam for sterilizing.* If there is not enough water, the safety valve will blow out. The equipment will burn. The cooker will be spoiled. Prevent this. Never let the cooker boil dry. Put in two cupfuls of water before you start. Don't let the cooker lose so much steam that this water is all lost.

SOME RULES

Start heating with the weight *off* the vent. Don't put it on again until there is a good flow of steam coming out. If you don't let the air out, you will be sterilizing in a mixture of air and steam.

Start counting the time for sterilizing *after* you have turned the heat low in step (4) above.

Don't take off the weight until the cooker is cool.

Only open the cooker after it is cool.

Never use the cooker more than half full of water, or two thirds full of equipment.

Keep the vent clean.

Take the plungers out of the syringes. If you don't do this, they may break.

Equipment inside a tin will sterilize better if you lay it on its side. Never sterilize anything in a tin or bottle with the lid on—take lids off.

A pressure cooker spoils some plastics.

LET OUT THE STEAM BEFORE YOU START STERILIZING

STERILIZING WITH A PRESSURE COOKER

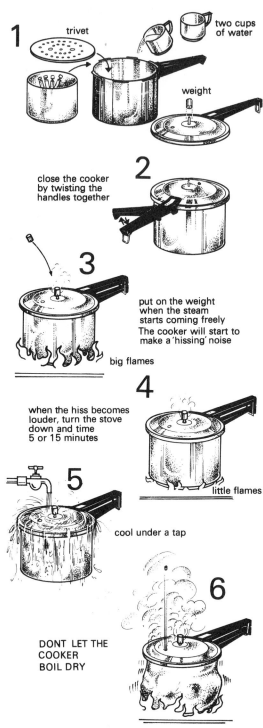

1 trivet   two cups of water   weight

close the cooker by twisting the handles together   2

3   put on the weight when the steam starts coming freely
The cooker will start to make a 'hissing' noise

big flames

when the hiss becomes louder, turn the stove down and time 5 or 15 minutes   4

little flames

5   cool under a tap

DONT LET THE COOKER BOIL DRY   6

Fig. 6–9   Sterilizing with a pressure cooker.

86

7 The malnourished child

7.1 Growth

Children must grow. So they must have plenty of food. Unfortunately, many children do not get enough food, or they get the wrong food. So they become malnourished and don't grow. We can prevent malnutrition in several ways. We can teach a child's mother how to feed him better (nutrition education). We can give him extra food, such as dried skim milk (supplementary feeding). We can also prevent and treat his infections.

We must know if a child is well nourished or not. We must also know if his nutrition is becoming better or worse—we must monitor his growth with a weight chart.

The weight chart. If a child is growing his weight increases each month. We can weigh him and record his weight on a chart (N 1.3, 6.2). A weight chart is printed on strong card and has a graph on it. The child's age in months is written along the bottom of the graph. His weight in kilos is written up the side. When we weigh him we put a dot (mark) on his chart opposite his weight and his age.

If we weigh a child once, we can make one dot on his chart. But we do not know if he is growing, or losing weight, or if his weight is staying the same. To find this out we must weigh him two or more times, so that there are two or more dots on his chart. We join up all the dots to make a line called a **growth curve**. If his growth curve is rising (going up), he is growing and *he is healthy*. If his

GROWTH CURVES

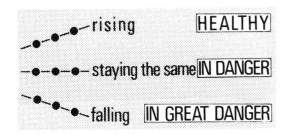

growth curve is flat, his weight is staying the same. If his growth curve is falling (going down), he is losing weight.

HEALTHY CHILDREN HAVE RISING GROWTH CURVES

There are two thick curved lines on the chart. The **upper line** shows the weight of well-fed children. Malnourished children weigh less than well-fed children of the same age. We need a line to tell us when to worry about children who weigh less than they should do for their age. So the weight chart has a second thick curved line called the **lower line**. The space between these two lines is called **the road to health**. Children should be on the road to health. A child below the road to health is **underweight**.

A child *anywhere on the chart* is in danger if he is not growing. So a child's growth curve should always be rising. A child *on or above the road to health* is sick if his growth curve is flat or falling. *Children grow in different ways*. A child below the road to health is healthy *if his growth curve is rising*. Where a child's growth is moving (up or down) is more important than where his curve is on the chart. Growing is more important than being on the road to health. All healthy children grow. If a child's growth curve is flat or falling, he is not healthy and is becoming malnourished. He is in danger. He may be on the road to health now or above it, but because he is not growing, he will soon fall off it. So growth is more important than position (where a child is) on the weight chart.

NOT GROWING IS THE FIRST SIGN OF MALNUTRITION

USING A WEIGHT CHART

Ask the child's mother the month and year of his birth. If she does not know these, you will have to use a local events calendar (N 1.6e).

Write the month of the child's birth, say March, in all the thick black lined boxes on the child's weight chart. These are the first boxes for each year.

Write the other months in the other boxes.

Put the year (for example '79) opposite each January, and each birth month.

Weigh the child.

Make a dot for the child's weight opposite the month you are in. Make a big dot, about 3 mm. If you are near the beginning of the month, put the dot at the left of the column for that month. If you are in the middle of the month, put the dot in the middle of the column. If you are at the end of the month, put the dot at the right of the column.

The solid lines across the chart are for whole kilograms. The lines with dots are for half kilograms. For example, if your child weighs a little less than 6·5 kg, put your dot a little below the dotted half kilo line for 6.5 kg.

When a child has several dots, join them up with *thick* lines to make a growth curve.

Fill in ALL the other parts of the card. Does he need special care (6.3)? If he needs it, write in the reasons. Record what his parents think about family planning. If you cannot do all these things at his first visit, do them at his later visits.

GROWTH IS MORE IMPORTANT THAN POSITION ON THE WEIGHT CHART

The arm circumference. This is a useful quick way to diagnose if a child is malnourished. A child's arm circumference is the distance round the middle of his upper arm. During his first year his arm circumference increases rapidly as he grows. *But it stays about the same from his first birthday until his fifth birthday.* If he becomes malnourished his muscles waste, his arm becomes thin, and his arm circumference becomes

THE INSIDE OF MULENGA'S WEIGHT CHART

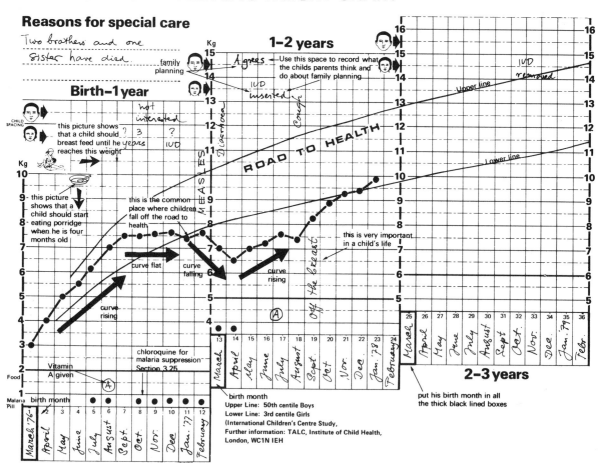

Fig. 7–1 The inside of Mulenga's weight chart.

88

smaller. If his arm circumference is less than 14 cm during this time, he is malnourished. The arm circumference is useful because we do not need to know a child's exact age. We only need to know that he is somewhere between one year old and five years old.

The arm circumference does not show small changes in a child's nutrition, but the weight chart does. So the arm circumference shows less clearly if a child is growing.

THE ARM CIRCUMFERENCE

(1) Use a tape measure. Measure the child's left arm. Let it hang by his side with his elbow straight. Measure his arm circumference half way between the point of his shoulder and his elbow.

Put the tape gently, but firmly, round his arm. Don't pull so tight that folds come in his skin.

(2) You can also measure a child's arm circumference with a 1 cm strip of old X-ray film.

Soak the film in hot soda for a day. Wash off the 'picture' with hot water. Make a scratch down the film at 0 cm. Make two more scratches at 12·5 cm and 14 cm. Colour the film below 12·5 cm red with a spirit pen. Colour the film yellow between 12·5 and 14 cm. Colour it green above 14 cm. Put the red colour close to the scratches, but don't let it touch them. Cut the film into 1 cm strips.

A child with an arm circumference below 12·5 cm is severely malnourished. If his arm circumference is between 12·5 cm and 14 cm, he is moderately malnourished. If it is above 14 cm, he is normal.

You can also use a piece of coloured string to measure the arm circumference. It is not so good because it stretches.

The arm circumference is NOT helpful in children under one year or over five years.

A CHILD WITH AN ARM CIRCUMFERENCE OF LESS THAN 14 CM BETWEEN THE AGES OF ONE AND FIVE IS MALNOURISHED

Nutrition Education

7.2 Five rules for good nutrition

Here are some rules for feeding children so that they grow.

First rule. Breast-feed until at least eighteen months. If possible a mother should breast-feed her child until he weighs about 10 kg. A picture on the weight chart shows this (7–1). Breast-feeding is always best. A rich mother with plenty of money, fuel, and water can make a safe bottle-feed, if she wants to. But it is not so good as breast-feeding (N 8.1). A poor mother cannot make a safe bottle-feed, and she cannot buy enough milk. A badly made bottle-feed contains so many micro-organisms that a child gets diarrhoea (9.8). It has so little milk that he becomes malnourished. So,

MEASURING THE ARM CIRCUMFERENCE

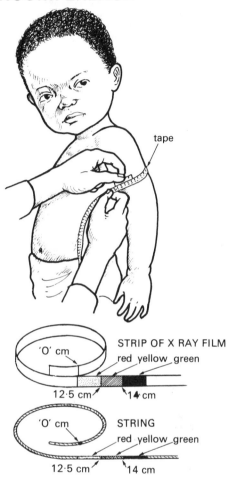

Fig. 7–1b Measuring the arm circumference.

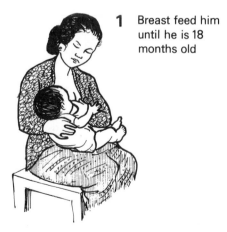

1 Breast feed him until he is 18 months old

7.2

Fig. 7–2 The first rule for good nutrition.

89

mothers should breast-feed their children until they are at least a year old. If possible they should breast-feed their children until they are eighteen months or two years old. A child needs his mother's milk all this time. Even if she is pregnant, she should go on breast-feeding him for a few months. Her milk is still safe for him and he needs it. But she must eat plenty of food herself. She now has three people to feed—herself, the child inside her, and the child at her breast.

IF THERE ARE ADVERTISEMENTS FOR BOTTLE FEEDING IN YOUR CLINIC, TAKE THEM DOWN

Second rule. Start porridge at four months. Breast-milk alone is enough for a child for the first four months. After that he needs porridge also. Tell mothers not to give their children foods like rice or bananas too early, because they may cause diarrhoea. These foods may fill up a child's stomach so that he does not want to suck. Four months is the best time for a child to start eating other foods. Some mothers give children fruit or fruit juice (vitamin C) much earlier than this. A child needs fruit juice if he is bottle-fed. But he does not need it if he is breast-fed. Breast-milk contains all the vitamins a young child needs.

Make a child's porridge from a good staple. This will give him most of the protein he needs. Rice, maize, millet, wheat, and Irish potatoes are good staples. They contain about 8 per cent of body-building protein. Cassava, yams, bananas, and sago are poor staples. They only contain 1 per cent of protein.

When a child is a year old he should eat all the foods his family eat. But they must be soft or well cut up. He needs a plate and spoon of his own, and his mother must help him to feed himself.

GOOD STAPLES MAKE THE BEST PORRIDGE

Third rule. Add protein foods to porridge. Even porridge made from a good staple does not contain enough protein for a young quickly growing child. His mother must add some protein food to it. **Legumes** are good cheap protein foods. Legumes are any kind of peas or beans, especially soya beans, or groundnuts. They contain 20 per cent of protein or more. Fish is also useful, and dried fish is sometimes cheap. Milk, eggs, meat, or liver are very good protein foods, but they are too expensive for most families.

Fourth rule. Give children four good meals a day. Children need much food and have small stomachs, so they must eat often. One meal a day is not enough—a young child needs four. Not eating often enough is a common cause of malnutrition. Most of the mothers of malnourished children could feed them more often.

2 Give him porridge when he is four months old

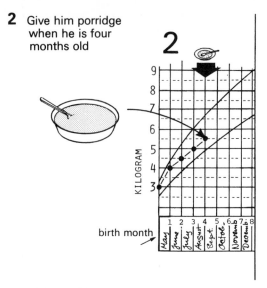

Fig. 7–3 The second rule for good nutrition.

3 Add protein foods to his porridge

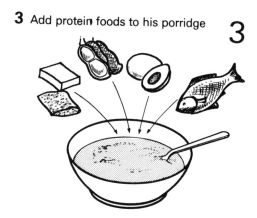

Fig. 7–4 The third rule for good nutrition.

4 A child needs four meals a day

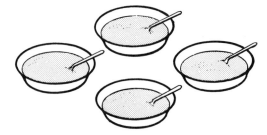

Fig. 7–5 The fourth rule for good nutrition.

90

Fifth rule. Give protective foods to children over four months old. These are the fruits and vegetables which contain minerals, and vitamins, such as vitamin A (16.13) and folic acid (22.6). Teach mothers to give their children yellow or orange fruit or vegetables, such as carrots, or papaya, or any kind of dark green leaves, such as spinach. Children need some of these foods every day.

5 A child needs some protective foods every day

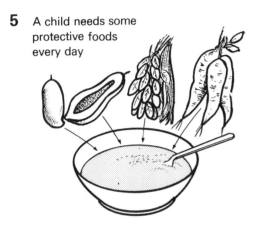

Fig. 7–6 The fifth rule for good nutrition.

Sixth rule. Sick children need feeding. A child's body is made of protein. This protein is slowly being destroyed all the time (N 3.3). If he eats enough protein food he can repair his body, and have enough protein for growing. But, if he has a fever his body protein is broken down faster than normal. So he needs more protein to repair his body when he is ill. But many diseases stop him wanting to eat, and some diseases (such as measles) make his mouth sore, so that eating hurts. So sick children often eat very little food or no food. They lose more protein than they eat and become malnourished.

Energy food is important also. A child's body burns energy food to keep warm. A child with a fever burns more energy food to heat his body and make his fever. If he does not eat enough energy food, he burns his body and becomes thin. So a sick child can become very malnourished, if he is sick for several weeks. He can also become malnourished if he has several shorter illnesses.

The mother of a sick child must make sure that he does not become malnourished, especially if he has fever or diarrhoea. He may not want to eat, so she must try hard. Tell her to give him any food he likes, especially any soft protein food. Tell her that when his symptoms are gone he is only half recovered. *He is not completely recovered until he has regained the weight he lost when he was ill.* While he is regaining this weight he needs extra food, especially energy foods such as oil. If he is young, his mother must breast-feed him extra often.

If mothers follow these rules, there will be no malnourished children. Unfortunately the rules are often broken.

6 Sick children need feeding

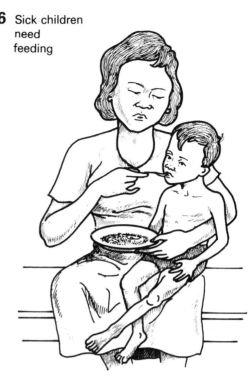

Fig. 7–7 The sixth rule for good nutrition.

7.3 Falling off the road to health

If children are breast-fed, they usually climb up the road to health for the first six months of their lives. But after this time the growth curves of some children become flat, and they fall off the road to health. They fall off because they do not start eating porridge at four months. They fall off because there is not enough protein food in their porridge, and because they don't eat often enough. They fall off because their mothers don't feed them when they are sick. This is what has happened to the child in Figure 7.7b. *So falling off the road to health is a sign that the rules of good nutrition have been broken.* It is usually a sign that our nutrition education has failed. One of our most important jobs is to prevent children falling off the road to health.

PREVENT CHILDREN FALLING OFF THE ROAD TO HEALTH

7.4 Teaching mothers and fathers to follow the six rules

When you teach a mother by herself, find out which of the five rules she is breaking (7.2). Find out why she is breaking them. Then think about the easiest way in which she could stop breaking them. This is not easy. Before you can help her you must know about her and her children. You must also know about how useful each food is, and how much it costs. To do this you should go to the market and make 'best buy lists' for protein (N 6.4) and joules (N 6.5). Teaching, or explanation is the eighth step (5.24), and is the best way to help a malnourished child. Here are some of the things you can teach her.

FALLING OFF THE ROAD TO HEALTH

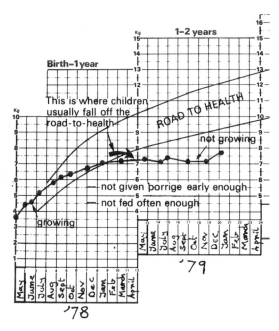

Fig. 7–7b Falling off the road to health.

NUTRITION TEACHING

Teach a mother something at each visit. Don't try to teach her too much at once.

Teach her about the weight chart.

Teach her any of the six rules of good nutrition (7.2).

Teach her that 'a good food is a mixed food'. Mixed foods are better than one food only. Many children are given plain porridge only. Any other food added to the porridge makes it better.

Teach mothers about body-building foods and energy foods. Teach them how to buy the most protein and energy for the money they spend.

If mothers can buy oil, teach them that it is a good energy food for preventing or treating malnutrition. Tell them to add a teaspoonful to a child's porridge and cook his food with it.

If any nutritional diseases, such as kwashiorkor or pellagra are common in your district, teach mothers about them.

How can we find out if our nutrition education is working? We can watch children's growth curves. Our education is working if they climb up towards the road to health (7–7b). In a good clinic most of the children's weight curves are climbing. Few of them have fallen off the road to health.

CLIMBING WEIGHT CURVES ARE A SIGN OF A GOOD CLINIC

7.5 'Musonda is often sick and is becoming thin'—malnutrition and infection

Malnutrition makes infections worse. It weakens a child's body so that harmful organisms can infect him more often, and more severely. Also, a malnourished child is more likely to get complications when he is infected. He is more likely to die and he recovers more slowly. Measles and TB, for example, are much more serious in malnourished children.

Infections make malnutrition worse. If a child is ill with an infection, he does not want to eat. If he has diarrhoea, he cannot absorb his food normally. If he has fever, his body protein is broken down faster than normal (7.2). If he has measles, his mouth is so sore that he does not want to eat. So he loses weight and becomes malnourished. Because malnutrition and infection make each other worse, they make a **vicious circle**, like that in Figure 7–8.

This vicious circle explains why so many children have both malnutrition and infections. They more often come to the clinic because of their infections than because of

THE VICIOUS CIRCLE OF MALNUTRITION AND INFECTION

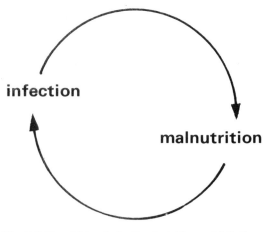

Fig. 7–8 The vicious circle of malnutrition and infection.

their malnutrition. You will find that many of the children who have diarrhoea, malaria, measles, chest infection, and TB are malnourished also. A child whose growth curve is flat may be malnourished only. But if his growth curve is falling, he probably has an infection also. There is only one way to help malnourished children, and break this vicious circle. We must treat both their malnutrition and their infections.

MANY CHILDREN NEED TREATMENT FOR MALNUTRITION AND INFECTION

Supplementary feeding

7.6 Dried skim milk

This is a common supplementary (extra) food for malnourished children. It is cheap and contains much protein (about 36 per cent). Unfortunately, there is not enough of it in the world, and many clinics do not have any. But, if you have milk, use it in the best way, and don't waste it. Give it only to children over six months with flat or falling weight curves. If you only have a little milk, give it to the children who need it most. Don't give it to healthy children to try to make their mothers bring them to the clinic. NEVER give it to children under six months who are breast-feeding normally, because their mothers may start bottle-feeding.

DON'T WASTE SUPPLEMENTARY FOOD ON CHILDREN WHO DON'T NEED IT

We can use other supplementary foods. One of them is CSSM, or Corn (maize), Soy (soy bean), and Skim Milk. Use them in the same way as dried skim milk.

EXPLAINING THE USE OF DRIED MILK

Tell the child's mother to add some of the milk to all his porridge. *Don't* **let her feed it to him in a feeding bottle or give it to him as a drink. If his mother says it causes diarrhoea, see Section 9.29. Explain that it is for him only and not for the rest of the family, or their visitors. He needs about two level teaspoonfuls of milk each day for each kilo of his body weight. Give him enough milk to last him until he comes to the clinic again.** *Remember—education is as important as milk.*

DON'T LET DRIED SKIM MILK START BOTTLE-FEEDING

Malnutrition

7.7 Protein–energy malnutrition

A child becomes malnourished if he does not eat enough body-building protein, or enough energy food. He gets **protein–energy malnutrition** or **PEM**. He can also become malnourished if he does not get enough vitamins. But lack of vitamins is usually less important than lack of protein and energy food. Most protein foods contain vitamins, so if a child eats enough protein foods, he gets enough vitamins also.

A CHILD WHO GETS ENOUGH PROTEIN AND ENERGY FOOD USUALLY GETS ENOUGH VITAMINS ALSO

7.8 'Mutiani's growth curve is flat'—mild malnutrition

The commonest kind of malnutrition is mild PEM. If a child is not given enough food, he stops growing, and his weight stops increasing. He runs about and plays less because he lacks energy. He is thin with mild muscle wasting, but has no other signs. He looks like a healthy child some months younger. There may be so many underweight children in the district that you and his mother think he is normal. This is why you must weigh all children. Mildly malnourished children have flat or falling growth curves. Most of them are below the road to health. *They get more infections than healthy growing children.* Underweight children *usually* come to the clinic with some other symptom such as a cough. Weigh an underweight child a few times, so that he has a growth curve. Then you know if he is growing or not.

The underweight child

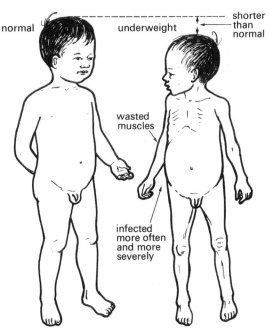

normal   underweight   shorter than normal

wasted muscles

infected more often and more severely

Fig. 7–9 The underweight child.

7.5

7.8

7.6

7.7

93

Although these children don't look sick they are already malnourished. They need more food and treatment for any infections they have. Their parents need nutrition education by themselves and in groups. Some children may need supplementary food for a few months.

GROWING CHILDREN GET FEWER INFECTIONS

Severe PEM

7.9 'Abdul is only skin and bone'—marasmus

Marasmus means starvation and is easy to diagnose. A marasmic child eats so little energy and protein food that he is very thin. His muscles are **grossly wasted**, and there is almost no fat under his skin. His face is so thin that he looks like a little old man. He is only about half the weight that he should be for his age. His arm circumference is much less than 14 cm (7.1, N 1.5). Sometimes, he has chronic diarrhoea (9.12). He is hungry, and anxious (worried).

Marasmus and dehydration (9.17) can both cause some of the same signs. They can both cause loss of skin elasticity (9.18), sunken eyes, and a sunken fontanelle. In a child with marasmus lack of fat, not lack of water causes these signs. So, to find out if a marasmic child is

dehydrated, *look for other signs*, such as thirst and a dry mouth.

Marasmus is common in babies. Some difficulty with breast-feeding usually causes it. A child's mother may have had too little breast-milk, or she may have died. She may have tried to bottle-feed him, but not been able to buy enough milk. Or she may not know how to sterilize his bottle, so that he often has diarrhoea. Or, he may have had diarrhoea, and she stopped feeding him, because she thought that this was the right treatment (9.31). Older children can also get marasmus if they do not eat enough food.

IF THE CHILD OF A POOR MOTHER IS NOT BREAST-FED, HE WILL PROBABLY DIE

7.10 'Ukeje's legs are swollen'—kwashiorkor

A child gets kwashiorkor because he has been eating too little body building protein. He may have been eating nearly enough energy food. Usually, he is underweight, but sometimes he is on the road to health. Occasionally he is even above it (N 1–15). He weighs less than before he was ill, but he may still have fat under his skin. Sometimes he has a round face like a full moon—a 'moon face'. His muscles waste and make his upper arms

Marasmus

Kwashiorkor

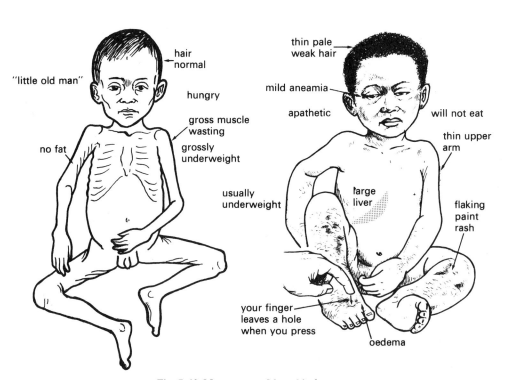

Fig. 7–10 Marasmus and kwashiorkor.

94

thin, so that his arm circumference is less than 14 cm (7.1, N 1.5). His buttocks waste, and his abdomen swells because his abdominal muscles are weak (20–8).

His legs and arms swell (19.8), and sometimes his face swells also. They swell because there is too much fluid (**oedema**) under his skin. If you press an oedema swelling, it feels like a ripe pawpaw and your finger makes a hole (7–10). All children with kwashiorkor have oedema. It is the most important sign of kwashiorkor. When a child's oedema comes, his weight rises about half a kilo. When his oedema goes his weight falls about half a kilo. You can see this on his weight chart.

OEDEMA

Press your thumb over the bone above his ankle. Take your finger away. If it leaves any mark or hole, he has oedema.

Oedema fluid falls slowly to the lowest part of a child's body. Look for it in the part that has been lowest during the last few hours. When you look for oedema always press with your thumb over a bone.

A child with kwashiorkor is unhappy, like the child on the cover of this book. He sits still, he does not move and is not interested in anything—**apathy**. Even though he is malnourished, he does not want to eat (18.15). Not running about and playing and not eating are important *early* signs of kwashiorkor. An important later sign is a '**flaking paint rash**' on his arms and legs (11.22).

THE MOST IMPORTANT SIGNS OF KWASHIOR-KOR ARE OEDEMA, APATHY AND A FLAKING PAINT RASH

A child with kwashiorkor has pale hair which is easy to pull out. Sometimes it is thin and pale, or slightly red. He is anaemic. He has a large liver (20.3). Often, he has chronic diarrhoea (9.12). Sometimes, he has signs of vitamin deficiency such as xerophthalmia (16.13), or sores at the corners of his mouth (18.10). Sometimes there is too little sugar in his blood (hypoglycaemia), so that he has drowsiness, coma (14.8), or fits (15.9).

Most children with kwashiorkor have most of these signs, but few children have all of them. Some children are very thin like the child with marasmus, and have oedema and the rash of kwashiorkor. Children like this have a mixture of both diseases called **marasmic kwashiorkor**.

Kwashiorkor and marasmus differ in several ways. Marasmus is more common. Marasmic children are much thinner than children with kwashiorkor. Marasmic children are more active and less apathetic. They don't have oedema. They are hungry and they don't die so easily. Marasmus comes on more slowly than kwashiorkor. Marasmic children take longer to recover.

Severe kwashiorkor is dangerous. If a child has muscle wasting, oedema, misery, and a flaking paint rash, he is seriously ill. If he cannot eat, he should go to hospital—soon. But, if he cannot go to hospital, you can help him in your clinic and at home.

7.11 Treating severe malnutrition

7.11

Food is the only cure for malnutrition. But if a child is to be cured, *he must be able to eat*, and his family must have enough food for him. If he does not want to eat we have to feed him through a tube. This is easiest in a hospital or health centre, but mothers can tube-feed children at home. The danger signs which show that a malnourished child needs treatment quickly are *oedema*, *apathy*, and *'not eating'*.

7.9

We can make a high-protein high-energy milk feed. This is the easiest way to give a severely malnourished child the food which he needs. Skim milk does not contain enough energy, so add sugar and cooking oil. Use any eatable cooking oil, such as cotton seed oil, or coconut oil. If you have no dried skim milk, you can use any other kind of milk or sour milk. You can also give him eggs or beans and maize, rice, or millet.

7.10

A severely malnourished child needs much treatment. You may not be able to do it all—do what you can.

SEVERE PEM

HIGH PROTEIN HIGH-ENERGY MILK FEED

Making the feed. **If possible weigh the things for the feed. If not, use dessert spoonfuls (Dsp). Take full spoons of oil and sugar. Take 'rounded' (not heaped or flat) spoonfuls of milk. Mix 80 g (6 Dsp) of dried skim milk, 60 g (7 Dsp) of cooking oil, and 50 g (3 Dsp) of sugar. If possible add 1 g of potassium chloride, and 0·5 g of magnesium hydroxide. This makes 1 litre of feed. It contains about 4 J (1 kcal) in each ml. Make the powder by mixing the milk and the sugar, then add the oil and mix again thoroughly. The mixture will keep for one month in a closed tin. Add seven rounded dessertspoonfuls of mixture to 500 ml of cold boiled water. Be sure everything you use is** *clean.*

Giving the feed. **If possible let the child drink his feed from a cup. If he will not drink from a cup, pass a thin plastic tube through his nose down into his stomach (9.24). Put the feed through the tube with a drip or with a syringe. Make sure the tube is in the stomach before you put feed through it (9.24).**

Don't sterilize the feed. Make it in cold boiled water. If you heat the feed the oil in it will come to the top. Don't keep liquid feed for more than six hours, or it will go sour. You can keep it longer in a refrigerator. If you cannot keep liquid feed cold, make it up only as you need it. Change the feed in a child's drip every six hours, or it too will go sour.

The dose of milk feed. **Give him 150 ml/kg/day. If he has oedema give him 100 ml/kg/day until his oedema has gone. Feed him 6 times a day.**

OTHER TREATMENT

Vitamin A. **Give him a capsule of vitamin A. Some mal-**

nourished children start to show signs of severe vitamin A deficiency while you treat them.

Rehydration. **A child can be dehydrated, and have oedema, so look for signs of dehydration (9.17). If necessary rehydrate him (9.20). The best way is usually to put glucose–salt solution into his intragastric drip (9.24). A dehydrated child with kwashiorkor is in special danger.**

Warmth. **Keep him warm, either close to his mother or well covered (10.1).**

Hypoglycaemia (drowsiness, coma, fits). **If possible, give glucose intravenously (sterile 20–50 per cent solution). And give glucose (or sugar) by mouth or by tube.**

INFECTIONS

Skin or chest infections. **Give all severely ill children tetracycline or chloramphenicol. These children often have septicaemia.**

Malaria. **In a malarious district give him chloroquine.**

Diarrhoea. **There is no need to treat mild diarrhoea. If it is severe, give chloramphenicol (3.18) or tetracycline (3.17) orally, or by tube, until 24 hours after the diarrhoea has stopped. Don't give either drug for more than five days.**

Hookworm. **If he is anaemic with a heavy hookworm load (21.1) give him children's iron mixture (3.33). When he starts to recover, give him TCE (3.27), or bephenium (3.27) to remove the hookworms. Don't give him TCE while he is ill.**

Other infections. **If he has an** *Ascaris* **infection, treat it (21.3). Treat any other infections you can find.**

LATER TREATMENT. **Give him protein foods by mouth as soon as he will eat them. Give him children's iron mixture until his haemoglobin is normal. If necessary suppress his malaria with chloroquine (3.25).**

EXPLANATION. **Explain to his mother why you are tube feeding him. Make sure she understands that** *food* **not medicine is curing him. Explain that when he is beginning to recover he will start to smile again. On that day you and she will both be very happy. Tell her to play with him as he recovers.**

If he cannot eat, and cannot go to hospital, his mother can tube-feed him at home. Mothers soon understand feeding tubes and soon see how useful they are. If many children need tubes, teach a helper how to put them in.

TREATING SEVERE MALNUTRITION AT HOME

If necessary lend the child's mother a 200 ml mug, and a teaspoon. Give her a 10 ml or larger disposable syringe. For babies use thin plastic tube. For older children use the tubing from old drip sets. Use whatever supplementary food powder you have.

Show her how to splint (hold) the child's arms, so that he cannot pull out the tube.

Put in the tube and fix it in place (9.24). Show her how to mix the food and inject it down the tube.

Write down the child's weight, the spoonfuls of feed he needs, and how many syringefuls of water to mix it with. Write down how many feeds he needs.

The child can suck or eat and drink with the tube in him. Ask his mother to come back to the clinic each day. When the child starts to eat normally (usually about two or three days), take out the tube. If the tube comes out, tell her to feed him with a spoon and come back to the clinic.

Give him any other treatment he may need.

EXPLANATION. **Explain carefully to the child's mother how seriously ill he is, and how the tube helps. Explain that you are putting food not medicine down his tube. As soon as he starts eating normally again, she must give him all the food he will eat.**

7.13 Caring for a malnourished child

Mildly malnourished children usually present with signs of infection, such as a cough or diarrhoea. Severely malnourished children can present like this. They can also present as apathy, swollen legs, 'not eating', loss of weight, or a rash. A diagnosis of 'PEM' is not enough by itself, and there are five things we need to know.

A. How severely malnourished is he? His weight chart is very useful, but you must examine him also.

B. What other diseases has he? Many children with PEM also have infections (7.5), and some lack vitamins.

C. Which of the six rules (7.2) of good nutrition have been broken?

D. Why have the rules been broken? Perhaps the child's father has too little land, or earns too little money, or has no job. So his mother cannot follow some of the rules. A child like this is difficult to help. Lack of knowledge is an easier block to remove. Often, a child's family have enough food, or money, but they do not know how to feed him. We can teach his parents how they should feed him.

E. How could his mother feed him? Try to find the easiest thing that she *could* do. Ask what good food she already gives him. Praise her, and tell her to give him more of it more often.

Here are *some* of the things you may need to do.

If a young baby is not growing, go to Section 26.21.

WEIGHING AND CHARTING. **Fill in his weight chart. Is he on the road to health or below it? Is his growth curve rising, staying the same, or** *falling*? **For how long has he not been growing? (Not growing is serious if it lasts more than a few weeks. It is always serious in babies).**

Can he eat? **(If he eats normally you can treat him at home. If he does not eat, he may need tube-feeding.)**

WHICH OF THE SIX RULES ARE BEING BROKEN?

First rule. **Is he breast- or bottle-fed? Is his mother going to breast-feed him until he is 18 months old? If he is bottle-fed, when did she stop breast-feeding and why is he bottle-fed? How is his bottle sterilized? What is put into it?**

Ask to have a look at the bottle. Is it clean? Does it smell? Is there too little milk in his feed? Is it sour?

Second rule. When did he start to have porridge? What kind of porridge is it? Does he have a plate and spoon of his own? Does anyone help him to feed?

FOOD CURES PEM

Marasmus

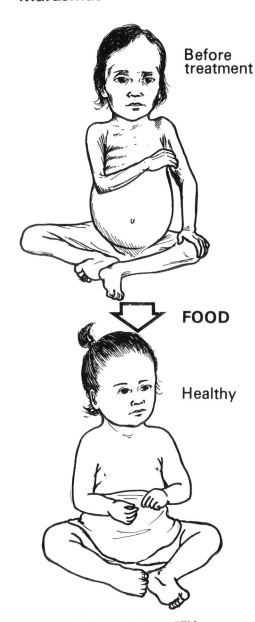

Before treatment

FOOD

Healthy

Fig. 7–11 Food cures PEM.

Third rule. Are any protein foods added to his porridge? What are they? How much of them does he eat?

Fourth rule. How often is he fed? *He probably needs more meals and more food at each meal.*

Fifth rule. Is he being given any protective foods, such as fruits and vegetables?

Sixth rule. Is he fed when he is sick?

WHY ARE THE RULES BEING BROKEN? **Does the family own land? How much land? Does his father work? How much money does he earn each day? How many people does this land or this money have to feed? How does the family spend the money they have? Are they in debt? Has the family enough fuel?**

PAST HISTORY. **Has the child been ill? Has he had measles?**

7.13

WHAT OTHER SYMPTOMS HAS HE? **Has he any symptoms that show he might have an infection, such as diarrhoea or a cough? Other symptoms of TB?**

EXAMINATION. **Unhappy?** *Apathetic* (kwashiorkor)? **Anxious (marasmus)?**

Is his body round and smooth, showing that there is still some fat under his skin, or is he thin? Look at his arms, shoulders, and buttocks. If he is between one and five years old, what is his arm circumference (7.1)? If this is less than 14 cm, he is malnourished.

Are his muscles wasted? Feel the muscle at the back of his upper arms. Feel his buttocks.

Oedema **(kwashiorkor)?**

Flaking paint rash **of kwashiorkor, or the rash of pellagra (11.23)?**

Anaemia?

Are his corneae dry? Bitot's spots (vitamin A deficiency, 16.13)?

Gums normal? (Infected gums are common in malnutrition)

What is his temperature (hypothermia, 10.1)?

Drowsiness, fits or coma (perhaps hypoglycaemia)?

DIAGNOSIS IN FIVE PARTS. **A. How severely malnourished is he? Mildly or moderately? If he is severely malnourished, has he got marasmus or kwashiorkor, or some of the signs of both of them?**

B. What other diseases has he? Infections? Vitamin deficiencies? Hypothermia?

C. Which of the six rules of good nutrition have been broken?

D. Why have these rules been broken?

E. How could his mother feed him better?

MANAGEMENT. **You can treat mild and moderate malnutrition at home. If he has kwashiorkor, try to send him to hospital. If he cannot go to hospital you may be able to treat him yourself. Be sure that each child has a weight chart and you observe carefully until he is on the road to health (N 2.10). If his growth curve stays flat or falls, go to Section 13.7 and examine him for TB.**

EXPLANATION. **This is the most important part of caring**

for a malnourished child. Be sure that his mother knows why he is sick. Explain that *only food can make him recover. If you give him a drug or injection, explain that it is not medicine, but food, that is curing him. Explain his weight chart. If he is underweight, don't make her feel ashamed.* Has she any questions to ask? Tell her when to come to the clinic again. When she comes again, ask her about his weight chart. What has she learnt about it?

RECORDS. If necessary, put him in the special care register (6.3).

8 Cough

8.1 'Rosa has a cough'

Viruses and bacteria often infect a child's respiratory system. Infections of its upper part are common, but are seldom serious. Infections of its lower part are less common, but they can be very dangerous. More children, especially babies, die from lower respiratory infections than from any other disease.

Most children with an upper respiratory infection have a cough as their most important local symptom. Infection of the lower respiratory system causes several other signs such as stridor (noise on breathing in), and fast breathing. All mothers can recognize a cough, but they cannot recognize these other signs so easily.

In adults, TB is the most important cause of a chronic cough. Children with TB also cough, but losing weight and being 'ill' (5.15) is more important. This is why there is a special chapter for TB (13.1).

**LOWER RESPIRATORY INFECTIONS ARE THE
MOST COMMON CAUSE OF DEATHS
IN CHILDREN**

8.2 The respiratory system

When a child breathes, air goes from his nose into spaces inside his head called his **nasal cavities** (1–6). These make the air warm and wet. The air then goes into his **pharynx**, which is the back part of his mouth. If you ask an older child to open his mouth, and say 'Ah . . .', you can see his pharynx (18–2). Below his pharynx is his **larynx**. This is a narrow space filled with air. It is at the top of the front of his neck.

There is a large tube below the larynx. This tube has strong walls and is called the **trachea** (wind pipe). It takes air to the **lungs**. The lungs are two organs filled with air, one on each side of the chest. In the middle of the chest the trachea joins two short thick tubes called the right and left **main bronchi**. One of the main bronchi goes to each lung and joins many smaller tubes called the **smaller bronchi**. The smaller bronchi join onto very small tubes called the **bronchioles**. There is smooth muscle round the walls of the smaller bronchi and bron-

chioles. This smooth muscle can contract and make them narrower (8–4), or expand to make them wider. The bronchioles take air to millions of small bags called **alveoli** (8–3), which are covered with capillaries (small blood vessels).

The tubes of the respiratory system are covered inside by thin wet tissue called **mucosa**. Another kind of mucosa covers the inside of the mouth and the nose. The mucosa keeps itself wet by making mucus.

The heart and lungs lie in a cage made of many curved bones called the **ribs**. Across the bottom of this cage

THE RESPIRATORY SYSTEM

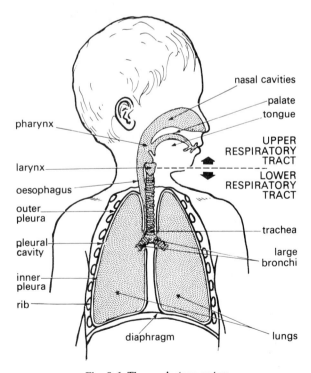

Fig. 8–1 The respiratory system.

there is a thin flat muscle called the **diaphragm**. The diaphragm is fixed to the inside of the lower ribs. It makes a wall across the body between the thorax (chest) and the abdomen.

Each time a child **inspires** (breathes in) his ribs move outwards and make his chest wider. His diaphragm moves downwards at the same time like the plunger of a syringe. A syringe sucks in air when you pull the plunger out. In the same way the diaphragm sucks fresh air into the lungs when it moves down. When a child **expires** (breathes out), his ribs move in, and his diaphragm goes up. The space inside his thorax gets smaller, and he pushes out waste air from his lungs.

The lungs are covered with very thin smooth tissue called the **pleura**. More of this tissue covers the inside of the ribs. The pleura around each of the lungs touches and slides over the pleura inside the ribs. The narrow space between these two layers of pleura is called the **pleural cavity**. There are two pleural cavities, one round each lung. They are empty, except for a few drops of fluid. Occasionally, when a lung is diseased, the pleural cavity around it fills with pus (empyema 8.16), or with fluid.

capillaries round the alveoli is very close to the air inside the alveoli. So oxygen in the air can easily go into the blood. Carbon dioxide can easily go out of the blood into the air. Blood coming to the lungs is more blue because it has little oxygen. After it has been through the capillaries of the lungs it has much oxygen, and it is red. If blood does not get enough oxygen while it goes through the lungs it stays blue.

Blood in the blood vessels makes some parts of a child's body red. A healthy child has red lips, a red tongue, and red conjunctivae. The skin under his finger nails is also red. If his blood is more blue than normal, then those parts of his body, which should be red, become blue. He is **cyanosed** (blue). This usually happens because (a) respiratory obstruction prevents oxygen going to his alveoli, or (b) because many of his alveoli are filled with pus (pneumonia) and have no air in them. Occasionally, cyanosis is caused by his heart not working well (heart failure). Cyanosis is a serious sign. It shows that his heart or respiratory system are not working normally. Extra oxygen will help him, but health centres do not usually have oxygen. So a cyanosed child should go to hospital.

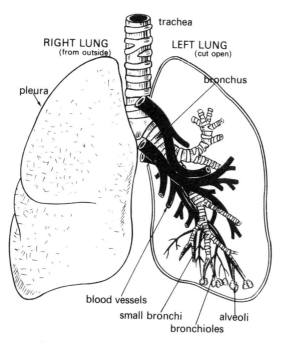

Fig. 8–2 The lungs, the bronchi, and their blood vessels.

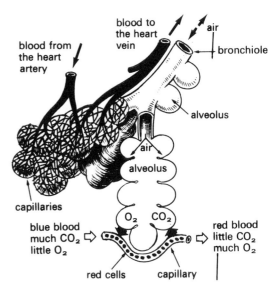

Fig. 8–3 How oxygen goes into the blood and carbon dioxide comes out.

CYANOSIS IS A SERIOUS SIGN

8.3 How infections harm the respiratory system.

Viruses cause most respiratory infections. They infect the mucosa of the nose, trachea, and bronchi. These primary (first) virus infections cause the mucosa to swell and make much mucus. The swelling of the mucosa and the extra mucus obstruct the flow of air through the tubes of the respiratory tract. Coughing is a sign that a

One of the gases in the air is called **oxygen**. A child's body uses oxygen to burn the food he eats. This gives him energy. He needs this energy to move and keep warm (N 4.1). When his body burns food with oxygen, another gas called **carbon dioxide** is made which he breathes out. Oxygen goes into the blood and carbon dioxide goes out through the alveoli of the lungs. The walls of the alveoli are very thin. So the blood in the

SOME LESIONS OF THE LARYNX TRACHEA AND BRONCHI

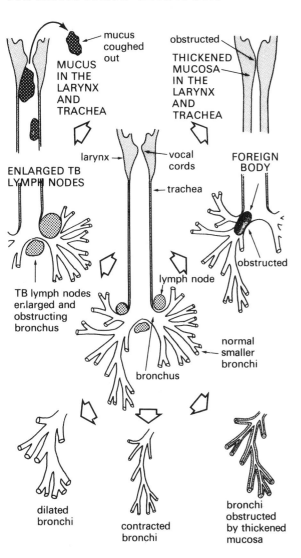

mucus coughed out

MUCUS IN THE LARYNX AND TRACHEA

obstructed

THICKENED MUCOSA IN THE LARYNX AND TRACHEA

larynx — vocal cords

FOREIGN BODY

ENLARGED TB LYMPH NODES

trachea

obstructed

TB lymph nodes enlarged and obstructing bronchus

lymph node

normal smaller bronchi

bronchus

dilated bronchi

contracted bronchi

bronchi obstructed by thickened mucosa

Fig. 8–4 Some lesions of the larynx, trachea, and bronchi.

child's lungs are trying to push out the mucus, and clear the tubes. Bacteria grow more easily in mucosa which has already been harmed by viruses. This secondary bacterial infection (2.6) causes pus to form and makes the disease worse. Unfortunately we have no drugs to treat a primary virus infection. But we have good drugs to treat secondary bacterial infection (3.13).

8.4 The upper and lower respiratory system.

The upper respiratory system is the part above the larynx. The lower respiratory system is the larynx, and everything below it. Diseases of the lower respiratory system are more dangerous, because the tubes in it are narrower, and more easily obstructed. If a child's nose is obstructed, he can breathe through his mouth. But if his larynx, bronchi or bronchioles are obstructed, air cannot get to his alveoli. This makes him seriously ill. All the tubes in a baby's respiratory system are very narrow, so respiratory infections are especially dangerous in babies.

LOWER RESPIRATORY INFECTIONS ARE MORE DANGEROUS

8.5 Symptomatic treatment for coughs

8.5

We can give a child with a cough curative treatment with antibiotics, or symptomatic treatment, or both. *Only a few children need antibiotics for their coughs*. Give antibiotics to the few children who are seriously ill with bacterial infections of their respiratory tracts. They may need symptomatic treatment also.

Most children with coughs have mild virus infections and recover without treatment. Antibiotics don't help these children and are wasted if you give them. These children need symptomatic treatment only.

SYMPTOMATIC TREATMENT FOR COUGHS

HISTORY. **Does his cough stop him sleeping?**
EXAMINATION. **Does he cough up much mucus (a 'wet' cough) or none (a 'dry' cough)? You can usually hear from the sound of a cough if it is 'wet' or 'dry'. Children swallow their sputum, so you will not see it.**

TREATMENT
Postural drainage. **This is useful for any child with a 'wet' cough. Show the child's mother how to bend him over her knee, or the edge of a bed. Put him with his head lower than his buttocks. Lie him first on one side and then on the other. Show her how to slap (gently hit) him all over his chest with her hand. This shakes the mucus in his respiratory tract and helps it to come out. He should cough out much mucus and pus while she does this. Afterwards he can breathe more easily.**

Promethazine (3.45). **Give this to the older child with a 'dry' cough who cannot sleep. Don't give it to children less than a year old. Don't give it to the ill child with a 'wet' cough who is coughing up much mucus and pus. We must not stop his cough. Coughing is useful because it helps to keep the tubes of his respiratory tract open. If pus and mucus stay in his respiratory tract, they make his disease worse.**

8.3

Placebo cough mixture. **If a child does not need any of the other treatments, but his mother wants something, give him 'Children's cough mixture' (3.46). Ask mothers to bring bottles with them to the clinic. Put 100 ml of cough mixture into a bottle. The dose for all children is 5 ml three times a day. If she wants an injection for him, immunize him (4.4).**

8.4

Disease of the upper respiratory system

8.6 Acute Upper Respiratory Infections—'URI'

The common infections of the upper respiratory tract are colds, pharyngitis, and tonsillitis. They can all cause a cough, fever, and a sore throat. They can all stop a child eating. Often, you will have difficulty deciding which of these diseases a child has. You will only be sure that he has an upper respiratory infection, or 'URI'. Tonsillitis and pharyngitis (18.11) are described in Chapter 18. But remember that they are both 'URIs' and often present as a cough.

Upper respiratory infections usually heal themselves, even without treatment. Sometimes, infection spreads below the larynx and causes laryngitis, or bronchitis (8.11), or pneumonia (8.15). Occasionally infection spreads to the middle ear and causes otitis media (17.9).

8.7 'My child has a cough and a discharging nose'—a cold.

Colds are infections caused by viruses which grow in the nose. Cold viruses are much more dangerous in babies. The same virus which causes a cold in an adult may cause bronchitis in a two year old child and pneumonia in a baby. Drugs cannot kill viruses, so there is no causal treatment for a cold. Antibiotics, such as penicillin, do not help.

A child with a cold, coughs and sneezes. His nose starts to discharge. For the first day or two the discharge is watery, then it becomes thick and yellow. After this it dries and forms crusts. Young children sometimes have a high fever (10.10). The infected mucosa swells and obstructs a child's nose, so that he has to breathe through his mouth. This is not important in older children. But a baby with a blocked nose cannot breathe and suck from the breast at the same time. So he may stop sucking. Then he does not get enough milk.

There are other causes of discharge from the nose. If there is blood in the discharge, or it is from one side only, go to Section 25.11.

COLDS

COUGH. **Give him children's cough mixture (3.46) or promethazine (3.45).**

FEVER. **Occasionally, you will need to treat this (10.3).**

EXPLANATION. **Tell his mother that there is no quick cure for a cold, but he will recover in a week. She must not stop breast-feeding. Some mothers and fathers suck out their babies' noses with their mouths. This is a good custom (2–7). Tell her to do this.**

ANTIBIOTICS DO NOT CURE COLDS

8.8 Chronic upper respiratory infection

Sometimes, a child's upper respiratory infection does not become better or worse. Instead, it stays the same, and becomes chronic. The mucosa of his nose swells, so that his nose is obstructed and he breathes through his mouth. Mucus runs from the front of his nose, and drips from the back of it into his pharynx (post-nasal drip). This makes him cough, especially at night. He is only mildly ill and does not usually have fever. If you cannot find a more serious cause for a child's cough, see if his nose is blocked. Look into his pharynx (18.2). Is mucus dripping down it from the back of his nose?

CHRONIC URI

SECONDARY INFECTION. **If his secretions are purulent, give him a course of sulfadimidine (3.14), or penicillin (3.15), or tetracycline (3.17).**

EXPLANATION. **Tell his mother that his cough is not serious, and that it will probably go slowly.**

Disease in the lower respiratory system

8.9 The six signs of lower respiratory disease.

These are helpful for diagnosing lower respiratory disease. You will not find them in upper respiratory infections.

1. Cyanosis. This is blueness of a child's lips and conjunctiva. Cyanosis is the least common, but the most serious sign. It shows that not enough oxygen is going into a child's blood (8.2). Examine children in a good light, because cyanosis is not an easy sign to find. Anaemia hides cyanosis, so you won't see it in anaemic children.

2. A moving nose. The sides of the nose of a healthy child stay still when he breathes. But, if he has difficulty breathing enough air into his lungs, his nose opens wider each time he breathes in. It closes each time he breathes out. So, look for movement of the nose whenever you see a child with a cough.

3. An increased respiratory rate. A healthy child breathes slowly when he is quiet or asleep. When he is angry, or moving about, he breathes faster. He also breathes faster when he has disease of his lungs, especially pneumonia. The speed of his breathing—whether it is fast or slow—is called his **respiratory rate**. An increased respiratory rate is a very useful sign. But you *must* count it before a child becomes angry, or starts moving about.

COUNTING THE RESPIRATORY RATE
Count while the child is quiet or asleep *before* you start examining him, and if possible, before you undress him. Use a watch with a second hand. Count his breathing for 30 seconds. Multiply your answer by two. Babies do not breathe evenly, so count a baby's breathing for a whole

minute. If your watch has not got a second hand, count the respirations of every child for a whole minute.

A person's normal respiratory rate depends on his age. If he is older, he breathes more slowly. A healthy adult breathes about twenty times a minute—he has a respiratory rate of about 20. A healthy sleeping new-born baby has a respiratory rate of about 40. Faster rates than this are abnormal in a quiet child. Lower respiratory disease is the commonest cause of abnormally fast breathing. But, dehydration, or severe anaemia, or any high fever can cause fast breathing. Pneumonia causes the fastest breathing. If a child has a respiratory rate above 60 when he is quiet, he probably has pneumonia.

OVER 40 ABNORMAL, OVER 60 PNEUMONIA (IF THE CHILD IS QUIET)

---

4. Inspiratory stridor. A healthy child makes no noise as he breathes. So any kind of noisy breathing (stridor) is abnormal. *Mild stridor* (a 'rattling' noise in the throat) is common in lower respiratory infections. A piece of mucus moving in a child's trachea or bronchi causes it. Mild stridor is not serious. *Severe stridor* is a dangerous sign of laryngeal obstruction. You will not hear it with other kinds of lower respiratory disease. It is usually worse when he breathes *in*, so it is called inspiratory stridor.

If stridor is severe there is always insuction also. If there is no insuction, stridor is not serious.

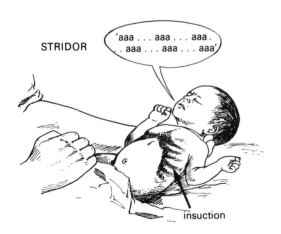

STRIDOR

'aaa . . . aaa . . . aaa. . . aaa . . . aaa . . . aaa'

insuction

Fig. 8–5 Stridor and insuction in a young child.

5. Expiratory wheezing. When a child has asthma, the muscles round his smaller bronchi contract, so that they become narrow. His bronchi become even more narrow when he tries to breathe out. So air has difficulty coming out of his alveoli, and breathing out takes longer than normal. As he breathes he makes a noise called a wheeze. This noise is worse as he breathes *out* (expires), so it is called an **expiratory wheeze**.

Babies are not strong enough to make much noise when they have respiratory obstruction. The noise they make on expiration sounds like a little pig. We call it **grunting** (26.1).

8.6

6. Insuction (retraction). A child with respiratory obstruction has to breathe in very strongly to get enough air. As he breathes in, he sucks in the skin between his ribs and at the bottom of his neck. This sucking in of the skin is called **insuction**. It shows that air cannot get into his alveoli normally.

A young child's lower ribs are soft and can bend easily. The edge of his diaphragm is fixed to them inside. If his obstruction is severe, his diaphragm has to contract very strongly each time he breathes in. This pulls in his whole lower chest, and not only the skin between his ribs. His chest looks as if a string has been tied tightly round it each time he breathes in.

8.7

EXAMINING FOR INSUCTION IN OLDER CHILDREN

8.9

In older children insuction is less easy to see. If you are not sure about it, examine for it like this.

Put a finger each side of a child's chest and watch your fingers moving. In a healthy child your fingers will move *outwards* as he breathes in. But if a child has respiratory obstruction, your fingers will move *inwards* as he breathes in.

You will see the most severe insuction in laryngeal obstruction in young children. Insuction is moderate in bronchitis and asthma and mild in pneumonia.

Teach mothers to recognize the first four of these signs—going blue, moving nose, fast breathing, and noisy breathing.

8.10 Acute lower respiratory diseases

8.10

Lower respiratory infections usually start with an infection of a child's upper respiratory system, such as a cold, or measles. After he has been ill for a few days with an upper respiratory infection, he becomes more 'ill'. He

SEVERE INSUCTION IN A YOUNG CHILD

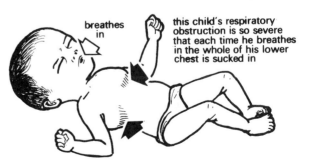

breathes in

this child's respiratory obstruction is so severe that each time he breathes in the whole of his lower chest is sucked in

8.8

Fig. 8–6 Severe insuction in a young child.

has fever and shows some of the 'six signs'. The signs he has depend on the part of his lower respiratory system that is most seriously infected. Often, his most severe lesions are in his bronchi and he has bronchitis. Occasionally, his most severe lesions are in his larynx, and he has laryngitis. Sometimes there are lesions in a child's larynx, trachea and bronchi. If the infection is mostly in his alveoli, he has pneumonia.

Other lower respiratory diseases are asthma, bronchiolitis, whooping cough, TB, and a foreign body in the bronchus. All these diseases are infections, except for a foreign body and the allergic kind of asthma.

8.11 Obstructive laryngitis (croup)

A child's larynx is very narrow. So, when infection makes its mucosa swell, the swollen mucosa easily obstructs his larynx. A child with obstructive laryngitis has a dry cough, which sounds like the barking of a dog. He has severe inspiratory stridor, and *very severe insuction*. Sometimes he becomes cyanosed. He breathes much more deeply than normal. Breathing is so difficult that he may suddenly stop breathing and die.

Obstructive laryngitis is sometimes caused by diphtheria. So look for a diphtheritic membrane (18.9) in his throat.

INSUCTION IN AN OLDER CHILD

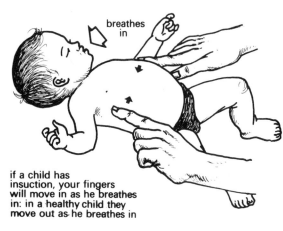

breathes in

if a child has insuction, your fingers will move in as he breathes in: in a healthy child they move out as he breathes in

Fig. 8–7 Examining for insuction in an older child.

OBSTRUCTIVE LARYNGITIS

MANAGEMENT. **If a child's obstruction becomes severe, he may need a tracheotomy (making a hole in his trachea). This lets air go into his trachea below the obstruction. This is usually only done in a hospital, so try to send him there quickly. Cyanosis is serious and shows that he must go to hospital as an emergency. If you have to treat him yourself, care for him like this —**

TREATMENT

Curative. **Give him chloramphenicol (3.18), for his secondary bacterial infection. If he vomits this, give him penicillin *and* streptomycin (3.21).**

Symptomatic. **He will breathe more easily if you bend his head backwards slightly. He will also breathe more easily if the air is wet. So hang wet cloths in the room near him. Don't give him drugs to make him sleep, because he needs to breathe as strongly as he can. These may make him breathe less strongly.**

Treat his fever (10.3).

EXPLANATION. **If his mother has to treat him at home, show her how to wet the air in his room. Ask her to stay with him and try to keep him quiet. This is very important, because breathing is more difficult if he cries or moves about too much.**

8.12 Bronchitis

The child with bronchitis has fever and a noisy 'wet' cough. Often, he has moderate insuction. He breathes faster than normal (40 to 60), but not as fast as in pneumonia (8.15). Bronchitis is much more common and much less dangerous than obstructive laryngitis. You can easily treat bronchitis. Viruses usually cause it, so antibiotics don't help. But if a child is 'ill' he may have a secondary bacterial infection, so treat it.

BRONCHITIS

CAUSAL TREATMENT. **If the child has a temperature of less than 38·5°C, he probably needs nothing. If his temperature is more than 38·5°C, give him penicillin (3.15) or sulphadimidine (3.14). If he is severely ill, give him chloramphenicol (3.18).**

SYMPTOMATIC TREATMENT. **Treat his cough (8.5), and his fever (10.3). Don't give him promethazine, because this may dry his sputum; then he cannot cough up the sputum easily.**

EXPLANATION. **Tell his mother that he should recover in a week. Ask her to bring him back quickly if he becomes worse, or has stridor or fast breathing. Show her how to give him postural drainage (8.5).**

8.13 'Salim is wheezing'—asthma

Asthma usually starts with a cough and a discharge of mucus from a child's nose. His breathing becomes difficult and noisy. His cough gets worse, he becomes irritable and restless, and he begins to wheeze. The smooth muscle round his smaller bronchi contracts. Their mucosa swells. Both these things make the space inside his bronchi narrower, so that air has difficulty going in and out. They make the child wheeze and make his breathing difficult.

Infection in the bronchi (bronchitis) often causes asthma. Then the child has fever.

A child's bronchi can become allergic (3.2) to small

pieces of protein from animals and plants. This causes asthma. These small pieces of protein are in dust, and go into the air he breathes. They are harmless to most children, and only a few unfortunate children are allergic to them. There is no fever in this kind of asthma, but all the other signs are the same.

Some children have one or two attacks of asthma and then never have asthma again. They are fortunate. A few unfortunate children have many attacks, and are 'asthmatic'. Don't say a child is asthmatic until he has had several attacks, because, if this is his first attack, he may never wheeze again. Children less than about a year old do not have asthma, because they do not have enough smooth muscle round their bronchi. Children who are going to be asthmatic usually get their first attack when they are about two years old. They then have several attacks a year. These become fewer as they grow older.

A child with asthma needs symptomatic treatment with ephedrine or adrenaline to make his bronchial muscle relax. These drugs also help to reduce the swelling in his bronchi. If he has fever, give him sulphonamides or tetracycline. Don't give him penicillin, ampicillin, or aspirin, because some asthmatic children are allergic to these drugs. Don't give antihistamines, because they do no good. They may make his sputum thicker and more difficult to cough up.

Some other diseases also cause wheezing. Worm larvae can make a child wheeze as they move through his lungs. A foreign body in the bronchus (8.18), or a TB lymph node pressing on the bronchi (13.2) can also cause wheezing.

ASTHMA

MANAGEMENT. **Treat mild asthma at home. But if a child has had severe asthma for a day or more, give him adrenaline and try to send him for help, especially if he is cyanosed. He may need different injections, and perhaps oxygen.**

SYMPTOMATIC TREATMENT FOR BRONCHIAL CONTRACTION. **Is it mild or severe?**

Mild attacks. **Give ephedrine tablets (3.39).**
Severe attacks. **Give adrenaline by subcutaneous injection (3.40).**

CAUSAL TREATMENT FOR BRONCHIAL INFECTION. **If he has fever, give him tetracycline (3.17), or sulphadimidine (3.14) for his bronchitis.**

FLUID. **Give him plenty of fluids to drink, so that his sputum becomes more liquid, and he coughs it up more easily.**

EXPLANATION. **Tell his mother why you think he is having difficulty breathing. Explain that he must drink plenty of water or tea, and must stay quiet. If he has had several**

attacks, explain that these will become fewer as he grows older. Write 'ASTHMA' on his weight chart.

ASTHMA IS NOT THE ONLY CAUSE OF WHEEZING

8.14 'My ten month old baby is wheezing'—bronchiolitis

8.14

Babies less than about a year old have a disease of their own called bronchiolitis. This causes wheezing and insuction. Viruses cause it. It needs different treatment from asthma. Antibiotics don't kill the viruses, but they may kill the bacteria causing the secondary infection. Small babies have very little muscle round their smaller bronchi, so ephedrine or adrenaline don't help.

8.11

8.12

BRONCHIOLITIS

MANAGEMENT. **The only useful treatment is oxygen, so try to send the baby somewhere he can have it, especially if he is cyanosed.**

TREATMENT. **If you have to treat him yourself, put him in a quiet room with wet towels near his cot (8.11).**
Don't give him adrenaline, or ephedrine. Give him penicillin (3.15) or sulphadimidine (3.14).
Make sure he is fed, if necessary by tube (26.18).

EXPLANATION. **Tell his mother why he is sick and how she can care for him.**

DON'T GIVE EPHEDRINE TABLETS OR ADRENALINE TO A BABY LESS THAN A YEAR OLD

8.15 'Ahmad has a fever and is breathing fast'—pneumonia

8.15

Pneumonia is an acute septic infection of the lungs. Bacteria usually cause it. Pus forms in some of the alveoli, so that air cannot go to them. Pneumonia usually begins with an infection of a child's upper respiratory tract, such as a cold or measles. Then this infection spreads down into his lungs. He has fever and becomes 'ill'. His nose moves as he breathes. If his pneumonia is severe, he becomes cyanosed. He has mild or moderate insuction. His pleura become inflamed. This makes his breathing painful, so that it is more shallow than normal. He also breathes faster than normal, which is very useful for diagnosis. If a child has a respiratory rate of 60 or more, he probably has pneumonia (or, rarely, heart failure). The respiratory rate of a child with pneumonia is usually 80 or 100.

8.13

THE RESPIRATIONS IN PNEUMONIA ARE FAST AND SHALLOW

DIAGNOSING PNEUMONIA BY COUNTING THE RESPIRATORY RATE

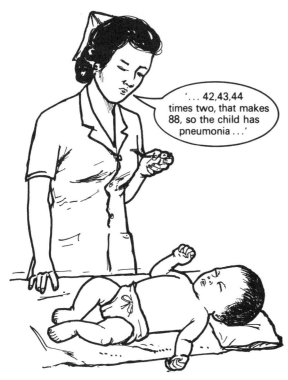

'... 42, 43, 44 times two, that makes 88, so the child has pneumonia ...'

Fig. 8–9 Diagnosing pneumonia by counting the respiratory rate.

Dehydration can also cause fast abnormal breathing. But the breathing of dehydration is *deep* (acidotic breathing, 9.18)—the child takes big breaths. Pneumonia causes fast *shallow* breathing—the child takes small breaths. A child with acidotic breathing has no other signs of lower respiratory infection, such as insuction. But he does have signs of dehydration, such as sunken eyes.

PNEUMONIA

If the child is less than three months old go to Section 26.26

MANAGEMENT. **Send him for help if he is very ill, or cyanosed.**

TREATMENT. **Give him penicillin (3.15), or sulphadimidine (3.14), or ampicillin (3.16) for not less than three days. 'Depot penicillin' (3.15) is very useful for treating pneumonia.**

If he comes from a malarious area, give him chloroquine (3.25).

If he has stridor, wet the air in his room (8.11).
Treat his fever (10.3).

EXPLANATION. **Tell his mother that he has a disease of his lungs. Explain that he is severely ill, but will recover in a few days. He must have all the drugs that you give her. Explain that he needs plenty of fluids and as much soft protein food as he will eat.**

DIAGNOSE PNEUMONIA BY WATCHING A CHILD BREATHE

8.16 'Ahmad is not recovering from pneumonia'

If a child with pneumonia has the right treatment, he should start to recover in one or two days. If he is not recovering, or is becoming more sick, ask yourself these questions —

Has he been having his drugs? Perhaps his mother has not been giving him his sulphadimidine tablets.

Has he got some other disease? Other diseases sometimes look like pneumonia. He may have TB (13.7) or typhoid (10.8). A foreign body, such as a nut, may be in his bronchi (8.18).

Send the child for help if he has not *started* to recover after three days of antibiotic treatment. He may have pus in his pleural cavities (empyema). This is difficult to diagnose and treat. If you cannot send him for help, stop the drugs he is having, and give him chloramphenicol, or tetracycline.

Sometimes, pneumonia harms a child's lung so that he has a cough for the rest of his life.

8.17 'Bayo is whooping'—whooping cough (pertussis)

Bacteria cause whooping cough. They grow in the bronchi, and spread by droplet infection. These bacteria cause the mucosa of the bronchi to make very sticky mucus. So a child coughs in a special way. He coughs out many times without breathing in. Then, when he breathes in again, he breathes so strongly that he makes a noise called a whoop. He goes 'Cough—cough—cough—cough—whooooop ...'. He becomes cyanosed, and he looks as if he is going to choke to death. After whooping he vomits, and thick sticky mucus hangs from his mouth. When he is not coughing, he looks healthy, and has no abnormal signs. Diagnose whooping cough from the sound of the whoop—it is diagnostic (5.20).

Whooping cough starts with a nasal discharge, fever, and a cough. The cough gets worse for ten days. After a few days it starts to come in spasms (lots of coughing together). Diagnosis is difficult at this time before the whoop has started. Ask his mother if her child has been near any other child with whooping cough. Whooping cough causes special signs in the blood, so a laboratory may be able to help in the diagnosis (L 7.21). After a child has coughed for about ten days, he starts to whoop, and diagnosis is easy. Children usually whoop for another three months and then recover. It is sometimes called '100 days cough'. The Yoruba call it 'wukotititi'. This means the cough that goes on and on. The Hausa call it 'tarin jaki'. This means the cough like a donkey. A child with a mild attack coughs for a few days only and never whoops.

The bacteria causing whooping cough are sensitive to chloramphenicol. But, by the time a child has started to whoop, it is too late for chloramphenicol to be helpful. Sometimes a child who has recovered from whooping cough starts to whoop when he has another respiratory infection. This is *not* a second attack of whooping cough. If he needs an antibiotic, give him penicillin or sulphadimidine. He does *not* need chloramphenicol.

Complications. Sometimes a piece of sticky mucus blocks one of a child's smaller bronchi and causes **pneumonia**. This may harm his lungs, so that he coughs for the rest of his life.

A child who is having his primary TB infection (13.2) sometimes gets whooping cough at the same time. Most children recover from their primary TB infection. But, if they have whooping cough at the same time, TB bacilli can cause more disease. So a child may start with whooping cough, and then go on coughing and losing weight for several months, because he now has **TB**.

CONJUNCTIVAL BLEEDING IN WHOOPING COUGH

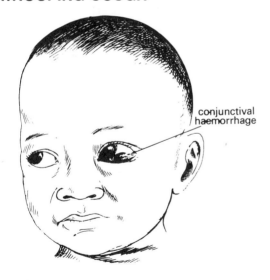

Fig. 8–10 Conjunctival bleeding in whooping cough.

If a child with whooping cough vomits too much, he loses weight, even if he is eating well. If he was already underweight before he got whooping cough, he may become very malnourished. He may get **marasmus** or **kwashiorkor** (7.10). Sometimes he has **oedema** without the other signs of kwashiorkor.

Sometimes, a child has a **fit** while he whoops. If this happens more than once, give him phenobarbitone (3.43). Occasionally, he **bleeds from his nose**. Sometimes he **bleeds into his conjunctivae**. This may cause a bright red lesion in his sclera. It is useful for diagnosis (8–10), but is not serious. His **eyelids may swell**. Sometimes he gets a **sore tongue,** because his tongue comes out over his lower teeth as he coughs. Lastly, he may cough so much that he gets a **hernia** (20.4).

Whooping cough in babies. Babies less than a year old seldom whoop. Instead, they have spasms of coughing, stop breathing for a minute or two, become cyanosed, and then vomit mucus. Sometimes they die in one of these attacks. Whooping cough is especially dangerous in babies less than six months old. It is difficult to diagnose, because there is no whoop. If an older child has whooping cough and his baby brother has nasal discharge, he may be infected also. In these first few days of the illness, chloramphenicol can cure a child, and perhaps save his life. So give babies ampicillin, chloramphenicol or tetracycline if they are ill when their older brothers are whooping.

Prevent whooping cough with DPT vaccine (4.9).

8.16

WHOOPING COUGH

MILD CASES. **There is no useful causal treatment, so give the child cough mixture (3.46).**

MORE SEVERE CASES, **especially in malnourished children.**

Treat the infection. **Chloramphenicol is only helpful during the first week of the disease. If he gets pneumonia, treat it (8.15).**

Sedation. **If his cough keeps him awake, give him promethazine (3.45).**

8.17

EXPLANATION. **Explain to the child's mother that his cough will last several weeks and cannot be cured quickly. Explain that this is a dangerous time for his nutrition. Tell her to feed him again after he has vomited. If he vomits after large meals, tell her to give him small meals more often. Ask her to bring him regularly for weighing. Explain that immunization can prevent whooping cough in her younger children.**

FOLLOW UP. **If his cough is not becoming less after three months, look for TB (13.7), especially if he is also losing weight.**

8.18 'Chichi has inhaled a groundnut'—foreign body

8.18

If a piece of food goes into a child's larynx, it causes sudden respiratory obstruction called **choking** (25.4). Usually, he coughs the food out or swallows it. Sometimes it goes through his larynx into one of his bronchi. A foreign body in the bronchus is easy to diagnose if his mother saw him choke. But it is difficult if she did not see him. Think of a foreign body if you see a child with sudden severe coughing, wheezing, and cyanosis. Sometimes a child is well for a few hours or days and then has another sudden severe coughing attack. This is called the 'silent interval' (time without coughing) and is useful for diagnosis. A foreign body is very dangerous. It obstructs a bronchus, so that the child gets pneumonia caused by secondary infection. Foreign bodies can only be removed in hospital. If we don't remove a foreign body, he will probably die.

8.19 Cough with other symptoms

Many of the children in a clinic have coughs. Most of them have mild upper respiratory infections caused by viruses, and recover by themselves. For many of these children the best diagnosis is a cold or 'URI'. They need cough mixture NOT an antibiotic. Some children have early measles, others have tonsillitis, and a few are whooping or wheezing. Be sure to diagnose the few children with lower respiratory infections. They do need an antibiotic and it may save their lives.

MOST CHILDREN WITH COUGHS DON'T NEED AN ANTIBIOTIC

Ordinary coughs are very common, so we do not want to spend too much time diagnosing and treating them. So it is helpful to have two 'Caring for . . .' sections. Section 8.20 is for the *many* children with an ordinary cough, who have none of the six signs of lower respiratory disease. Section 8.21 is for the *few* children who have any of these signs.

Any mother can recognize a cough, but the signs of lower respiratory infection are more difficult for her. She may see that her child's breathing is abnormal. But she may not be able to tell you anything more about it than this. For example, when she says he is 'sneezing', she may mean stridor, or fast breathing, or wheezing. So ask her what she means.

'Patson has a cough, fever, and mild diarrhoea.' Many children present with these three symptoms. Diseases of the gut which cause diarrhoea do not cause coughs. But infections of the respiratory tract which cause coughs can also cause *mild* diarrhoea and fever. Usually, children with cough, fever, and diarrhoea have upper respiratory infections. Their mild diarrhoea does not need treatment. Sometimes they have chronic diarrhoea caused by malnutrition (9.12). If a child has a cough, and *moderate* or *severe* diarrhoea, go to Section 9.31. You may need to use the next two sections also.

8.20 Caring for a child with an 'ordinary cough'.

Quickly look for the six signs of lower respiratory infection. (1) Are the child's lips cyanosed? (2) Does his nose move when he breathes? (3) Is he breathing fast? (4) Does he make a noise when he breathes? Stridor is sometimes a difficult sign to be sure about. (5) Is he

wheezing? (6) Is there insuction? For this you must undress him. You can look for all these signs in a few seconds. If he has any of them, go to Section 8.21. If he has none of them, use this section.

HISTORY. **How long has he been coughing? (This tells us if his disease is acute or chronic.)**

How old is he? (Babies do not whoop. Measles is uncommon children under six months.)

If he has only been coughing for one or two days, has he had measles, or been near a child with measles? Has he been immunized against it?

If he has been coughing for ten days, has he started to whoop? Has he been near a child with whooping cough?

If he has a chronic cough, has he been losing weight (TB)? Look at his weight chart.

EXAMINATION. **Discharge from his nose (URI)?**

Nose blocked so that he has to breathe through his mouth (acute or chronic URI)?

Tonsillar lymph nodes large or tender (18.2) (tonsillitis, URI)?

Look at his breathing, if this is abnormal go to Section 8.21.

Examine his mouth. Koplik's spots (measles)? Red throat (URI)? Tonsils large and red? Pus on the tonsils (tonsillitis)? Mucus or pus coming from the back of his nose into his pharynx (postnasal drip from a chronic upper respiratory infection)?

Ears discharging? Ear drums normal? (Children with middle ear disease often cough.)

Common

DIAGNOSIS. **A cold (8.7)? Acute 'URI' (18.11)? Tonsillitis (18.11)? Measles (10.6)? Chronic 'URI' (8.8)? Whooping cough (8.17)? TB (13.7)? Otitis media (17.9)? Typhoid (10.8)?**

Rare

EXPLANATION. *The four danger signs in a coughing child.* **Teach mothers that an 'ordinary cough' is not serious. Explain that if disease spreads down to a child's chest, it is dangerous. Tell her to bring him back to the clinic if he goes blue, if his nose starts moving, or if he breathes fast or with difficulty.**

MANAGEMENT WHERE DIAGNOSIS IS DIFFICULT. **If he is not seriously ill, weigh him, give him cough mixture, and ask his mother to bring him back in a few days. He may start to whoop, or the measles rash may come. Examine him again. If he is 'ill', try giving him sulphadimidine or an antibiotic. If he is not well in a few weeks and is losing weight, he might have TB. So go to Section 13.7.**

8.21 Caring for a child who has a cough and any signs of a lower respiratory infection—cyanosis, moving nose, fast breathing, stridor, wheezing, or insuction.

Table 8:1 Diagnosing lower respiratory infection

	Respiratory rate	Depth of respiration	Insuction or inward movement of the chest	Other signs
Lower respiratory infections				
Laryngitis	40–60	Deeper than normal	+++++	Stridor
Bronchitis	40–60	Normal	++	——
Asthma	40–60	Deeper than normal	+++	Expiratory wheeze
Pneumonia	More than 60	shallower than normal	+	——
Two other diseases which may cause difficulty				
Anaemia	40–60	Normal	None	Grossly anaemic
Dehydration (acidotic breathing)	40–60	Much deeper than normal	None	Sunken eyes etc.

The diagnostic signs have boxes round them. Only some of the many 'other signs' are shown.

8.19

Most of these children are seriously ill and need antibiotic treatment for *at least three days*. We have put severe anaemia, severe dehydration, and high fever among the diagnoses. They don't cause a cough but they do cause fast breathing. TB does not usually cause any signs in the lungs. It only causes signs after a child's lungs are partly destroyed.

If he is less than a year old, wheezing, and cyanosed go to Section 8.14.

HISTORY. Has he inhaled anything, such as a bead or a groundnut (foreign body)?

Are there times when his breathing seems to be normal ('silent interval') before he has another severe attack of cough and cyanosis (foreign body)?

Has he been immunized with DPT (diphtheria)?

EXAMINATION. Cyanosis (a serious sign)?

Count his respirations (if they are more than 60, he probably has pneumonia). Is he breathing more deeply, or less deeply than usual? (Acidosis causes deep breathing, pneumonia shallow breathing.)

Any signs of dehydration (acidotic breathing)?

Grossly anaemic?

Noise when he breathes *in*? (Severe stridor is usually caused by laryngitis, sometimes diphtheria.)

Wheeze, when he breathes *out*? (Usually asthma, occasionally TB, or foreign body or worms.)

Insuction (any lower respiratory disease)? Bronchitis is the most common cause of insuction. Obstructive laryngitis causes the most severe insuction.

Examine his throat (18.2) and feel for enlarged tonsillar lymph nodes (tonsillitis, diphtheria).

Temperature? (A high fever may cause fast breathing.)

DIAGNOSIS. Bronchitis (8.12)? Pneumonia (8.15)? Asthma (8.13)? Obstructive laryngitis (8.11)? The acidotic breathing of dehydration (9.18)? Late TB (13.1)? Anaemia (22.9)? High fever? Diphtheria (18.12)? Foreign body (8.18)?

MANAGEMENT IF DIAGNOSIS IS DIFFICULT. If he is seriously ill or cyanosed, he may need oxygen, so try to send him for help. If this is not possible, treat him for pneumonia. If penicillin or sulphadimidine does not cure him in two or three days, give him chloramphenicol, or tetracycline.

8.20

8.21

A CHILD WITH A LOWER RESPIRATORY INFECTION NEEDS AN ANTIBIOTIC FOR AT LEAST THREE DAYS

9 Diarrhoea

9.1 'Yani has diarrhoea'

Diarrhoea is common. Many children die from it and it is especially dangerous in babies. Fortunately, we can prevent diarrhoea. If you treat children with diarrhoea carefully, few of them will die.

The stools of a normal *baby* are described in Section 26.29. A healthy *older* child passes stools once or twice a day, or sometimes only once in two days. His stools are brown and solid. If he passes many fluid stools he has diarrhoea. Sometimes there is blood and mucus in diarrhoea stools, or the stools may be green. Stools become green if they are passed so quickly that the green bile does not have time to become brown.

Diarrhoea has many causes, but infection and malnutrition are the most important causes. They often work together. Bacteria or viruses *inside* the gut cause infectious diarrhoea. Often, these organisms are not dangerous enough to harm adults. But sometimes they are especially dangerous and can cause diarrhoea at any age. Sometimes, diarrhoea is caused by infections *outside* the gut, such as malaria or tonsillitis.

Infections inside the gut

9.2 The flora of the adult gut are dangerous to a baby

A healthy baby is born with no organisms on him, or in his gut—he has no flora (2.2) and is sterile (2.2b). During the first few months of his life he meets many organisms for the first time. They come to him from the skin, the hands, or the breasts of his mother. A few of them are helpful. Some organisms (lacto-bacilli) grow well in digesting breast milk and help to keep the harmful organisms away. As a child grows older other organisms come to live in his gut. They come to him in his food and water from the faeces of healthy adults. Some of them can grow in him and cause diarrhoea, because he has not yet become immune to them. As he grows older his body learns to live with the organisms he meets. This is why older children and adults get diarrhoea less often.

Gut micro-organisms, which are not dangerous enough to harm adults, often cause diarrhoea in young children. *You will probably see about ten children with*

this kind of diarrhoea for every one child with one of the 'special' organisms in the next section.

Some specially dangerous organisms

9.3 'Olu has bloody diarrhoea'—dysentery

Dysentery is the name for any diarrhoea with blood and mucus in the stools. Bacillary and amoebic dysentery are the most common kinds, but some worms can cause it.

Bacillary dysentery. Bacilli are pencil-shaped bacteria. The child has bloody diarrhoea and fever. Often,

THINGS YOU MIGHT SEE IN THE STOOLS OF CHILDREN WITH DIARRHOEA

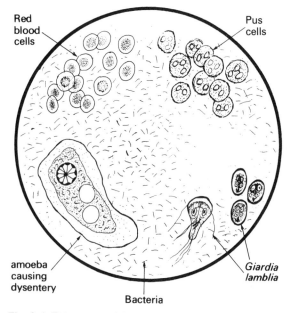

Fig. 9–1 Things you might see in the stools of children with diarrhoea.

110

he becomes severely dehydrated. If you examine his stools with a microscope, you will see blood and pus cells. But you cannot recognize dysentery bacilli, because they look like the ordinary bacteria of the faeces.

BACILLARY DYSENTERY. **Give him tetracycline (3.17), or chloramphenicol (3.18). Sulphonamides do not usually help (3.12). If necessary, rehydrate him (9.20).**

9.4 Amoebic dysentery

This is common in some districts. Organisms called amoebae cause it. Amoebic dysentery does not make a child so 'ill' as bacillary dysentery and seldom causes dehydration. He has soft faeces with blood and mucus. Amoebae are larger than bacteria. You can usually find them if you examine *warm* faeces with a microscope (L 10.7).

AMOEBIC DYSENTERY. **Metronidazole (3.26) is the best drug, but you can treat amoebic dysentery with tetracycline (3.17).**

9.5 Dysentery caused by worms

Heavy infections with some kinds of worm sometimes cause dysentery. You can treat these worms, so try to examine all dysentery stools with a microscope (L 10.2). Heavy infections with *Strongyloides* (21.6), *Trichuris* (21.7), *H.nana* (21.4), and *Schistosoma mansoni* (23.8) can cause dysentery. But *Ascaris* does not cause it.

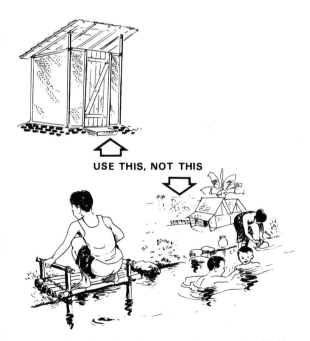

USE THIS, NOT THIS

Fig. 9–2 Organisms from the gut are dangerous in drinking water.

9.6
9.6 'Aleya has diarrhoea with bubbles in her stools'—giardiasis

In this kind of diarrhoea a child's stools are yellow and full of bubbles. They smell bad but there is no blood or mucus in them. Stools like this are caused by an organism called *Giardia* or by malnutrition. *Giardia* are usually easy to find. Examine the stools with a microscope. *Giardia* are very common in some districts. Look for them if a diarrhoea stool has bubbles and the child is losing weight. Treat him with mepacrine (3.26), or metronidazole (3.26).

9.4

9.7
9.7 'Ramon's stools look like rice water'—cholera

9.1
Bacteria called *Vibrio cholera* cause this very serious diarrhoea. It is uncommon under the age of one year. Mild cholera is just like any other diarrhoea. A child with severe cholera passes stools which look like the water in which rice has been cooked ('rice water stools'). Severe cholera starts suddenly with severe diarrhoea and sometimes vomiting. It quickly causes gross dehydration (9.18). If there is cholera in your district, and a child has rice water stools, he probably has cholera. He needs rehydrating quickly in the same way as any other child with severe dehydration. Give him tetracycline (3.17), or chloramphenicol (3.18).

9.3

9.5

9.8
9.8 Preventing gut infections

Infectious diarrhoea is usually caused by organisms which spread from faeces to mouth by Path A, in Figure 2–6. Prevent it. Make sure that everything that goes into a child's mouth is clean. This is difficult, but here are some of the things that parents can do.

Breast-feed. Milk from a healthy breast is sterile and never causes infectious diarrhoea, even if the mother is pregnant. It contains antibodies which help to kill harmful bacteria, and prevent diarrhoea. Milk from a dirty feeding bottle often contains many micro-organisms and causes diarrhoea. The micro-organisms grow in the bottle because it has not been cleaned and sterilized. Many mothers do not know that they should sterilize feeding bottles. They do not have enough time or enough money for fuel. They cannot buy enough dried milk, so their babies become malnourished. Prevent this kind of diarrhoea. Teach mothers to breast-feed their children. If they have no breast-milk, teach them how to make a *safe* artificial feed (26.15).

9.2

BREAST-FEEDING PREVENTS DIARRHOEA

Keep faeces away from drinking water. Some people pass their faeces into rivers. Then they take their drinking water from the same river. The water from these rivers is mixed with faeces, and is especially dangerous for a young child. Prevent diarrhoea. Teach people to use latrines. If a child must drink dirty water, boil it.

BREAST FEEDING IS BEST

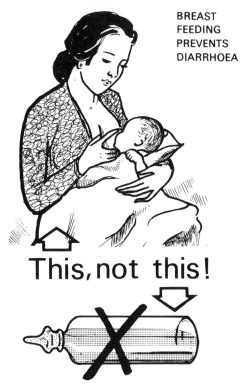

BREAST
FEEDING
PREVENTS
DIARRHOEA

This, not this!

Fig. 9–3 Breast-feeding is best.

Wash hands. We must prevent the organisms in our own gut infecting the food we touch. We can do this by *always* washing our hands after going to the latrine and *before* touching food. All mothers must wash their hands when they cook their children's food.

Keep flies away from food. A fly's feet can easily carry harmful organisms from faeces to a child's food. Cover his food and keep flies away from it.

Stop dirt going into a child's mouth. There are many harmful organisms on the ground. Do not let a child eat food which has fallen on the ground. Wash spoons or toys which he has dropped before he puts them in his mouth again. If possible, find a clean place for young children to play.

EVERYTHING THAT GOES INTO A CHILD'S MOUTH MUST BE CLEAN

Make sure *your* clinic has a tap or a well where mothers can get clean water. It should also have a clean, safe latrine with a small hole which children can use without being frightened.

Infections outside the gut

9.9 Malaria (10.7)

The parasites of *falciparum* malaria can harm the wall of the gut and cause diarrhoea. The diarrhoea is usually mild and there is seldom any blood or mucus in the stools. In malarious districts many children have both malaria and harmful organisms inside their gut. So we do not know which infection is causing the diarrhoea. If a child has malaria, we must treat him, or he may die. The safe rule is this—*in a district where falciparum malaria is common, give chloroquine by mouth to all children with diarrhoea and fever. If they are vomiting, give them chloroquine or quinine by injection.* Look for parasites in a blood slide. If a child has diarrhoea and many parasites in his blood, malaria is probably causing his diarrhoea.

A CHILD'S DRINKING WATER SHOULD BE BOILED

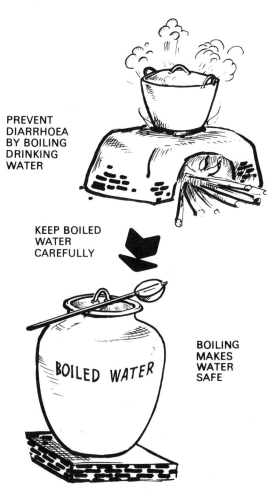

PREVENT
DIARRHOEA
BY BOILING
DRINKING
WATER

KEEP BOILED
WATER
CAREFULLY

BOILED WATER

BOILING
MAKES
WATER
SAFE

Fig. 9–4 A child's drinking water should be boiled.

If he has few parasites, there is probably some other cause.

9.10 Other infections

Severe measles (10.6) often causes diarrhoea, sometimes with blood in the stools. A child may have mild diarrhoea when he has a cold, otitis media, pneumonia, a urinary infection or thrush (18.5). In older children these infections don't usually present as diarrhoea. Older children have other symptoms, such as ear pain or cough. These symptoms help us to make the right diagnosis. But, in babies, diarrhoea and vomiting can be the presenting symptoms of many infections (26.32). So, when a child, especially a baby, has diarrhoea *and fever*, look for an infection in *some other part of his body*.

IF A YOUNG CHILD HAS DIARRHOEA LOOK FOR AN INFECTION OUTSIDE HIS GUT

9.11 Malnutrition—PEM

Malnutrition causes diarrhoea in this way. Food is digested by substances called enzymes. These enzymes are special proteins that the body makes in the gut (N 3.7). If a child is malnourished he cannot make enough enzymes, and cannot digest his food normally. Malnutrition also weakens the wall of his gut, so that he

FLIES SHOULD NOT GET TO A CHILD'FOOD

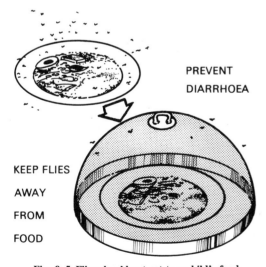

PREVENT DIARRHOEA

KEEP FLIES

AWAY

FROM

FOOD

Fig. 9–5 Flies should not get to a child's food.

CHILDREN SHOULD PLAY IN A CLEAN PLACE

9.9

PREVENT DIARRHOEA BY KEEPING DIRT OUT OF A CHILD'S MOUTH

9.10

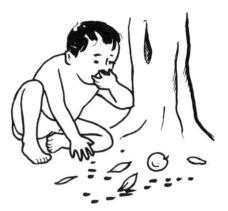

Fig. 9–6 Children should play in a clean place.

cannot absorb food. Food which he cannot digest and absorb goes out of him in diarrhoea stools. Micro-organisms grow more easily in this undigested food, and make his diarrhoea worse.

9.11

MALNUTRITION CAUSES DIARRHOEA. DIARRHOEA CAUSES MALNUTRITION

Diarrhoea causes malnutrition in this way. Diarrhoea stops a child eating. Also, the organisms which cause diarrhoea harm the wall of a child's gut. This prevents him from digesting and absorbing his food normally. Diarrhoea makes his food go through his gut too quickly, so that he does not have time to absorb it. Because he does not absorb his food normally, he becomes malnourished.

So malnutrition helps to cause diarrhoea, and diarrhoea helps to cause malnutrition. When two things make one another worse in this way, they make a **vicious circle**. This is the vicious circle of malnutrition and diarrhoea. It is one example of the vicious circle of malnutrition and infection (7.5).

PREVENT DIARRHOEA BY PREVENTING MALNUTRITION. PREVENT MALNUTRITION BY PREVENTING DIARRHOEA

Malnourished children have acute infectious diarrhoea more often than well-nourished children (7.5). They are also more likely to die, because their bodies are weaker. Help children to be well nourished. This is one of the best ways of preventing diarrhoea, and the deaths from diarrhoea. Teach mothers to treat diarrhoea *early*. This keeps them eating and prevents them losing weight. It also prevents malnutrition.

MOST CHILDREN WITH CHRONIC DIARRHOEA ARE MALNOURISHED

9.12 'Carmen is thin and always has diarrhoea'—chronic diarrhoea in an underweight child

Many children are ill for a few days with acute diarrhoea. These children become dehydrated, and need rehydration (9.20).

Many other children have moderate diarrhoea which lasts for weeks or months. They may not have it every day, but they have it most days. Their stools may be watery or liquid, bubbly, and bad smelling, but they contain no blood. They lose a little water with each loose stool. But they are only passing a few liquid stools, so they do not become dehydrated. They also lose some food with each stool, and this is important. They may be given very little food, and may not want to eat. So, if they lose even a little food in their stools, they become malnourished. They are being harmed by the vicious circle of malnutrition and diarrhoea. You can break this vicious circle and cure them. Give them more energy and protein food. They are not dehydrated, so fluids do not help them.

More food sometimes makes a child pass more stools, but *he also absorbs more food*. Tell his mother that this is much more important than the number of stools he passes. The *worst* thing she can do is to stop feeding him. If he stops eating, his stools may be less, but his malnutrition will get worse. Finally, when he is better nourished, his diarrhoea will stop.

FOOD IS THE BEST TREATMENT FOR CHRONIC DIARRHOEA IN AN UNDER-WEIGHT CHILD

THE VICIOUS CIRCLE OF MALNUTRITION AND DIARRHOEA

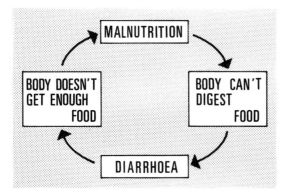

Fig. 9–7 The vicious circle of malnutrition and diarrhoea.

Sometimes, a child who has chronic diarrhoea gets acute diarrhoea also. He is acutely dehydrated and malnourished. He has **acute-on-chronic diarrhoea**. This is a very serious kind of diarrhoea and you must diagnose it. These children need treatment for their dehydration first. As soon as that is better, they need more food.

9.13 Food and diarrhoea

Breast-milk is the only food most children need for the first four months of their lives. If a mother gives her newborn child other foods, he may get diarrhoea. He does not normally need foods until he is at least four months old (26.21, N 7.3).

A child sometimes has diarrhoea if he eats a lot of a new food. Or too many beans with their skins on, or if he is given medicines. This kind of diarrhoea is usually mild. Sometimes a mother says that an important protein food, such as groundnuts, gives her child diarrhoea. Tell her to give him a little of the new food for a few days. It will soon stop causing diarrhoea and he can then eat more of it.

If food stays in a warm place, organisms grow in it, and it spoils. If children eat this food they get diarrhoea and vomiting (20.14) (food poisoning). They must only eat newly cooked food. Sometimes milk causes diarrhoea because it is given in a dirty bottle (26.15), or because of lactose intolerance (9.29).

A child with acute diarrhoea should start eating again as soon as possible. This is especially important if he is malnourished, or his malnutrition will get worse. So a baby with diarrhoea should go on breast-feeding. If he stops, he should start again as soon as possible. An older child should go on eating, or eat again as soon as he can.

A CHILD WITH DIARRHOEA NEEDS FOOD AS SOON AS HE WILL EAT

One more cause of diarrhoea

9.15 Surgical diseases

A few children have diarrhoea because they have a serious abdominal disease (acute abdomen, 20.2) which needs a surgical operation in hospital. In the disease called **intussusception** a part of the gut is pushed into a part lower down. It causes a swelling in the abdomen. The child has pain, vomits, and passes blood and mucus, with very little faeces. He needs an operation quickly.

Diagnosis

9.16 Diagnosis may be difficult

Often, we cannot diagnose why a child has diarrhoea. He may have no blood or mucus in his stool, so he has not got dysentery. He may be well-nourished, so his diarrhoea is not caused by malnutrition. He may be breast fed, so it is not caused by badly managed bottle feeding. He is probably infected by ordinary gut organisms (9.2), but we cannot be sure. Fortunately, a sure diagnosis of why a child has diarrhoea is seldom important. When we treat his dehydration, he usually recovers.

Dehydration

9.17 Diarrhoea causes dehydration

There is much water inside a child's body. If his body loses water and becomes too dry, he is dehydrated. He is ill with **dehydration** (de- means without, hyd- means water). He can become dehydrated slowly during several days, or very quickly in a few hours.

The stools of a healthy child contain little water. The stools of a child with diarrhoea contain a lot of water—they may look like dirty water. A child with acute diarrhoea easily becomes dehydrated. If he is vomiting also, he becomes dehydrated faster, because he is losing water from both ends of his gut. Vomiting makes treatment difficult, because a child vomits up the fluid he drinks. *So, diarrhoea with vomiting is a more dangerous cause of dehydration than diarrhoea alone.*

There are mineral salts in diarrhoea stools. So a child with diarrhoea also loses mineral salts. He loses **sodium chloride**, which is ordinary salt, and another important mineral called **potassium**. He also loses **bicarbonate**. We have to put all these salts back into him.

A child who dies from diarrhoea is not killed by the organisms in his gut. He dies because they make him lose water and salts. He dies from dehydration.

**A CHILD WHO DIES FROM DIARRHOEA
DIES FROM DEHYDRATION**

9.18 The signs of dehydration

Loss of weight. When a child loses water and becomes dehydrated, his body becomes lighter. A severely dehydrated child may have lost 10 per cent of his normal body weight. If he weighed 10 kg before, he may have lost a kilo of water and may now weigh only 9 kg. He loses this weight quickly *during a few hours or days*. A malnourished child loses weight slowly during several weeks or months.

Thirst. Dehydration causes no signs, except thirst, until a child has lost 5 per cent of his body weight (500 g for a 10 kg child). So thirst is the first sign of dehydration. A young child cannot tell you he is thirsty, except by crying. Find out if he is thirsty. Give him water to drink.

**THIRST IS THE EARLIEST SIGN
OF DEHYDRATION**

If a child has *any* other signs, he has lost at least 5 per cent of his body weight. He may have lost much more weight.

Sunken eyes. This is a very useful sign. A child's eyes lie in soft wet fatty tissue. If he becomes dehydrated this tissue gets drier and smaller, and his eyes sink (fall back) into his skull. His eyes also lose their shine, they look dull, and stay half open when he sleeps. The eyes of a marasmic child are also sunken, because he has lost the fat behind them. So, in a child with marasmus, sunken eyes are *not* a sign of dehydration.

9.12
9.13

9.17

Dry mouth. A dehydrated child cannot make enough saliva, so his mouth and tongue become dry and red. This is an important early sign.

Little urine. A healthy child passes urine about every three hours. The body of a dehydrated child tries to save water. It makes less urine. Mothers usually know how much urine their children have passed, so ask them if there has been less than usual. When a dehydrated child is treated, he passes plenty of urine again. This is a sign that he is recovering.

Sunken fontanelle. The fontanelle is the soft place between the bones of the top of a baby's skull. It is large when he is born, and is closed by the time he is about eighteen months old. When he is a year old, it is already quite small. When a baby sits up, you can see his fontanelle move with the beating of his heart. It also moves as he coughs or cries.

When a baby becomes dehydrated his brain becomes dry, and becomes smaller. This makes his fontanelle sink down between the bones of his skull. In a dehydrated baby, you can see and feel that his fontanelle has sunk. You can feel the edge of his skull bones around it. Dehydration also stops it pulsating, or makes it pulsate less.

Marasmus also makes the fontanelle sink, so a sunken fontanelle is not helpful for diagnosing dehydration in marasmic children.

9.18

The fontanelle is also useful for diagnosing meningitis. In meningitis there is too much fluid inside the skull, so the fontanelle swells (15.6).

9.15

**SIGNS IN THE FONTANELLE ARE ONLY
USEFUL IN THE FIRST YEAR**

Loss of skin elasticity. When we stretch a rubber band and then let go, it goes back immediately to the shape it was before—it is elastic. The skin of a healthy child is elastic also. If you pinch the skin of his abdomen, and then let go, his skin quickly goes flat again. Dehydration makes a child's skin dry and less elastic, so it sticks up for some seconds before it goes flat.

9.16

TESTING FOR SKIN ELASTICITY—FIGURE 9–8
Pinch up a fold of skin at the side of a child's abdomen between your finger and thumb. Hold it for a few seconds, and then let go. Normally, the fold of skin goes back immediately. If the fold stays up for two seconds, he is severely dehydrated.

When diarrhoea begins, a child's skin takes several hours to lose its elasticity. If he has sudden severe diarrhoea, he may become very dehydrated while his skin elasticity is still normal. If this might have happened, look for *other* signs of dehydration.

If a child is very fat, or very thin, loss of skin elasticity is not helpful for diagnosing dehydration. A marasmic child has no fat, so his skin is not elastic, even though he is not dehydrated. A very fat child does not lose his skin elasticity, even if he is dehydrated.

MALNUTRITION (AND TOO MUCH FAT) HIDE SOME OF THE SIGNS OF DEHYDRATION

A dehydrated child becomes 'ill'. At the first he is only mildly or moderately ill (Stage C, Table 5:2). He cries and will not be comforted, he is weak and hypotonic, irritable and restless, or drowsy. As his dehydration gets worse he becomes severely ill (Stage D). He may seem to be asleep, but can only be partly awakened. Later, you cannot awaken him he is in coma (Stage E). This is a sign of gross dehydration—he *must* have intravenous fluid quickly.

Fast weak pulse. Dehydration makes a child's pulse faster and weaker. When he becomes grossly dehydrated it may be so weak that you cannot feel it at his wrist. You may have to feel for it in his groin, or listen to his heart. A pulse of more than 140 is a sign of severe dehydration. With very severe dehydration the pulse sometimes slows.

COUNTING THE PULSE
Movement increases a child's pulse rate, so count it while he is still. Use a watch that counts seconds. Count his pulse for half a minute and multiply the answer by two. Feel it with the ends of your index and middle fingers in one of these places. Record whether it is strong or weak.

Wrist. **Feel for the pulsing of his radial artery on the thumb side of the front of his lower arm above his wrist.**

In front of his ear. **Feel for his temporal artery at the side of his face in front of his ear.**

Groin. **Feel for his femoral artery in the middle of the fold of his groin (1–7).**

Foot. **Feel the artery (dorsalis pedis) that goes along the top of his foot.**

Heart. **If you cannot count his pulse in any other way, count the beating of his heart with a stethoscope.**

A PULSE OF MORE THAN 140 IS A SIGN OF SEVERE DEHYDRATION

A SEVERELY DEHYDRATED CHILD

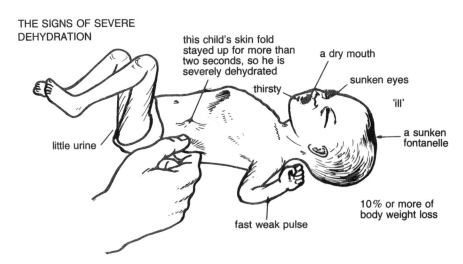

THE SIGNS OF SEVERE DEHYDRATION

this child's skin fold stayed up for more than two seconds, so he is severely dehydrated

a dry mouth

thirsty

sunken eyes

'ill'

a sunken fontanelle

little urine

10% or more of body weight loss

fast weak pulse

Fig. 9–8 A severely dehydrated child.

Acidotic breathing. Sometimes, a severely dehydrated child breathes fast (40–60 times a minute) and *deeply*. He takes larger breaths than normal. This kind of breathing is called **acidotic breathing**. It happens when a child has been dehydrated for some days, or has been rehydrated with the wrong fluids. Don't mistake acidotic breathing for the faster (over 60) *shallow* breathing of pneumonia. A child with pneumonia takes many very small breaths. A child with acidotic breathing needs intravenous fluids, not antibiotics.

Shock. Very severe dehydration causes shock (14.2). A child lies quiet. His skin is pale and cold. Shock is a very serious sign, and shows that a dehydrated child needs intravenous fluids immediately.

**A DEHYDRATED CHILD WITH SHOCK OR
FITS NEEDS INTRAVENOUS FLUID NOW**

Fits. There is a special kind of dehydration in which a child's body lacks water, but has enough or too much salt (**hypernatraemic dehydration**). Children get this kind of dehydration if they are given too much salt in their rehydration fluid. They can also get it if they are given artificial feeds which are too strong. These children have fits, are irritable, and have a dry mouth, *but their skin elasticity may be normal*. So fits in a child with severe diarrhoea are a sign that he has hypernatraemic dehydration. Fits show that he is more seriously ill than is shown by his skin elasticity. A dehydrated child with fits needs intravenous fluid quickly.

Fever. A child may have a fever because he is dehydrated. More often, fever is a sign of infection. Sometimes the infection is in his gut. Often, the infection is outside the gut, so if you see a child with diarrhoea and fever, think of malaria, otitis media or tonsillitis. Sometimes the fever is so high that a child has hyperpyrexia (10.4).

9.19 How severe is his dehydration?

When you have seen many sick children, you will be able to diagnose very quickly how dehydrated they are. But when you are beginning, make a 'dehydration score'. This may help you. To make the score easier, use only six of the signs. Look how 'well' or 'ill' a child is, feel his skin elasticity and look at his eyes. Count his breathing, look at his mouth and count his pulse.

Add up the points to make a score. The lowest score a child can have is 6. But he is not normal, *because all children with acute watery diarrhoea are dehydrated*. If his score is 6 his dehydration is mild. He has lost less than 5 per cent of the weight of his body. If his score is between 7 and 12, his dehydration is moderate. He has lost about 8 per cent of his body weight. If his score is 13 or more, his dehydration is severe. He has lost 10 per cent or more of his body weight. If he is in *shock*, or has *fits,* or is *too weak to drink*, you must rehydrate him intravenously.

**ALL CHILDREN WITH WATERY
DIARRHOEA ARE DEHYDRATED**

Rehydration

9.20 Rehydration is more important than drugs

A child who dies from diarrhoea, dies from dehydration. But we can treat him before he dies. We can put back the

Table 9:1   The dehydration score

Where to look	Points to score for the signs you find		
	1	**2**	**3**
The whole child (well or 'ill' 5.15)	'Well'	Restless, irritable, or abnormally quiet, drowsy, or 'floppy'	Delirious, comatose or shocked, very 'ill'
Skin	Normal elasticity	Moderately reduced elasticity	Severely reduced elasticity
Eyes	Normal	Moderately sunken	Severely sunken
Respiration	20–30	30–40	40–60
Mouth	Normal	Dry	Dry and cyanosed
Pulse	Strong, less than 120	120–140	Over 140

water and salt he has lost. This is called **rehydration**, and it is much more useful than drugs. The cheapest and easiest way to do this is to give him water, salt and sugar to drink—**oral (by mouth) rehydration**. But he must be able to drink. So the most important question is—CAN HE DRINK? If he cannot drink, we can give him fluids down a tube through his nose into his stomach—**nasogastric rehydration**. This often helps him, even if he is vomiting. The fluids we give him by mouth are called **oral rehydration fluids**.

Oral rehydration fluids are absorbed from a child's gut in the same way as his food and drink. Like food, these fluids must be clean, but they need not be sterile. A few 'ordinary' organisms in a child's rehydration fluid will not harm him. This is useful, because non-sterile rehydration fluids are cheap and easy to make.

WAYS OF REHYDRATING A CHILD

You can put fluid into a child
in all these ways

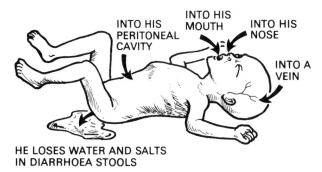

INTO HIS MOUTH
INTO HIS PERITONEAL CAVITY
INTO HIS NOSE
INTO A VEIN

HE LOSES WATER AND SALTS IN DIARRHOEA STOOLS

Fig. 9–9 Ways of rehydrating a child.

If a child is severely dehydrated, we *must* give him fluid into one of his veins—**intravenous rehydration**. This is the best way to put fluid into his body quickly and stop him dying. Sometimes, we put fluid into his peritoneal cavity (20.1)—**intraperitoneal rehydration**.

When we put fluid into a child's veins or into his peritoneal cavity, it is going inside his body. So it must be sterile and have *no* organisms in it. Sterile fluids are more expensive, because we cannot make them in the clinic.

When we give fluids down a tube, we call it a **drip**, because fluid drips down it. A child can have a 'nasogastric drip' into his stomach, or an 'intravenous drip' into a vein. The tubes and needle which we use are called a **drip set**.

CAN HE DRINK?

He can drink—oral rehydration

9.21 Two kinds of oral rehydration fluid—glucose–salt solution, and salt and sugar water

Glucose–salt solution. This contains sodium chloride (ordinary salt), sodium bicarbonate (baking soda), potassium chloride, and a special sugar called glucose. Glucose is better than ordinary sugar at helping the gut to absorb salt and water. We cannot store the solution, because it goes sour in a few days or weeks. Instead we have to use the dry powders and add them to water. We cannot mix large weights of the dry powders unless we have a special machine. If they are badly mixed, they are dangerous. For example one child might get too much potassium chloride, and another child none. The best way is to make small packets of powders. These contain enough salts and glucose for 200 ml or 1000 ml of solution. These packets are best made in a pharmacy, or a factory, but you can make them yourself.

MAKING ONE-LITRE PACKETS OF GLUCOSE–SALT SOLUTION

Get many small polythene bags and put these weights of chemicals into each of them. If you cannot get glucose, use sugar.

Sodium chloride (ordinary salt) 3·5 g or 1 *level* teaspoonful

Sodium bicarbonate (baking soda) 2·5 g or $\frac{3}{4}$ of a *level* teaspoonful

Potassium chloride 1·5 g or $\frac{1}{3}$ of a *level* teaspoonful

Glucose (or sugar) 20 g or 8 *level* teaspoonfuls

Water 1 litre

If possible, use the special scoops in the equipment list (3:2, 9–10b). If you have not got these, use a spoon. You can measure $\frac{3}{4}$ of a teaspoon easily like this. Fill it with salt, and press the salt flat with a knife. Then take away $\frac{1}{4}$ of the salt from the tip of the spoon (9–10b). Or you can make your own measures from old bottle tops which hold about the right amount of chemicals. Find how much they hold. Weigh them full and empty. You can also measure chemicals in a syringe. Tap (gently hit) the syringe until the top of the powder is flat. Use the volumes shown in Figure 9–10b.

Seal up the bags with a heat sealing (closing) machine, or with a flame.

In damp (wet) districts the mixed powder for glucose–salt solution does not store well. If you do not keep it in tightly closed tins, it becomes damp. So keep the chemicals separately, and make the powder when you need it. Sometimes damp powder goes brown or yellow. It is not harmful and you can use it.

Salt and sugar water. *This fluid is not so good as glucose–salt solution.* But it is useful because mothers can easily make it at home. Tell a mother to add *one level teaspoonful of salt* to a *litre of water*. Then she should add

118

eight level teaspoons of sugar. These are 5 ml spoons (3–1).

Most cups hold about 200 ml, so a litre is about five cupfuls. There may also be some local measure that a mother can use, such as a coconut shell. Show her a measure which holds about a litre. Teach everyone how to make this fluid.

Oral rehydration fluids *must* have the right amount of salt and sugar in them. Too *little* salt does not make such a good rehydration fluid. The fluid is not so dangerous. But *too much salt* is very dangerous.

You can make a better kind of salt and sugar water. Add eight level teaspoonfuls of sugar, one level teaspoonful of salt, and $\frac{3}{4}$ of a level teaspoonful of sodium bicarbonate to a litre of water. *Measure carefully*. If a mother makes this kind of salt and sugar water, she can easily make it too strong. So, if she uses sugar, *baking soda* and salt, tell her to add them to *one and a half litres of water*.

You should boil the water for a rehydration fluid. If you cannot boil it, use clean drinking water.

TOO MUCH SALT (OR SUGAR) IN A REHYDRATION FLUID IS DANGEROUS

9.22 Using an oral hydration fluid

You can treat most dehydrated children with an oral rehydration fluid. It is the best treatment for the many children with mild diarrhoea. It stops them becoming more dehydrated later.

MAKING GLUCOSE SALT SOLUTION

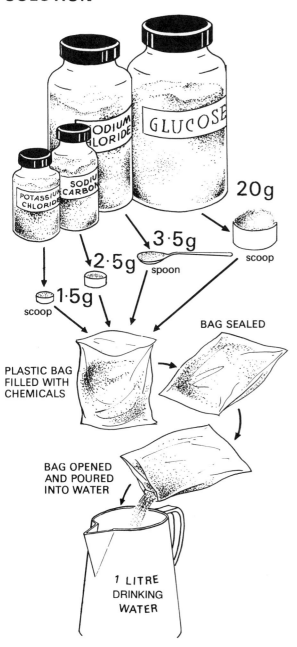

Fig. 9–10 Making glucose–salt solution.

TEACHING A MOTHER HOW TO REHYDRATE HER CHILD

Sit the child on his mother's knee in a quiet corner of the clinic.

USING GLUCOSE–SALT SOLUTION. **Get a bucket or a large jug of clean boiled water, a smaller jug, a clean mug or cup, a teaspoon, and a packet of glucose–salt solution for one litre. Ask her to measure five cupfuls of water (one litre) from the bucket into the jug. If some local measure, such as a coconut shell, four 'Coke' bottles, or two beer bottles, is easier, use this. If you use local measures, show her which size of local measure she must use. There are different sizes of coconut shells, Coke bottles, and beer bottles. Ask her to empty the packet into the litre of water she has measured and mix well. Teach her the name 'glucose–salt solution'. (Some packets are for different volumes of water, such as 200 ml. So read the writing on the packet carefully.)**

USING SALT AND SUGAR WATER. **Show her how to measure a litre of water. Give her a bowl of sugar, and a bowl of salt. Ask her to measure *one level teaspoonful* of salt, and eight *level* teaspoonfuls of sugar to the litre of water. Tell her to mix it well. Make sure she understands what a teaspoon is. Explain that she must NOT add too much salt or sugar. Let her taste it to see how salty it should be.**

FLUIDS OF BOTH KINDS. **Ask her to let her child drink the fluid she has made. He may be very thirsty, and she may** have come a long way on a hot day. If he is very dehydrated he will probably only be able to drink a little fluid at a time. *But she must go on trying.* Tell her that he will only recover, *if she can make him drink, and go on drinking.* Don't try to make him drink all the time. Give him some fluid, then wait a few minutes. Then give him some more.

A dehyrated child needs fluids at least six times a day, and more often if possible. During 24 hours he needs as many cupfuls (200 ml) of fluid as there are kilos in his weight. A ten kilo child thus needs ten cupfuls of fluid in 24 hours. Too little is harmful. He cannot drink too much, so give him plenty.

Bottles are *not* a good way of feeding children (N 8.1), and a bottle may have caused his diarrhoea. But *if* he is bottle-fed, give him his oral rehydration fluid from his feeding bottle.

Measuring

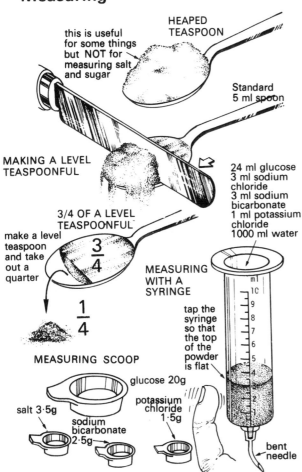

this is useful for some things but NOT for measuring salt and sugar

HEAPED TEASPOON

Standard 5 ml spoon

MAKING A LEVEL TEASPOONFUL

24 ml glucose
3 ml sodium chloride
3 ml sodium bicarbonate
1 ml potassium chloride
1000 ml water

3/4 OF A LEVEL TEASPOONFUL

make a level teaspoon and take out a quarter

$\frac{3}{4}$

MEASURING WITH A SYRINGE

tap the syringe so that the top of the powder is flat

$\frac{1}{4}$

MEASURING SCOOP

glucose 20g

salt 3·5g

sodium bicarbonate 2·5g

potassium chloride 1·5g

bent needle

Fig. 9–10b Ways of measuring glucose and salt to make glucose–salt solution.

As soon as he has had a good drink of fluid and passed urine, he can go home. Tell her to make a rehydration fluid for him at home. He needs it for as long as he has liquid stools. Give him a cupful of fluid every time he passes a stool. Ask her to give him food as soon as he can eat.

Explain that oral fluids do not stop liquid stools immediately. Oral fluids prevent liquid stools harming a child, so that he can recover from his diarrhoea by himself.

Teach her to give her child a rehydration fluid whenever he has liquid stools again. This will help to stop serious dehydration when he next has diarrhoea.

HE WON'T DRINK. **Try giving him 60 ml/kg of fluid through an intragastric tube (9.24) during one hour. He will usually drink after that.**

HIS EYELIDS ARE SWOLLEN. **This is not serious. Stop giving him fluids until the swelling goes.**

LET MOTHERS MAKE THEIR OWN REHYDRATION FLUIDS IN THE CLINIC

Many dehydrated children drink fluids thirstily, and recover while you watch them. But, if a child has only had one or two diarrhoea stools, he may not be thirsty and may not want to drink. Even so, fluids are the best treatment for him, and good education for his mother. A severely dehydrated child is too ill to drink. But try to make him drink some fluid, especially while he is on his way to hospital.

Mothers can also give tea to children with diarrhoea. But they should add glucose-salt powder or salt and sugar. They should add *one level teaspoonful* of salt and eight level teaspoonfuls of sugar to a litre (five cupfuls) of tea. Some mothers think that the best way to treat diarrhoea is to *stop* giving their children fluids by mouth. This is the *worst* thing they can do! If a mother cannot give her child salt and sugar water, let her give him plain water—he *must* have extra fluid!

THE WORST TREATMENT FOR DIARRHOEA IS TO STOP GIVING FLUID

In districts where mothers know about oral rehydration and treat dehydration early, severe dehydration is very rare. So a *severely dehydrated child* is a sign that our community needs more teaching about oral rehydration—SEVERE DEHYDRATION IS PREVENTABLE. We must teach mothers to treat diarrhoea early.

TREAT DIARRHOEA EARLY

MAKING SALT AND SUGAR WATER

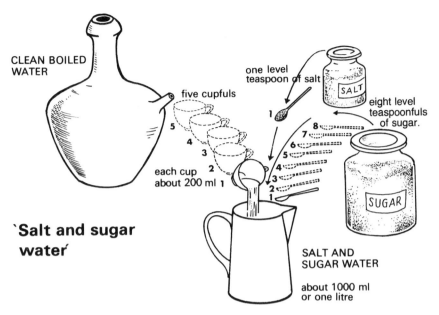

CLEAN BOILED WATER

five cupfuls

one level teaspoon of salt

SALT

eight level teaspoonfuls of sugar.

SUGAR

each cup about 200 ml

`Salt and sugar water`

SALT AND SUGAR WATER

about 1000 ml or one litre

Fig. 9–11 Making salt and sugar water.

9.23 'Yoyo vomits her oral fluids'

Some children vomit their oral fluids. When you see a child like this, try to find the answer to these questions.

How often and how much fluid is he vomiting?

How much fluid is he drinking?

Is his dehydration getting better or worse?

Give him a little fluid often. If he drinks more than he vomits, most of the fluid is staying inside him. He can go on with his oral rehydration. But *observe him carefully* to make sure that he is not becoming more dehydrated. Examine his eyes, his mouth, and his skin, and count his pulse. A pulse of over 140, with other signs of dehydration is serious.

DON'T STOP ORAL FLUIDS BECAUSE A CHILD VOMITS

If a child vomits everything he drinks, or if he is becoming more dehydrated, you must rehydrate him in some other way. An intraperitoneal drip, or an intravenous drip is best. Even if you have not got these, you may be able to help him. *Give him a slow nasogastric drip of about 20 drops a minute.* Be sure to try a nasogastric drip, if this is all you have.

A NASOGASTRIC DRIP OFTEN HELPS A VOMITING CHILD

LET MOTHERS REHYDRATE THEIR CHILDREN IN THE CLINIC BEFORE THEY GO HOME

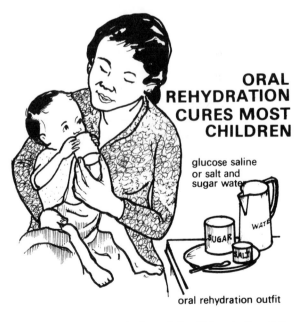

ORAL REHYDRATION CURES MOST CHILDREN

glucose saline or salt and sugar water

SUGAR

WATER

oral rehydration outfit

Fig. 9–12 Let mothers rehydrate their children in the clinic before they go home.

121

Nasogastric rehydration with glucose–salt solution

9.24 A very useful method

In this method glucose–salt solution or salt and sugar water runs down a thin tube. It goes through a child's nose into his stomach. Every health centre must be able to give a nasogastric drip. Children can also have these drips at home. If you cannot give a severely dehydrated child intravenous fluids, a nasogastric drip may save his life. This method is easy and often helps children who are vomiting. You can use a cheap non-sterile fluid, and you can use the bottle and tube again.

For small children use 'tubing, plastic, general purpose child care (3:1)'. For older children, you can use the tubes from old drip sets. For sterilizing these, see Section 9.27. Sterilization is much less important than with intravenous rehydration. You can also use a thin rubber catheter (tube).

A child soon gets used to a tube in his nose. If you fix it carefully to his face, he will probably not pull it out. If necessary, you can give him fluids like this for a week.

**EVERY HEALTH WORKER SHOULD BE ABLE
TO GIVE A NASOGASTRIC DRIP**

REHYDRATING A CHILD WITH A NASOGASTRIC TUBE

Weigh him.

PUTTING IN THE TUBE. **If possible make glucose–salt solution (9.21). If you cannot make this, make salt and sugar water (9.21). Put it into an empty intravenous fluid bottle, and use an old 'drip set' (9–16).**

Measure the length of the tube that is needed to go from the bridge of the child's nose to his xiphisternum (9–15). Mark it with a piece of tape. Leave an *extra* 15 cm of tube outside his nose so that you can fix it to his face.

Smooth the end of a new tube. Hold it for a moment in the flame of a match. Put a little oil on it, so that it slides easily, and then push it slowly down his nose. Stick the end of the tube to his face with tape.

Examine his throat with a torch and spatula to make sure the tube has not coiled up and stuck there.

The bottom end of the tube *must* be in his stomach. If he coughs a lot it is in his trachea. If by mistake you put fluid into his trachea he will die. Here are two ways of making sure that a tube is in the stomach. Try both of them.

(1) Suck the top end of the tube with a syringe. If fluid comes, its bottom end is in the stomach.

(2) Inject about 10 ml of air down the tube. Listen over the stomach with a stethoscope. If you can hear air coming out of the bottom end of the tube, it is in his stomach.

If you think the tube *might* be in his trachea, take it out and try again. When you are *sure* that it is in his stomach, fix it with adhesive strapping from his nose to his ear. Join its top end to the needle of a drip set, and start the fluid dripping.

THE DOSE OF INTRAGASTRIC FLUID. **During the first 12 hours give him fluid like this—**
    6 kg child—25 drops per minute (75 ml an hour)
    9 kg child—35 drops per minute (100 ml an hour)
    12 kg child—50 drops per minute (150 ml an hour)
If he is better after 12 hours, slow the drip. If he is not better, go on at the same speed. Watch his eyes. Swelling of the eyes is a sign that he is having too much fluid.

If he vomits, slow his drip to 20 drops a minute, or less if he is very small. There are about 20 drops in a ml, so this is about 60 ml in an hour. Observe him carefully. Take the drip down as soon as he can drink. If his dehydration gets worse, he needs intravenous fluids.

EVERY HEALTH WORKER SHOULD BE ABLE TO GIVE A NASO GASTRIC DRIP

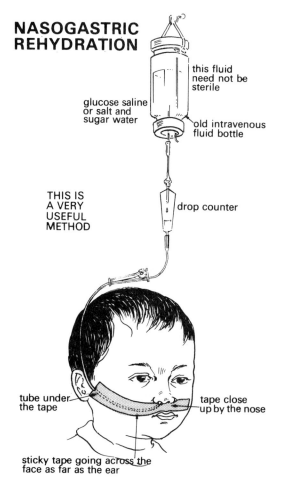

NASOGASTRIC REHYDRATION

this fluid need not be sterile

glucose saline or salt and sugar water

old intravenous fluid bottle

THIS IS A VERY USEFUL METHOD

drop counter

tube under the tape

tape close up by the nose

sticky tape going across the face as far as the ear

Fig. 9–13 Every health worker should be able to give a nasogastric drip.

EXPLANATION. **Tell his mother why you are putting a tube down his nose. If you are busy and have to look after other children, teach her to watch the drip. Show her where the level of the fluid should be each hour. Ask her to give him food as soon as he can eat.**

Intraperitoneal rehydration

9.25 Half-strength Darrow's solution in 2·5 per cent glucose

The best fluid for intraperitoneal or intravenous rehydration is half-strength Darrow's solution in 2·5 per cent glucose. This contains the right amount of glucose and salt that dehydrated children need. 'Normal' ('physiological') saline contains too much salt, and 5 per cent glucose contains no salt. Every health centre should keep bottles of half-strength Darrow's solution in 2·5 per cent glucose. If hospitals make their own fluids, this is the most useful fluid to make. You can use Darrow's solution for oral rehydration, but it is expensive. Glucose–salt solution is much cheaper.

9.26 Intraperitoneal rehydration

This method uses expensive sterile fluids, and does not put fluid into tissues fast enough to help a severely dehydrated child. But it is easy, and it only takes ten minutes. A child can go home soon afterwards, because there is no drip to watch. It is useful for the *moderately* dehydrated vomiting child, if we cannot observe him in the clinic.

Most of the organs in the abdomen lie in a bag called the peritoneal cavity (20.1). This bag contains very little fluid. We can easily put more fluid into it through a needle. We push the needle through the soft front of his abdomen. This fluid does not go into his gut, but into the

empty peritoneal cavity around it. If the fluid stayed in the peritoneal cavity it would be no use. But during the next four hours it is *slowly* absorbed and goes into the blood. Because fluid takes a few hours to be absorbed, intraperitoneal rehydration is not useful for treating severely dehydrated children. We must put fluid into their veins. **9.24**

If you put fluid into the peritoneal cavity, the fluid must be sterile. You must give it in a sterile way with a sterile needle and tube. If harmful bacteria get into a child's peritoneal cavity, he may get peritonitis (20.2). **9.25**

INTRAPERITONEAL REHYDRATION

Weigh the child.

PUTTING IN THE FLUID. **Warm a bottle of half strength Darrow's solution in 2·5 per cent glucose to body heat. Stand it in hot water. Don't make it too hot.**

Lie the child across a couch. Put one of the needles of the drip set through the cap of the bottle of fluid. Hang the bottle from a hook, or from a drip stand. Run a little fluid through the drip set.

Examine his abdomen to make sure that his liver and spleen are not enlarged, or his bladder distended (20.3). If they are large, the needle might cut them. **9.26**

Clean the skin of his abdomen with iodine. Push the needle of the drip set through the skin of his abdominal wall 2 cm *below* his umbilicus. If his spleen or liver are very large, put the needle into some other part of his abdomen far away from them.

When the needle is through his skin, open the clip (tap) of the drip set. It will not start dripping yet. Hold the needle vertically (straight up) and push it slowly through his abdominal wall into his peritoneal cavity. As soon as the needle is in the cavity, the fluid will begin to drip fast. If fluid is coming out of the needle, it will push the gut away

INTRAPERITONEAL REHYDRATION

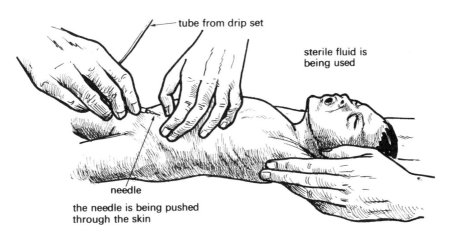

tube from drip set

sterile fluid is being used

needle

the needle is being pushed through the skin

Fig. 9–14 Intraperitoneal rehydration.

123

from its sharp point. As soon as fluid is flowing well, fix the needle to his skin with tape. When he has had the dose of fluid he needs, take out the needle and put a piece of adhesive tape over the hole. Send him home in an hour.

THE DOSE OF FLUID. **Give him 40 ml/kg during ten minutes. If necessary you can give him up to 70 ml/kg. If he is still dehydrated, he can have more fluid four hours later.**

EXPLANATION. **Tell his mother why you are putting a needle into him. Teach her about the 'danger signs of dehydration' (9.31). Tell her to bring him back quickly if he shows them. Make sure she gives him oral fluids also.**

Intravenous rehydration

9.27 The best method for severely dehydrated children.

If a child is severely dehydrated, we should give him fluid into a vein, especially if he is shocked (14.2), or in coma (14.8). Intravenous fluid is the surest way to save the life of a *severely* dehydrated child.

You can put fluid into any vein where a needle can go. Older children usually have large veins on the backs of their hands, or in their elbows. Use any of the veins in Figure 9–15. Babies usually have good veins on their scalps. 'Scalp vein drips' rarely become infected and are better than 'cut downs'(cutting into a vein on the leg). They are quick and safe, and easy to put in when you have learnt how.

You need a **scalp vein set**. This is a piece of thin plastic tube (about 1·5 mm bore) with a needle on one end which goes into the baby. The sterile disposable scalp vein sets in Figure 9–17 are the easiest to use, but you can make your own.

WHERE TO LOOK FOR VEINS

any of his other veins can be
used if you can get a needle into them

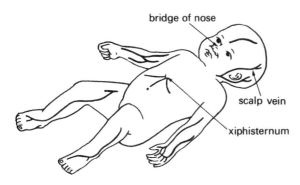

Fig. 9–15 Where to look for veins.

MAKING A SCALP VEIN SET

STERILIZING. **Try to sterilize the tube by boiling. Five minutes' boiling is enough. If boiling spoils it, put it in hypochlorite (or other antiseptic) for several hours. If necessary keep it in antiseptic. Draw the antiseptic inside with a syringe. Before you use it wash it through with boiled water. New tube from a roll will probably be sterile enough inside to use.**

A DRIP SET

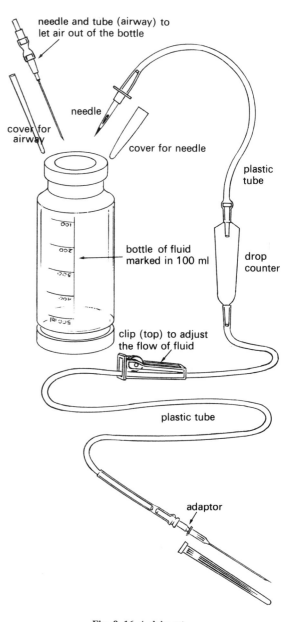

Fig. 9–16 A drip set.

124

THE SET. **Break off the adaptor of a short bevel needle (0·7 × 3·5 mm). If you have not got a short bevel needle, use an ordinary one. Put the broken end of the needle into the tubing. If the tube fits loosely, heat it in a match flame to soften it. Squeeze it tighter round the needle. Put an ordinary intramuscular needle into the other end of the tubing. Its adaptor must join onto the drip set, so make sure they fit together. Be careful. Don't tear the fine tube, and make sure that no fluid comes through the joins. Needles like this are too small to hold in your fingers, so use artery forceps. (Picture 5, Figure 9–19.)**

The scalp vein set must be full of fluid when it goes into a vein. If there is air in the set, the blood in the vein clots. There are two ways of filling the set with fluid. You can fill it with fluid from a drip set, or from a syringe. Use whichever way you find easiest. The syringe way is probably the easiest when you are beginning. If the needle becomes blocked with blood, you can remove it more easily with a syringe.

INTRAVENOUS REHYDRATION THROUGH A SCALP VEIN

Get or make a scalp vein set (9–17).
   1. **Weigh the child.**
   2. **In older children, try to find a vein on the hand or ankle before using a scalp vein. Veins swell and become easier to see if you make the skin warm in water. Ask a helper to squeeze the arm or leg and pull the skin upwards while you pull it downwards. This holds the vein while you put in the needle. The child in Picture 2 had no good veins on his arms or legs, so we used a scalp vein.**
   3. **Put the needle of the drip set into the bottle of fluid. Fix the scalp vein set to the drip set.**
   4. **Run fluid through the drip set and the scalp vein set to remove the air in them.**
   5. **Ask a helper to hold the child. Shave the hair from the side of his head, and look for a good vein. The best ones are usually just above his ears. Make sure that you have found a vein, and not an artery. Feel it with your finger. If it is an artery, you can feel it pulsating. If you cannot find a good vein, make the child cry, or rub his skin with spirit, or warm it with a hot wet cloth.**
   If you are using an ordinary needle, hold it in a pair of artery forceps. Press with a finger of your left hand just below the place where you want to put the needle, so as to make his vein swell. Put the needle flat on his skin. Push it through his skin *along* the side of the vein. When it is through the skin, push it carefully into the vein. As soon as it is in the vein, blood goes slowly up the needle into the tube. If by mistake the needle is in an artery, blood goes quickly up the tube. Take the needle out, press hard with gauze to stop bleeding, and try again in another place.
   6. **Put a piece of gauze with a cut in it round the needle.**
   7. **Put several pieces of adhesive tape over the gauze. Cut them as shown and make sure that they stick to the tube of the scalp vein set and hold it firmly. Fixing it is**

SCALP VEIN SETS

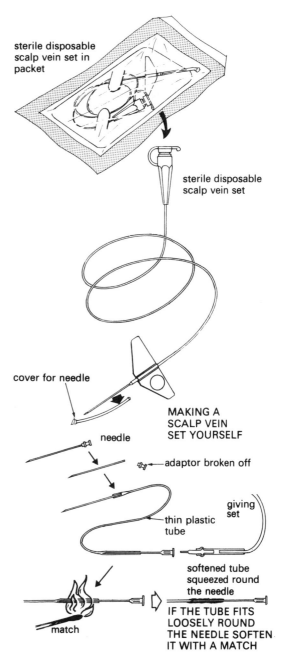

sterile disposable scalp vein set in packet

sterile disposable scalp vein set

9.27

cover for needle

MAKING A SCALP VEIN SET YOURSELF

needle

adaptor broken off

giving set

thin plastic tube

softened tube squeezed round the needle

IF THE TUBE FITS LOOSELY ROUND THE NEEDLE SOFTEN IT WITH A MATCH

match

Fig. 9–17 A scalp vein set.

important, or it will soon fall out. Don't cover its point with tape. You will need to see if fluid is coming out of the needle and making a swelling in the tissues.
   8. **Use more adhesive tape to hold the drip set with a loop**

(turn) so that it will not be pulled out. Ask the child's mother to stay with him and watch him, so that he does not pull out the needle.

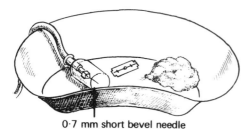

0·7 mm short bevel needle

Fig. 9–18 Some health workers can give a child a scalp vein drip with no more equipment than this.

USING A SYRINGE. **Fill a syringe with fluid from the bottle. Fix the syringe to the scalp vein set. Inject fluid through the scalp vein set to fill it with fluid. Keep the syringe fixed to the scalp vein set while you put the needle into the vein. If you are not sure if the needle is in a vein, inject some fluid from the syringe. If the needle is in a vein, the fluid will flow easily. If the needle is not in a vein, the fluid will make a small swelling. When you are in a vein, take off the syringe and join the scalp vein set to the drip set.**

9.28 The dose of intravenous fluid.

You cannot give a child too much fluid by mouth, because he will not drink more than he needs. But the dose of intravenous fluid is as important as the dose of a drug. You must also give it at the right speed. If a child gets too little fluid too slowly, he will die from dehydration. Too much fluid too quickly will kill him.

NO CHILD SHOULD DIE BECAUSE HE HAS NOT HAD THE FLUID HE NEEDS

THE DOSE OF INTRAVENOUS FLUID

A severely dehydrated child has lost 100 ml for every kilo he weighed before his diarrhoea started (10 per cent of his body weight). First give him 20 ml for every kilo he weighs (2 per cent of his weight) as fast as the drip will go. Thus a 12 kg child needs 12 × 20 = 240 ml, as fast as possible. This is *fast replacement*.

After this make the drip go more slowly. This is *slow replacement*. Give children:

Under 5 kg	25 ml per hour
Between 5 and 9 kg	50 ml per hour
Between 10 and 14 kg	75 ml per hour
Over 15 kg	100 ml per hour

Fix a piece of paper to the side of the bottle. Write on it the times and the places where the level of fluid should be at each hour. Watch the fluid level carefully. If necessary,

INTRAVENOUS REYHDRATION- ONE

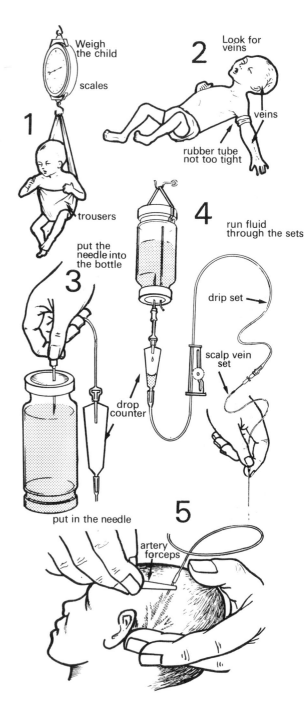

Fig. 9–19 A scalp vein drip—One.

126

INTRAVENOUS REHYDRATION - TWO

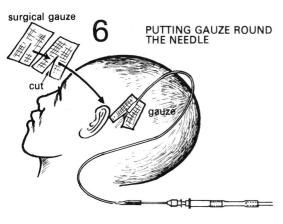

surgical gauze

6 PUTTING GAUZE ROUND THE NEEDLE

cut

gauze

7 PUTTING TAPE ROUND THE NEEDLE

sticky tape

tape pinched

point of needle not covered

scalp vein

these marks show where the fluid should have got to each hour

8 THE DRIP COMPLETE

loop of tube

drip set

more tape to hold tube

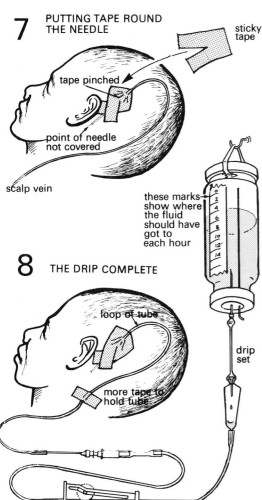

Fig. 9–20 A scalp vein drip—Two.

change the speed of the drip, so as to give the right amount of fluid. On most bottles the level of the fluid falls 2·5 cm for each 100 ml that is given.

Examine him every hour and count his pulse. As you rehydrate him, his pulse becomes stronger and slower and his eyes become less sunken. His skin becomes more elastic, his mouth becomes wet again and he passes urine. Watch his eyelids. Swollen eyelids are a sign that you have given *too much fluid*, so stop the drip immediately.

If after two hours he still has signs of dehydration, AND his pulse is still more than 140, give him ONE more dose of fluid fast—his weight in kg × 20 ml—again.

Don't stop giving him fluid by mouth because he is on a drip. Give him milk, glucose–salt solution, or salt and sugar water. Often a child wants to drink when he has improved a little.

Stop his drip when *all* these things have happened—he is no longer dehydrated, *and* he is drinking well, *and* he is not vomiting, *and* his stools are not watery.

Most children recover in less than six hours. They start drinking and can go home. If, after six hours a child is not drinking, or if he has severe diarrhoea, go on with the slow replacement drip.

EXPLANATION. Tell his mother that his diarrhoea has made him dry. Explain that you must put back the water and salt he has lost. Tell her that he should recover in a few hours. Ask her to watch the bottle. Show her where the level of the fluid should be at different times during the day. Let her nurse him on her knee.

Give her some oral rehydration fluid. She can give him this as soon as he can drink. Tell her to go on giving it as for long as he has watery stools. Give him food as soon as he can eat.

9.29 'Ako still has watery diarrhoea, treatment has not helped'—lactose intolerance.

Breast-milk and cow's milk contain a sugar called lactose. Some children cannot digest this lactose. They have watery diarrhoea when they drink milk. These children have **lactose intolerance**. This is common in malnourished children between the ages of six and eighteen months. Often it follows infectious diarrhoea. It is important in two ways—

(1) Dried skim milk causing diarrhoea. Dried skim milk contains much protein, but it also contains 50 per cent lactose. If a malnourished child drinks it he may have diarrhoea. Prevent this. Tell his mother to add a *little* of it to *all* the food he eats. If he eats a little in all his food, it is less likely to cause diarrhoea.

(2) Not recovering from acute infectious diarrhoea. Sometimes a child has acute infectious diarrhoea, or measles with severe diarrhoea. His diarrhoea stops when he is treated, and then starts again when he drinks milk. His infection has made him intolerant to lactose. Usually, the intolerance only lasts a short time. In a few days he can start drinking milk again. Lactose intolerance is *not* a good reason for stopping breast-feeding, except for a few days. So we must prevent the mothers of these children from stopping breast-feeding.

LACTOSE INTOLERANCE

SPECIAL TEST. **You must use fresh stool. Get a specimen by putting a rectal tube, or your little finger into his anus. Usually, if a child has lactose intolerance, watery stool pours out when you do this. Catch the stool on a plastic sheet so you have the watery part. You cannot do the test on stool from a nappy. The cloth absorbs the watery part with the lactose.**

Add eight drops of fresh liquid stool to 5 ml of Benedict's solution, and boil for five minutes. If the mixture goes yellow, orange, or red (+++ or ++++) the child has lactose intolerance. You can also use 'Clinitest' tablets but *not* methods which only test for glucose ('Clinistix', 'Combistix' etc.).

TREATMENT. **Stop breast- or bottle-feeding for one to three days. Show the child's mother how to express her breast milk, so she can feed him again later. Give him glucose–salt solution and any food he will eat.**

When diarrhoea stops try breast-feeding again. If this causes diarrhoea again give him glucose–salt solution and food only. If necessary try this several times. Usually, after 3 days to two weeks the diarrhoea stops and he can drink milk.

If milk goes on causing diarrhoea, stop giving him ordinary milk. Instead give him food or lactose free milk. Foods made from soya bean, or coconut cream are useful.

9.29b Some more difficulties

'There is not enough intravenous fluid.' If you have many dehydrated children and not enough intravenous fluid, give each severely dehydrated child some of it. Give, say 20 ml/kg, and then treat them by nasogastric drip.

'He is a baby' (26.32). Too much intravenous fluid can easily kill a small baby. Never give a baby weighing less than 5 kg more than 20 drops of fluid a minute, or 60 ml an hour.

'He is having shivers (rigors).' Even a very little dirt in the fluid or the drip set may cause rigors (10.1). If these are severe, they may kill him, so take down the bottle and the drip set and put up another one.

'He is drowsy or in coma.' A severely dehydrated child wakes up slowly when he is rehydrated. He may not be completely awake for 24 hours. If he is still drowsy or in coma after this time, send him for help.

FLOW CHART FOR INTRAVENOUS REHYDRATION

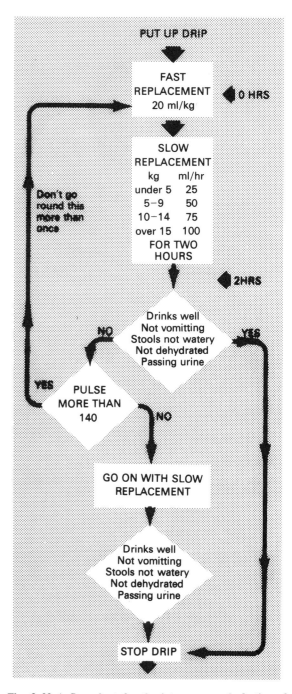

Fig. 9–22 A flow chart for the intravenous rehydration of severely dehydrated children with half strength Darrow's solution.

128

'His abdomen is swollen.' A child's abdomen may swell if he has had diarrhoea for a long time. The wrong fluids also cause swelling, especially if they contain no potassium. Swelling is a dangerous sign. Pass a soft rubber catheter (tube) into his rectum to let out the gas in his gut. This gas is causing the swelling. Give him chloramphenicol or tetracycline and send him for help.

9.30 Drugs for diarrhoea

We can use two kinds of drugs for treating diarrhoea, causal drugs and symptomatic ones (3.1). *Neither of them is as useful as rehydration.* Tetracycline and chloramphenicol are causal drugs which sometimes kill organisms causing gut infections. But, often they don't work, because the organisms are resistant to them (3.12). Sometimes these drugs cause diarrhoea. They harm the normal gut flora. Many bacteria which cause diarrhoea are now resistant to sulphadimidine and other sulphonamide drugs. Streptomycin and neomycin seldom help. So, only give a causal drug, *if there is a special reason for it,* such as amoebic or bacilliary dysentery, cholera, giardiasis, tonsillitis, malaria, or pneumonia.

ONLY GIVE A CAUSAL DRUG WHEN YOU CAN FIND A CAUSE

There are many symptomatic drugs for diarrhoea, but they do not help children and are not necessary. Don't use opium, papaveretum, morphia, diphenoxylate, kaolin, pectin, bismuth, tannalbumin, chalk, enterovioform, purgatives, 'heart tonics' such as adrenaline or coramine, steroids, charcoal, oxygen or liver. These drugs often *seem* to work with adults, because most adult patients with diarrhoea cure themselves. Many children have diarrhoea and you can waste much money giving them drugs which do not help.

MOST CHILDREN WITH DIARRHOEA DON'T NEED DRUGS

9.31 Caring for a child with diarrhoea, or with diarrhoea and vomiting—long case.

There are four parts to the diagnosis of diarrhoea—(1) hydration, (2) nutrition, (3) hyperpyrexia and (4) special infections. A few children are dehydrated, *and* malnourished, and have hyperpyrexia, and have some special infection, such as bacillary dysentery. Many children are malnourished and have acute dehydrating diarrhoea.

Many infections cause mild diarrhoea. Often a child has a cough, fever, and mild diarrhoea. An upper respiratory infection can cause all these symptoms. So, if a child has *mild* diarrhoea, and other symptoms also, go to the sections for them.

If he has a cough and *severe* diarrhoea use Section 8.20 and this one.

If he is less than about two months old, go to Section 26.32.

If he has vomiting only, go to 20.15.

WEIGHING
Is his growth curve flat or falling (malnutrition)?

Has he suddenly lost weight during the last few days (dehydration)?

9.30

HISTORY
How many stools has he passed today? (This tells us how severe his diarrhoea is.)

What do his stools look like? Is there blood in them (dysentery)?

How long has he had diarrhoea? When were his stools last normal? Has he had it before? (This tells us if his diarrhoea is chronic.)

Has he had measles? (Diarrhoea may last for some weeks after severe measles.)

OTHER IMPORTANT SYMPTOMS. **Has he been vomiting, and if so, how much? (Vomiting makes oral rehydration more difficult.) When did he last pass urine? (Dehydrated children pass little urine.)**

OTHER TREATMENT. **How has his mother treated him? Has she given him fluids? (Oral fluids may be all he needs.)**

NUTRITION. **Is he bottle-fed? Why is he bottle-fed? How is his bottle sterilized? What is put into it? Ask to have a look at his bottle. Is it clean? Does it smell? Is the milk watery?**

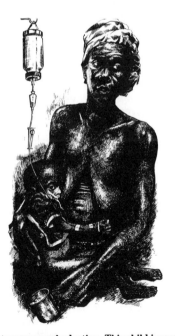

9.29b

9.31

Fig. 9–23 Intravenous rehydration. This child is severely dehydrated. His mother has some glucose–salt solution to give him as soon as he can drink.

129

Is it sour? (Badly managed bottle-feeding is an important cause of diarrhoea.)

If he is below the road to health, what is his nutrition history (7.13)? (He may have the chronic diarrhoea of malnutrition.)

EXAMINATION

Is he 'well' or 'ill' (5.15)? Is his skin less elastic than normal? Are his eyes sunken or dull? Has his fontanelle sunk? Is his mouth dry? How fast and how strong is his pulse? Is he cold (shocked)? (These are all signs of dehydration.)

Is his breathing normal? Or fast (40–60) and *deep* (acidotic breathing)?

Look at his stool. Blood or mucus (dysentery)? Bubbly (malnutrition or giardiasis)?

Signs of malnutrition (7.13)?

Are there any signs of an infection outside his gut, which might be causing diarrhoea, such as tonsillitis, pneumonia, or otitis media, or measles?

Take his temperature (infection perhaps with hyperpyrexia).

Examine his abdomen for tenderness, guarding, and rigidity (20.3). This is especially important if he is vomiting also. (Commonly, severe diarrhoea makes the abdomen tender all over, occasionally with rebound tenderness, but *without* guarding or rigidity. Acute abdomens are rare. Occasionally, they cause *mild* diarrhoea. Usually, they also cause vomiting, abdominal tenderness which is usually local, guarding, and rigidity.)

Give him some water. *CAN HE DRINK?* (Thirst is the earliest sign of dehydration. If he will drink, you can probably rehydrate him by mouth.)

SPECIAL TESTS

If he has a fever, are there any malaria parasites in his blood slide (L 7.31)?

Examine his stool with a microscope (L 10.2). If he has fever, pus cells in his stool show that he has a gut infection. If he has fever and no pus, look carefully for an infection outside his gut. If his stool is frothy, look for *Giardia*. If there is blood or mucus, look for amoebae, or worms.

If he has watery diarrhoea and is drinking milk, test for lactose (9.29, lactose intolerance).

THE FOUR PARTS OF THE DIAGNOSIS

(1) *Dehydration.* All children with acute *watery* diarrhoea are dehydrated. Is his dehydration mild, moderate, or severe?

(2) *Nutrition.* Has he got chronic diarrhoea because of malnutrition? Or acute-on-chronic diarrhoea (9.12)?

(3) *Fever.* Hyperpyrexia (10.4)?

(4) *Special causes.* Amoebae (9.4) or *Giardia* (9.6) or heavy loads of some worms can all cause diarrhoea. Sometimes it is chronic. If he has acute diarrhoea, has he got some infection outside his gut such as malaria (10.7)? or measles (10.6)? If he has had fever and diarrhoea for a week or more, has he got typhoid (10.8)? Has he been given broad-spectrum antibiotics which have *caused* his diarrhoea?

MANAGEMENT

If a dehydrated child will drink you can treat him at home. If he cannot drink, or is vomiting all he drinks, he must have fluids in some other way, either in the health centre or in hospital. Sometimes, you can give a child fluids by nasogastric, intraperitoneal, or intravenous drip, and then send him home with fluids by mouth. Tell his mother to bring him back if he gets worse.

If a dehydrated child has oedema (kwashiorkor), or fits, or stays in coma after rehydration, send him for help.

If you send a severely dehydrated child to hospital, *start* rehydrating him first, or he may die before he gets there.

TREATMENT

MALNUTRITION. See Section 7.13.

HYPERPYREXIA. See Section 10.4.

REHYDRATION. All dehydrated children need fluids. The kind of fluid he needs depends on: Can he drink? How severely dehydrated is he? Is he vomiting?

Mild dehydration. Show his mother how to start rehydrating him with glucose–salt solution (9.22), or salt and sugar water (9.22). If you show her in the clinic, she can go on doing it when she goes home. It will prevent his diarrhoea getting worse.

Moderate dehydration. If he can drink, give him oral fluids. If he cannot drink, he needs fluid in some other way as soon as possible.

Severe dehydration, especially if he is shocked or in coma. Give him intravenous fluid immediately. If you cannot do this you *might* be able to save his life with intraperitoneal fluid, or a nasogastric drip.

Vomiting. Try oral rehydration (9.22), or an intragastric drip (9.23). Observe him carefully. If dehydration gets worse, give intravenous fluids.

TREAT THE INFECTION

Mild or moderate diarrhoea. Drugs don't help.

Severe diarrhoea. If there is blood in his stools, give him chloramphenicol (3.18), or tetracycline (3.17). He probably has bacillary dysentery.

Other special gut infections. If necessary, treat him for amoebiasis (9.4) or giardiasis (9.6). If he has the 'rice water stools' of cholera, give him tetracycline (3.17).

Malaria and other infections outside the gut. Where malaria is common, give him chloroquine, especially if he has fever and a large spleen (3.25). If he is vomiting, give him chloroquine or quinine by injection. If he has an infection outside the gut such as tonsillitis treat him for it.

EXPLANATION

Acute dehydrating diarrhoea. If he is breast-fed, tell his mother that she must go on breast-feeding. If he wants to, he can suck while he is having a nasogastric or an intravenous drip. Explain that he needs extra fluids until his stools have become normal again.

If he is bottle-fed show her how to feed him with a cup and spoon, or a jug.

THE EXAMPLE OF THE LEAKING POTS FOR TEACHING MOTHERS ABOUT REHYDRATION

1 A CHILD WITH DIARRHOEA IS LIKE A POT WITH A LARGE HOLE

2 TREAT HIM BY FILLING UP THE POT FASTER THAN THE WATER FLOWS OUT

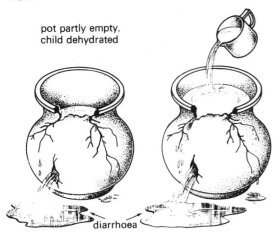

pot partly empty, child dehydrated

diarrhoea

glucose-salt solution or salt and sugar water

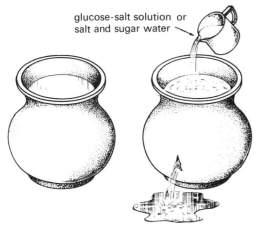

3 PREVENT DIARRHOEA BY MAKING THE POT STRONG. GIVE A CHILD PLENTY OF FOOD

4 IF HE HAS DIARRHOEA AGAIN, START TREATMENT IMMEDIATELY. THIS WILL PREVENT HIM BECOMING DEHYDRATED

Fig. 9–24 The example of a leaking pot for teaching mothers about rehydration.

Tell her that an older child can eat as soon as he wants to. If his mother wants to stop giving him solid food, she should only do this for one day.

If a baby has to stop sucking for a day or two (9.29), teach his mother how to express her milk. Her milk may decrease, but it will increase again when he starts sucking.

Chronic diarrhoea in an underweight child. **He needs more** food, so tell her about the easiest ways to give food to him. Put him on the special care register (6.3). He needs plenty of energy food, so oils, such as coconut oil, help him.

The four danger signs of dehydration. **Tell her to bring him** back immediately, if his *diarrhoea gets worse*; or if he starts *vomiting*, or if he *stops drinking*, or if he has *sunken eyes.* Explain that sunken eyes are caused by his body becoming too dry. If necessary, she must come at night, because he may need intravenous fluid quickly.

Health education lessons. **Tell mothers why their children** have diarrhoea. Show them how they can prevent it. They should breast-feed and keep their children on the road to health. Explain that when a child has diarrhoea we must replace the food and fluid he loses. Teach mothers to give glucose–salt solution or 'salt and sugar water' whenever a child has liquid stools. Ask them to bring a child to the clinic soon, before his dehydration becomes severe. *Show them a dehydrated child. Show them that oral rehydration cures him.*

Look at Figure 9–24. (1) Explain to mothers that a child with diarrhoea is like a leaking pot. (2) When the pot empties, a mother must fill it up with fluid. (3) Explain that making the pot strong is like making a child's body strong with plenty of good food. (4) As soon as a child starts to have diarrhoea again (the pot starts emptying again), she must fill him up with fluid immediately.

Talk to mothers about chronic diarrhoea in an underweight child. Explain that, children who eat well and grow well have diarrhoea less often and are less harmed by it.

DON'T STOP BREAST-FEEDING BECAUSE A CHILD HAS DIARRHOEA

9.32 Caring for a child with diarrhoea, short case

9.32

Many children have diarrhoea. So it is useful to have a short 'Caring for . . . ' section for them. It is for the children *who do not look 'ill'*, and who *do not have sunken eyes*. It is very short, so *never do less than this*. You may need to do much more.

HISTORY AND EXAMINATION

Is the child 'well' or 'ill'?
Can he drink?
Is he vomiting?
Look at his weight-chart. Is his growth curve falling?
How long has he had diarrhoea?
Is there blood in his stools?

Feel the skin at the side of his abdomen to see if he is dehydrated. Is his mouth dry?

If possible feel his abdomen for tenderness (9.15) (20.3).

Take his temperature.

DIAGNOSIS

We have done enough to know that his diarrhoea is not serious, and that we can rehydrate him orally. He is not severely dehydrated. He is not vomiting. He is not a case of 'chronic diarrhoea in an underweight child'. He has not got dysentery, or hyperpyrexia, or an acute abdomen. If he has any of these things, go to Section 9.31.

EXPLANATION

Always tell a child's mother how important fluids are. Show her how to make salt and sugar water. Tell her to breast-feed him or give him food as soon as he can eat.

HAS *YOUR* CLINIC GOT A CLEAN LATRINE WHICH IS SAFE FOR CHILDREN?

---

10 Fever

10.1 Temperature

'Hotness of the body' is a common presenting symptom. A mother feels that her child is hot when she carries him. Or she may feel that his urine is hot when he wets her. If you take his temperature, you will find that he has fever (pyrexia).

We measure temperature with a **thermometer**. This is a small glass tube filled with a liquid metal called mercury. When mercury gets hot, it gets bigger and goes up the tube. There is a scale on the tube which measures temperature in degrees Celsius, or °C. The position of the mercury along the scale tells us how hot a child is. Ice is cold and has a temperature of 0° Celsius. Boiling water

is very hot, and has a temperature of 100°C. The temperature of a healthy child is always about 37°C, because at this temperature his body works best. His temperature is seldom exactly 37°C and is always going up or down a little. He is never less than 36°C or more than 37·5°C. If he is hotter than 37·5°C, he has a fever. If he is colder than 36°C, his temperature is abnormally low.

A child's body burns energy foods to keep itself warm at 37°C. If he gets too hot he sweats. As his sweat dries, it takes heat out of him and cools him. When he is hot, more blood goes through his skin. He loses heat from his skin and becomes cooler. When he is cold, less blood goes through his skin. His skin seems cold, but he saves heat and keeps warm inside. If an older child gets very

THERMOMETERS

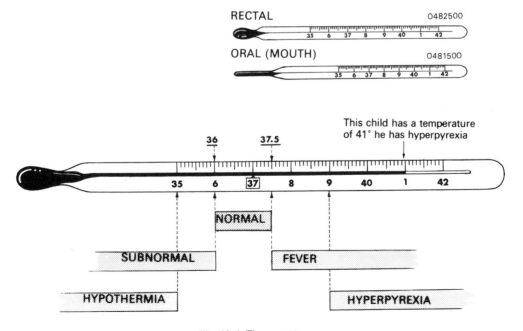

Fig. 10–1 Thermometers.

cold, his muscles contract and he shivers (shakes). Contracting muscles burn more energy food and make more heat, so this keeps him warm.

A child with a fever sometimes feels cold. He sits in the sun and shivers—he is having a **rigor**. This is a sign that his body is making heat, and that his temperature is going up. When he feels that he is hot and he sweats, his body is losing heat, and his temperature is going down.

A temperature of more than 39°C is dangerous. A child who is as hot as this has **hyperpyrexia** (very high fever). It may cause fits and harm his brain. So, if you find a child who is as hot as this, cool him quickly (10.4).

HYPERPYREXIA—MORE THAN 39°C
START COOLING A CHILD IF HIS
TEMPERATURE RISES ABOVE 38°C

Sometimes, a child with an infection is so sick that his body cannot make enough heat to cause a fever. If he is very sick, or very young, or very malnourished (7.9) his body cannot make enough heat to keep warm. So he gets cold. A temperature a little below 36°C is not serious. But a temperature below 35°C is called **hypothermia** and is very dangerous. Hypothermia is the opposite of hyperpyrexia. If you find a hypothermic child warm him up (10.4).

Young children cannot keep a normal temperature as easily as older children and adults. Newborn babies, especially low birth-weight babies cannot warm themselves by shivering. They become hypothermic very easily (26.25).

HYPOTHERMIA—LESS THAN 35°C
START WARMING A CHILD IF HIS
TEMPERATURE FALLS BELOW 36°C

Measure a child's temperature in his mouth, under his arms (axilla), or in his rectum. Use the rectum in children under one year, and the axilla between one and ten years. Use the mouth for older children and adults. The rectum is about half a degree hotter than the mouth. The mouth is about half a degree hotter than the axilla. All temperatures in this book are rectal. So when you read about a child's temperature being 35°C, this is his rectal temperature. It is the same as a mouth temperature of 34·5°C, or an axilliary temperature of 34°C.

ALL THE TEMPERATURES IN
THIS BOOK ARE RECTAL

You can use an oral (mouth) thermometer in all three places. But in the rectum a special rectal thermometer is better. This usually has a strong round blue bulb, which shows that it is for the rectum only. Most thermometers have a scale from 35°C to 42°C. Children die before they get to 42°C, so you will never find the mercury above the top of the scale. But you will find hypothermic children in whom the mercury stays below 35°C. It will not go up into the scale because they have a temperature of less than 35°C.

You can easily carry organisms from one child to another on a thermometer. So always keep thermometers in an antiseptic.

TAKING A CHILD'S TEMPERATURE

CARING FOR THE THERMOMETER. **Keep it in a small bottle of dilute lysol with some cotton wool at the bottom. Wash off the lysol before you use it.**

Hold the thermometer tightly in your thumb and first two fingers. Shake it quickly downwards with your wrist several times, so that the mercury goes below the end of the scale. Be careful. Don't let the bulb hit anything. It may break.

UNDER ONE YEAR—IN HIS RECTUM. **Make sure you have shaken the mercury down. Put some vaseline on the bulb of the thermometer. Lay the child on his back, hold his feet up, and put the thermometer 2 cm into his rectum. Hold it there for one minute, or until the mercury has**

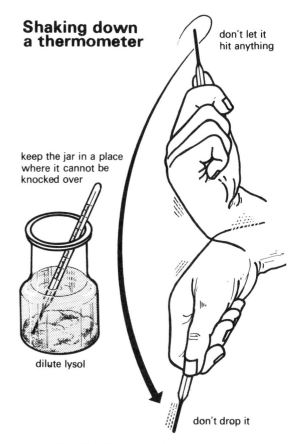

Shaking down a thermometer

don't let it hit anything

keep the jar in a place where it cannot be knocked over

dilute lysol

don't drop it

Fig. 10–2 How to care for a thermometer.

stopped moving. Take it out, wipe it with gauze, read it, wash it, shake it down, and put it back in its bottle of lysol.

ONE TO TEN YEARS—IN HIS AXILLA. **Put the bulb of the thermometer under his arm with its end deep in his axilla. Put his arm by his side, and ask his mother to hold it. Make sure that the bulb is inside his axilla. A thermometer takes longer to warm up under the arm, so leave it there for three minutes.**

OVER TEN YEARS—IN HIS MOUTH. **Put the thermometer under the side of his tongue. Ask him to close his lips and keep them closed. Tell him not to bite it with his teeth. Leave it in his mouth for two minutes. If his nose is blocked and he cannot keep his mouth closed, use his axilla.**

If the mercury will not go up into the scale, **take the child's temperature again, in his rectum. If it still does not go into the scale, he has a temperature of less than 35°C. He is hypothermic. Warm him (10.4).**

10.2 When to take the temperature

Measuring the temperature takes at least two minutes and is not necessary for most children. But you must diagnose hyperpyrexia and hypothermia, so take the temperature of every 'ill' child. This is especially important if he has severe diarrhoea, or if he is difficult to diagnose. Feeling his cheek or his arm is *not* enough, because you cannot always diagnose fever this way.

TAKING A RECTAL TEMPERATURE

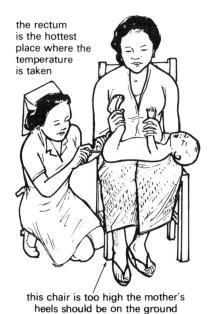

the rectum is the hottest place where the temperature is taken

this chair is too high the mother's heels should be on the ground

Fig. 10–3 Taking the rectal temperature.

Sometimes a child has a cold skin and is very hot inside. A good time to take his temperature is after you have examined him, while you are making his records.

TAKE THE TEMPERATURE OF ALL 'ILL' CHILDREN

10.3 'Ali feels hot'—the treatment of fever 10.3

The most important treatment for a child with fever is *causal* treatment (3.1) for the disease which is causing the fever. So, treat the fever of pneumonia or tonsillitis with penicillin. There is also some important *symptomatic* treatment for *all* children with fever.

FEVER

FLUIDS. **Children with fever sweat a lot. They must drink plenty of fluids, such as water, tea, or milk, or they may become dehydrated. If a feverish child is too ill to drink, give him fluids by intragastric tube (9.24), or intravenously (9.27).** 10.2

FOOD. **Children with fever need food. They need plenty of soft protein foods, especially if their fever has lasted several days.**

MOUTH. **If a child's mouth is sore and there are crusts on his lips, wash it out with saline. Put half a level teaspoonful salt in a cupful of water. Let him wash his mouth several times a day. Wash the crusts from his lips with a clean wet cloth, and put plain ointment on them. Fruit, such as orange, will also help to keep his mouth clean. See also Section 18.4.**

CHLOROQUINE. **If there is malaria in the district (10.7), give chloroquine (3.25) to all children with fever. Give them chloroquine and any other treatment they may need. If there is not enough chloroquine for every child with fever, give it to the seriously ill and anaemic children.**

ASPIRIN. **Give him aspirin (3.41) if he is over two years old, or paracetamol (3.42) if he is under two years.**

CLOTHES. **Teach mothers not to put too many clothes and blankets on children with fever (2–8). Clothes don't cause fever, but too many clothes may make an ordinary fever into hyperpyrexia.**

EXPLANATION. **Explain that he needs plenty of fluids and food, but few clothes and blankets. If his mouth is sore, show his mother how to care for it.**
Tell her to give him chloroquine when he has fever again.

10.4 Hyperpyrexia and hypothermia 10.4

If a child is hotter than 38°C, cool him, especially if he has fits (15.5). If he is cooler than 36°C, warm him up. Do both these things *soon*.

Cool a hyperpyrexial child with cool water. But *the water must not be too cold or he will shiver*. This is dangerous. In a hot district, where the tap water is warm, pour it over him. In a cold district where the tap water is very cold, wash him with a wet cloth. *Undress him*. Ice on his forehead will not help him if his body is wrapped in blankets.

TREATING A CHILD WITH HYPERPYREXIA - HOT DISTRICTS

Don't let the child shiver!

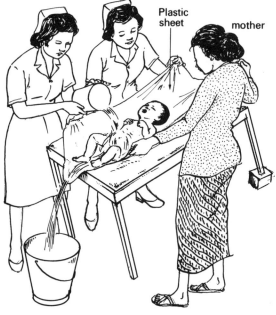

Don't worry! They will not let the child fall into the **bucket!**

Fig. 10–4 Treating a child with hyperpyrexia—hot districts.

HYPERPYREXIA—MORE THAN 39°C

IN VERY HOT DISTRICTS. **Take off his clothes. Lie him down on a plastic sheet on a couch (bed). Lift the sides of the sheet so that water will not run off the sides. Lift the head of the couch, and put a bucket of water at its foot. Pour water from the bucket over him with a jug. Do this until his temperature has fallen below 38°C. This should take less than 20 minutes. If it is not easy to cool him like this, take him outside and pour water over him.**

IN COLD DISTRICTS. **Take off all his clothes. Get a bucket of water and a cloth and make him wet all over. If you have a fan, let it blow air over him. Keep him wet and let the air blow over him until his temperature has fallen below 38°C.**

EXPLANATION. **Tell his mother why you are cooling him.**

TREATING A CHILD WITH HYPERPYREXIA-COLD DISTRICTS

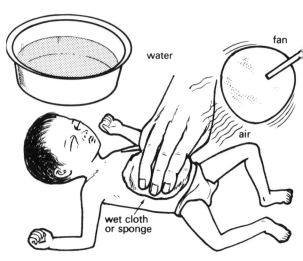

Fig. 10–5 Treating a child with hyperpyrexia—cold districts.

TEACH MOTHERS NOT TO PUT TOO MANY CLOTHES ON A CHILD WITH FEVER

HYPOTHERMIA—LESS THAN 35°C

If he is a small baby, let his mother warm him. Let her hold him close to herself with a blanket round them both.

If he is older, cover him with blankets. Fill some bottles with hot water. Close them well and cover them with cloth. Put them close to him, but do not let them touch him.

EXPLANATION. **Tell his mother why he needs warming, and explain that she can easily burn him with a hot bottle.**

10.5 Diseases causing fever

Almost any infection, except the common worms, can cause fever. Most infections with bacteria and viruses usually present with other symptoms, such as diarrhoea, a cough, or a sore throat. So they are in other chapters. But in some infections fever is usually the presenting symptom. These infections are measles (in the first three days), malaria, and typhoid. These are the diseases in this chapter.

10.6 Measles

Measles causes a cough, a rash, and sometimes diarrhoea, so it might be in several other chapters. We have put it here, because fever is usually its first symptom.

TREATING A CHILD WITH HYPOTHERMIA

Don't burn him!!

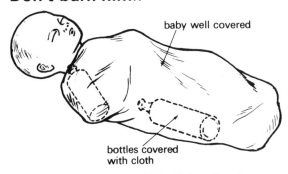

Fig. 10–6 Treating a child with hypothermia.

Table 10:1 Some infections causing fever
Infections which usually present as fever
Measles, malaria, typhoid
Young children—tonsillitis, urinary infections
Infections which usually present in other ways
Colds, stomatitis, 'URI' (18.11), otitis media
Bronchitis, pneumonia, TB
Most kinds of diarrhoea
Severe septic skin infections
Osteomyelitis
Meningitis, and poliomyelitis

Measles is a virus disease. It infects many parts of the body, but especially the skin and the respiratory tract. When an infected child coughs, small droplets go into the air with measles virus in them. When another child breathes in these droplets, he may get measles one or two weeks later.

Measles starts with a fever, a discharge from the nose, a cough, a sore mouth, and sore red eyes. The child becomes irritable and keeps his eyes closed. On the third day, his fever gets worse. On about the fourth day the rash comes and he begins to recover. Measles is not easy to diagnose before the rash comes, but red watery eyes are a useful sign. We can get more help by looking inside a child's cheeks. The measles rash starts here two or three days before it comes on the skin. The measles rash inside the cheeks is called **Koplik's spots**. These look like small white pieces of salt on the red mucosa of the cheeks. Always look for Koplik's spots if a child has fever, or a cough. Koplik's spots tell you that the measles rash is going to come tomorrow, or the next day.

THE MEASLES RASH COMES ON THE FOURTH DAY

LOOKING FOR KOPLIK'S SPOTS

3rd day

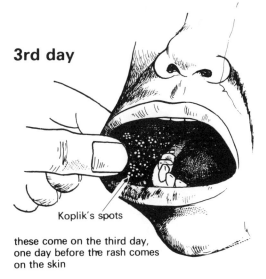

Koplik's spots

these come on the third day, one day before the rash comes on the skin

Fig. 10–7 Looking for Koplik's spots.

The measles rash is made of small red lesions. Some are flat (macules), and others are raised (papules). The rash first comes behind a child's ears. Then it comes on his neck, then on his face and body, and last on his arms and legs. It lasts about four days. About a week later, thin pieces of skin peel off (desquammation). In severe measles the rash is a darker red, and there is much more desquammation.

Immunity. A child who has had measles becomes immune (4.2). Most mothers have had measles when they were children. They are immune to measles so they give their babies a natural passive immunity to it (4.2). This immunity starts to get less as soon as a baby is born. But it protects him for the first six or nine months of his life. So few children get measles before this age.

In a large town there is always measles somewhere. Many children have it before they are a year old. Most children have measles before they are two years old. In a small village, measles only comes sometimes. So village children may grow much older and may even become adults before they have measles.

Complications of measles. Well-nourished children usually recover quickly. But in malnourished children the measles virus grows more easily and causes complications. The virus makes a 'rash' inside the gut and the respiratory system. Secondary bacterial infection makes some complications worse (2.6). If a child's symptoms might be a complication of measles, look for a peeling measles rash. Measles might have caused them.

Secondary infection of the conjunctiva sometimes causes blindness, especially if a child lacks vitamin A (16.13). Many children with measles have stomatitis

10.5

10.6

(sore mouth, 18.10). Sometimes they get a secondary infection with thrush, especially if they have had a broad-spectrum antibiotic. Some children have otitis media (17.9).

SOME COMPLICATIONS OF SEVERE MEASLES

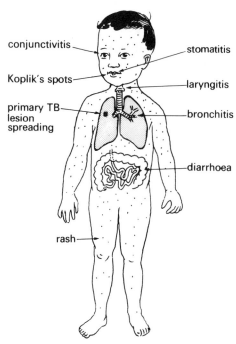

Fig. 10–8 Some complications of severe measles.

Measles can harm the respiratory system and cause laryngitis (8.11), bronchitis (8.12), or pneumonia (8.15). Some children have severe diarrhoea with blood and mucus in their stools (9.10). Their diarrhoea may last for several weeks. For a short time they may have lactose intolerance (9.29).

Most children with measles lose weight. Sometimes a child has a flat growth curve for several months and many infections of other kinds. If a child is already underweight, he may get kwashiorkor (7.10). Measles makes a child's nutrition worse in several ways. His sore mouth stops him eating. His diarrhoea makes him absorb less food. Measles harms his gut, so that he loses protein from his gut. So a child with measles must eat plenty of protein food. He must eat while he is ill, and while he is recovering. Making him eat is difficult, but his mother must try.

CHILDREN WITH MEASLES NEED FOOD

Measles makes a child less able to fight other infections. The bacilli in a primary TB lesion (13.2) may be able to multiply, and spread through him. So TB is a serious complication of measles.

We can prevent measles by immunizing a child (4.8) when he is about nine months old.

Antibiotics do not kill the measles virus, but they can kill the bacteria which causes secondary infection.

MEASLES

FEVER. **Treat this (10.3).**

SORE EYES. **Show his mother how to wash the crusts from his eyes. He may need antibiotic eye ointment if they are secondarily infected (16.8). He may also lack vitamin A, so give him a capsule of it (3.35).**

STOMATITIS. **Show his mother how to clean his lips and wash out his mouth (10.3).**

DIARRHOEA. **If necessary treat his dehydration (9.20). If his mother says breast-feeding causes diarrhoea, see Section 9.29.**

SECONDARY INFECTIONS. **If he shows signs of otitis media, or pneumonia, give him an antibiotic.**

COUGH. **If he cannot sleep because of his cough, give him promethazine (3.45).**

EXPLANATION. **Tell his mother that he will probably be ill for about a week. Explain that she must go on breast-feeding him. If his mouth is so sore that he cannot suck, show her how to express her breast-milk and feed it to him from a cup (26.18). Ask her to go on breast-feeding him after he has recovered. Teach mothers of older children to give them plenty of protein foods such as eggs, or beans.**

Don't forget to write 'MEASLES' on his weight chart (7–1).

MOST CHILDREN WITH MEASLES DON'T NEED AN ANTIBIOTIC

10.7 Malaria

Malaria is caused by parasites (organisms, 2.2) which live part of their lives in red blood cells. Malaria parasites are spread by the bite of mosquitoes. You can usually see parasites in the blood of a child with malaria. Take a drop of blood, spread it on a slide (a piece of glass), stain it (colour it), and look at it with a microscope. This special test is called a blood slide (L 7.31). Occasionally, you can find no parasites in a blood slide, even though the child has malaria.

There are four kinds of malaria parasite. *P. falciparum* is the most dangerous kind. It causes falciparum malaria (malignant tertian or MT malaria). *P. vivax* causes a milder more chronic malaria. The other two malaria parasites are less common.

Signs and symptoms. Malaria parasites cause fever. They destroy many red cells, and so they cause anaemia (22.7), and *mild* jaundice (22.10). The spleen removes things which are not wanted in the blood, such as malaria parasites. Removing many malaria parasites makes the spleen grow large. So a large spleen (20.3) is usually a sign that a child has malaria. His spleen does not become large until a few days after his fever has begun. If you treat him, his spleen becomes smaller again. It only becomes chronically enlarged after he has had several attacks.

In a district where malaria is common, it usually attacks children between the ages of three months and five years. An *acute* attack of malaria can be mild or severe. A mild attack of malaria causes mild fever, sweating, and not wanting to eat. A *severe* attack makes a child very ill with hyperpyrexia (10.4) and diarrhoea.

HOW MALARIA PARASITES DESTROY RED CELLS

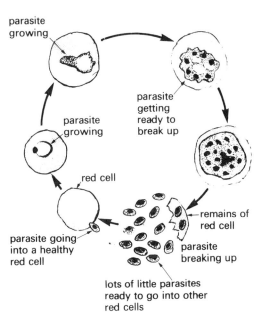

Fig. 10–9 How malaria parasites destroy the red cells.

Cerebral (brain) malaria. Malaria parasites can block the small blood vessels of the brain. This causes cerebral malaria. *P. falciparum* usually causes it. Cerebral malaria presents as sudden severe symptoms after a few days of ordinary malaria. A child may have hyperpyrexia (10.4), vomiting (20.15), severe diarrhoea (9.9), shock (14.2), or fits (15.9). He may go into coma (14.8) and have meningeal signs (15.6). A child with *any* of these signs might have cerebral malaria. If you don't give him a chloroquine or quinine injection quickly, he

will die. If you treat him too late, his brain may be harmed so that he becomes backward (24.16).

A CHILD WITH ANY SIGNS OF CEREBRAL MALARIA NEEDS A CHLOROQUINE OR QUININE INJECTION NOW

Malaria and other infections. In malarious districts most children have a few parasites in their blood (L 7.11, L 7.31). We can only be sure that they are causing a child's symptoms if he has very many of them (+ + + or + + + +, 1–8). If there are fewer than this, he probably has some other disease also. If malaria is common in your district, give chloroquine to all children with fever. Give them chloroquine *and* the drugs they need for other diseases. If, for example, a child has a fever, and the signs of pneumonia, give him penicillin *and* chloroquine.

IN A MALARIOUS AREA EVERY CHILD WITH FEVER NEEDS CHLOROQUINE AND HIS OTHER DRUGS

Immunity. An attack of malaria makes a child partly immune. But, unlike in measles, it is not a complete immunity for the rest of his life. He may get malaria again, but his next attack will not be so severe.

The age when a child becomes infected depends on how much malaria there is in his district. In districts which have malaria *for only a part of the year* people

A CHILD WITH MALARIA

Malaria

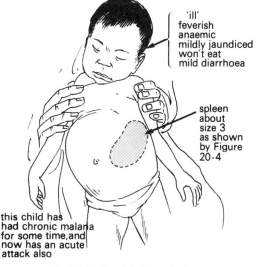

'ill'
feverish
anaemic
mildly jaundiced
won't eat
mild diarrhoea

spleen
about
size 3
as shown
by Figure
20-4

this child has had chronic malaria for some time, and now has an acute attack also

10.7

Fig. 10–10 A child with malaria.

seldom get a strong immunity. Children of any age may get severe malaria. In districts which have *malaria all the year* adults become immune. An immune mother can give her newborn baby a natural passive immunity (4.2). This protects him for the first three months of his life. It soon becomes weaker, and by the time he is six months old all his immunity has gone. In these districts children less than three months old seldom get malaria. After this age they get many attacks, they become anaemic, and some of them die. The children who do not die from malaria become immune by the time they are about five years old. These older children have a few malaria parasites in their blood. They sometimes have fever, but they are not seriously harmed. But, if they get another disease, such as malnutrition or pneumonia, the malaria parasites inside them may start multiplying again. This makes them very ill.

IN A VERY MALARIOUS AREA A CHILD IS IN THE GREATEST DANGER BETWEEN THE AGES OF THREE MONTHS AND FIVE YEARS

There is no malaria in mountain districts. The weather is so cold that parasites cannot grow inside the mosquito. There is no malaria in towns where mosquitoes have been killed. People living in these places do not get malaria, so they do not become immune. But, if they visit a malarious area, they may get severe malaria, so they are in special danger.

In some countries malaria parasites are becoming resistant to chloroquine. Fortunately, this has not yet happened (1977) in Africa. In districts where malaria parasites are becoming resistant, we must give a child quinine, or sulphadoxine with pyrimethamine, if he is severely ill.

MALARIA

TREATMENT

ORDINARY MALARIA. **Give him chloroquine tablets by mouth (3.25). If he comes from a district where malaria parasites are resistant to chloroquine, give him sulphadoxine with pyrimethamine.**

CEREBRAL MALARIA. **Weigh him and give him a chloroquine injection in the dose shown in Figure 3–17. Or give him quinine (3.25).**

Fits. **Treat these (15.9). If possible do a lumbar puncture to make sure meningitis is not causing his fits.**

Fever. **Treat this (10.3), especially if he has hyperpyrexia (10.4).**

Dehydration. **If necessary, rehydrate him (9.20).**

Shock. **Give him an intravenous drip of Darrow's solution (9.27).**

Coma. **Lie him on his front or his side, keep his airway clear and give him penicillin (3.15).**

DAILY CARE. **Observe carefully how 'well' or 'ill' he is (5:2). Take his pulse and temperature, and if possible his blood pressure. Record how much urine he is passing and look carefully for signs of dehydration.**

EXPLANATION. **Tell his mother about malaria. Explain how she can care for him. If he sleeps under a net, he will be less likely to have malaria again. Explain that you can prevent (suppress) malaria (3.25), but she must come regularly for the tablets.**

If you are not going to suppress his malaria, tell her to give him chloroquine when he has fever again.

Suppression. There is no vaccine for malaria. But we can prevent malaria. We can kill the mosquitoes which spread it. Or we can give children chloroquine or pyrimethamine, every week, or every month. We call this suppression (3.25).

10.8 Typhoid fever

Typhoid bacilli cause this. They grow in the gut and spread as a faeces-to-mouth infection (2.7). There are a few cases of typhoid in most districts. Sometimes many people have typhoid at the same time (an epidemic). It is more common in older children.

Typhoid usually presents as fever which lasts more than a week. Often, there are no other symptoms, or only mild ones. Sometimes a child is very ill with fever, diarrhoea, vomiting, a cough, drowsiness, headache, delirium, fits, and meningeal signs. He may be anaemic and have a large spleen. This is softer than the large spleen of malaria (10–10). His abdomen may be swollen and tender.

Typhoid is not easy to diagnose. Think of it if a child has fever for more than a week, especially if he has few other symptoms. Penicillin and chloroquine don't cure typhoid. So, if you have given him these, and he is not recovering, he may have typhoid. Think of typhoid if a child has had diarrhoea and fever for a week, and is very ill but not very dehydrated. If he has a headache (an older child), or fits (a younger child), and is drowsy and anaemic, with a large soft spleen, he probably has typhoid.

TYPHOID

MANAGEMENT. **If possible send him for help.**

TREATMENT. **If you have to treat a child yourself, give him 100 mg/kg/day of chloramphenicol for at least 10 days (3.18). He will recover slowly. His temperature may not be normal for a week.**
Treat his fever (10.3).

EXPLANATION. **Tell his mother why he is ill. Explain to her that he needs plenty of fluids and soft protein food.**

ONLY DIAGNOSE TYPHOID AFTER A CHILD HAS HAD FEVER FOR A WEEK

10.10 Caring for a child with fever

Fever is often difficult to diagnose. Many children have fever for a few days (sometimes as long as 10 days) and few other signs. So we cannot make a sure diagnosis. These children recover without any treatment, and we do not know what disease they had. Often, they never come back to see us. Perhaps they had a virus infection, or perhaps primary TB (13.2). We can only write in their records 'Fever? cause'.

Many children come with fever which has lasted one to two days. We cannot do all the examinations on all of them. But, if a child has had fever for longer than two days we must examine and observe him carefully. Signs often come during the first week of a fever and show us the diagnosis.

Signs come at special times in a disease. So, if a child has passed the special time for a sign, he has not got that disease. For example, if he has not had a measles rash by the fifth day, he has not got measles.

Many diseases such as otitis media and tonsillitis cause fever, but they usually present with other symptoms. But, in young children these diseases sometimes present with fever, so we must examine children for them.

SPECIAL PRESENTING SYMPTOMS. **If he has any of these symptoms go to the section for them:**
Cough, or cough and diarrhoea, go to Section 8.20.
Diarrhoea, go to Section 9.31.
Sore throat go to Section 18.13.
Ear pain, go to Section 17.14.
Frequency, or pain passing urine, go to Section 23.9.
Pain over a bone, go to Section 24.5.
Fits, go to Section 15.9.

HISTORY. **How long has he had fever? (If he has had fever for a week without other signs he may have typhoid or a urinary infection.)**
Does he live in a malarious district, or has he been to one?
Has he had measles, or been immunized against it? Has he been near any children with measles?

EXAMINATION. **Eyes, red and watery (measles)?**
Discharging nose (a cold)?
Breathing fast, noisily, or with difficulty? Is his nose moving (lower respiratory infection)?
Has he any meningeal signs (meningitis, 15.6)?
A rash or any skin lesions (measles, skin sepsis or lymphadenitis)?

Jaundiced (malaria, hepatitis)?
Anaemia (malaria, typhoid)?
Large tender liver and vomiting (hepatitis)?
Large spleen (malaria, typhoid)?
Tender over a bone, especially his thigh (osteomyelitis)?
Examine his throat (18.2). Tonsils large or red? Tonsillar lymph nodes large or tender (tonsillitis)?
Koplik's spots (measles)?
Ear drums red or opaque (otitis media)?
Take his temperature (hyperpyrexia).

SPECIAL TESTS. **Usually none will be necessary.**
If he might have malaria, look at a blood slide for parasites (L 7.31).
If he has frequency or pain when passing urine, examine it for pus cells (L 8.11).
If he has meningeal signs, he needs a lumbar puncture (15.3, L 9.1).

DIAGNOSIS. **A cold (8.7)? 'URI' (8.6)? Measles (10.6)? Malaria (10.7)? Tonsillitis (18.11)? Otitis media (17.9)? Lower respiratory infection (8.9)? Diarrhoea (9.31)? Hepatitis (22.11)? Skin sepsis (11.3)? Meningitis (15.6)? Urinary infection (23.4)? Typhoid (10.8)? TB (13.7)? Osteomyelitis (24.5)?**
Any of these diseases may also cause hyperpyrexia. If his temperature is over 39°C treat him for it (10.4).

MANAGEMENT WHEN DIAGNOSIS IS DIFFICULT. **In a malarious area, give every child with fever chloroquine. Give him symptomatic treatment for fever, and make sure he eats and drinks. Do not give him an antibiotic unless:**
You see signs of a bacterial infection.
OR he is very ill and you cannot get any help.
Observe him every day. Signs may come in a few days.

After seven days of fever. **If there are no signs, examine his urine to see if he has a urine infection. Think of typhoid, especially if he has several of these signs—diarrhoea, headache, dry cough, abdominal pain or swelling, anaemia. Think of TB. If he has no signs which help you make a diagnosis go on with symptomatic treatment and observation. Most children either have signs or recover in two weeks.**

MOST CHILDREN WITH FEVER DO *NOT* NEED AN INJECTION

---

11 Skin disease

11.1 'Carmen has spots'—skin lesions

A child's skin has a difficult job. It has to keep harmful organisms out of his body. If it is injured it has to heal itself quickly. But many children are malnourished, so they cannot fight skin infections easily (7.5). Families may have to pay for water, or carry it a long way. Soap is expensive. So mothers cannot wash children often enough to keep harmful organisms away from their skins. So many children come to see us with skin disease, and especially skin sepsis.

SOAP AND WATER PREVENT SKIN DISEASE

Some diseases, such as scabies and ringworm, harm a child's skin only, and the rest of him is healthy. Other diseases, such as measles and leprosy, cause lesions inside his body and on his skin. The lesions inside him are usually more important. Leprosy harms the nerves. Measles harms many parts of the body. The skin lesions of measles are only important as a sign to help us in diagnosis. When you see a child with skin lesions, always ask yourself—is there also disease inside him?

11.2 Ten questions to ask about skin lesions

Twenty-five skin diseases are described in this chapter. We diagnose them by looking at them, but the history is also helpful. Here are ten important questions to help you.

One. Where are the lesions? Each skin disease has its own special places where you will see it most often. The lesions of herpes simplex (cold sores) are on the lips. Scabies causes lesions between the fingers. Impetigo is most common on the face and scalp and around the ears.

Two. How many lesions are there? Measles and chickenpox cause many lesions. Ringworm and leprosy cause few lesions. A child with many skin lesions has a **rash**.

Three. How big are the lesions? Heat rash and measles cause many very small lesions. Scabies causes a smaller number of larger lesions. A large chronic lesion a centimetre or more across is called a **patch**. Leprosy and ringworm cause patches.

Four. Are the lesions symmetrical? Symmetrical means the same on each side of the body. Measles, pellagra, scabies, and ezcema cause lesions which are the same on the right and left sides of the body. They cause

TEN QUESTIONS TO ASK ABOUT A SKIN LESION

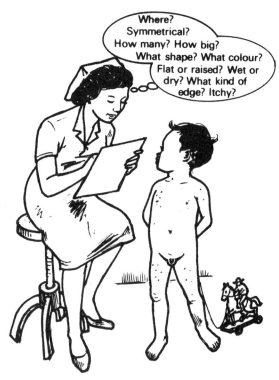

Fig. 11–1 Ten questions to ask about a skin lesion.

142

symmetrical lesions. Other diseases, such as impetigo, cause lesions which are different on each side of the body. The asymmetrical lesions are more on one side than the other, or in different places on each side.

Five. What shape are the lesions? Most lesions are round or nearly round. A few have special shapes. The lesion of creeping eruption, for example, is shaped like a worm.

Six. What colour are the lesions? Lesions may be darker, paler, or redder, than the healthy skin around them. Inflammation (2.4) makes them red, because the small blood vessels in the skin have dilated (opened wide) and contain more blood. This redness is called **erythema**. Stretch an erythematous lesion between two fingers, or press it with a piece of glass. It will become pale, because the blood is pushed out of the dilated vessels. Most red lesions are erythematous.

ARE THE LESIONS ERYTHEMATOUS OR PETECHIAL?

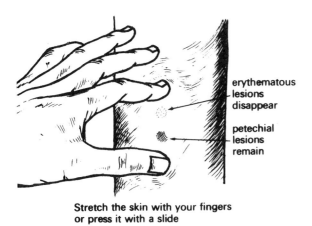

erythematous lesions disappear

petechial lesions remain

Stretch the skin with your fingers or press it with a slide

Fig. 11–2 Are the lesions erythematous or petechial?

There is another much less common kind of red skin lesion called a **petechia**. In petechial lesions the blood vessels have broken, so that the blood comes out of them into the skin. You cannot push the blood away, so these lesions do not become pale if you stretch the skin over them. Petechial rashes are rare. They are usually a sign of serious disease.

PETECHIAL RASHES ARE USUALLY SERIOUS

Sometimes a lesion is pale because it has lost its normal **pigment** (brown-coloured substance). It is **hypopigmented**. Severe burns, old ulcers, some fungus infections, and leprosy can cause hypopigmented lesions.

Seven. Are the lesions flat or raised? Are they solid, or is there liquid inside them? Flat lesions are called **macules** (spots). You can see them but you cannot feel them with your finger. A lesion which sticks up, so that you can see and feel it, is a **papule**. If there is clear liquid in it, it is a **vesicle** (blister). When the liquid in a vesicle becomes pus (2.4), it is a **pustule**. When the pustule heals, a dry **crust** is formed. Sometimes, when the crust goes, a **scar** is left.

The lesions of chickenpox and herpes go through all these stages one after the other. They start as macules, and then become papules, vesicles, pustules, crusts, and occasionally scars. In measles there are macules and papules, but not vesicles or pustules.

Eight. Are the lesions wet or dry? Some lesions are wet, such as acute eczma, or impetigo before the crusts form. Other lesions such as ringworm, are dry. Small pieces of dry skin called **scales** fall off some dry lesions when they are scratched.

Nine. What kind of edge has the lesion got? The lesions of ringworm and pellagra have an edge you can easily see. You can easily see where the lesions end and healthy skin begins. In other diseases, such as eczema and kwashiorkor, there is no edge. You cannot easily see where the lesions stop and normal skin starts.

11.1

11.2

SOME SKIN LESIONS GO THROUGH THESE STAGES

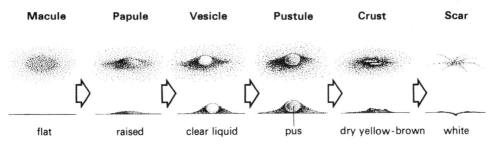

| Macule | Papule | Vesicle | Pustule | Crust | Scar |
| flat | raised | clear liquid | pus | dry yellow-brown | white |

Fig. 11–3 Macules, papules, vesicles, and pustules.

Ten. Do the lesions itch? Some lesions, such as scabies, itch, so that a child scratches them. Other lesions, such as those of measles and leprosy do not itch.

INFECTIONS

Septic infections caused by bacteria

11.3 Skin sepsis

Pyogenic (pus-making) bacteria often infect the skin. They cause acute inflammation called **pyoderma** (pus in the skin). Some kinds of pyoderma have special names, such as **impetigo**, and **boils**. Sometimes, as in boils, the pyogenic bacteria come first (primary bacterial infection). Often pyogenic bacteria come second, after the skin has already been harmed by insects (scabies), fungi (ringworm), viruses (chickenpox), or by a heat rash. They then cause secondary bacterial infection (2.6).

Pyogenic skin infections are dangerous, because they may spread and cause septicaemia. In Section 2.4 you read about the local signs of a spreading skin infection. These are increasing redness and swelling (cellulitis), red lines on the skin (lymphangitis), and swollen tender lymph nodes (lymphadenitis). The general signs of infection are fever and an 'ill' child. If a child has several of these signs, he needs antibiotic treatment quickly. Watch skin lesions carefully (2.4).

SPREADING SEPTIC SKIN INFECTIONS

TREATMENT. **The child needs drugs by mouth, or by injection. Ointment on his skin is not enough. Give him penicillin (3.15) or sulphadimidine (3.14). If necessary treat his fever (10.3).**

EXPLANATION. **Tell his mother that disease is spreading into his body. Tell her he needs tablets or injections, and also local treatment.**

SEVERE SKIN SEPSIS CAN KILL A CHILD

Lymphangitis is not common and is not easy to see in children with dark skins. Cellulitis and lymphadenitis may be the only signs that bacteria are spreading. Remember to feel the nearest lymph nodes when you examine a septic lesion. Sometimes a child presents with a swollen tender lymph node in his groin, for example. You may have to look carefully for the septic lesion which is causing it. Look for it in the part of the body which the swollen tender lymph node drains, as shown in Figures 19–1 and 19–1b.

**WHEN THERE IS A SEPTIC SKIN LESION,
LOOK FOR LYMPHADENITIS.
WHEN THERE IS LYMPHADENITIS,
LOOK FOR A SEPTIC SKIN LESION**

11.4 Impetigo

This is a common acute bacterial infection of the outer part of the skin. It is very infectious. The lesions are usually on a child's face, nose or ears, or on his head or buttocks. They start as red macules which become thin vesicles. Mothers often say they see these vesicles. Sometimes they are large (bullous impetigo). We seldom see vesicles because they break easily. The broken vesicles form red lesions which are wet with thin pus. Yellow crusts form, and these are what you see most often. As a lesion grows it may heal in the middle, so that the crusts form a ring, or part of a ring. Impetigo easily spreads to other parts of the skin.

The bacteria which cause impetigo sometimes spread inside the body and cause osteomyelitis (24.5) or septicaemia. Impetigo is much more dangerous in babies. It spreads quickly over his skin and causes many large vesicles. It may cause septicaemia, and kill the baby. Babies easily catch impetigo from older children and from each other (26.47).

Impetigo

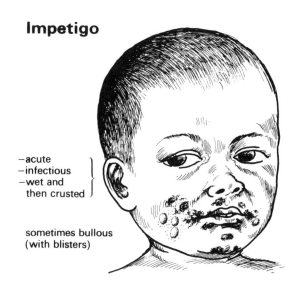

–acute
–infectious
–wet and
then crusted

sometimes bullous
(with blisters)

Fig. 11–4 Impetigo is an acute septic infection.

IMPETIGO

TREATMENT. **Bath the child twice a day using soap and water. If possible use an antiseptic, such as hypochlorite (3.48) or permanganate solution (3.48), in the water. Clean off the crusts. Impetigo is very infectious, so boil any instruments you have used, or other children may be infected.**

Cut away the child's hair from any lesions on his head. Sometimes you may have to cut it all off.

After each bath put gentian violet (3.48), or chlortetracycline ointment (3.17) on the lesions.

Give him penicillin (3.15) if there is cellulitis, or vesicles, or if the infection is spreading, or if he is less than a year

old. One injection of 'depot' penicillin (3.15) will usually cure him.

EXPLANATION. **Tell his mother that washing him and soaking his lesions is the most important part of the treatment. Show her how to do this as described in Section 11.6.**

11.5 Boils and abscesses

A small septic lesion close to the top of the skin is a pustule. The skin over it is thin, so the pus in it can easily get out. Boils are deeper, and usually start in the place where a hair grows. A larger lesion full of pus is called an **abscess**.

BOILS

TREATMENT. **Small boils in a well child need no treatment. Try covering a larger boil with a dry dressing for a few days, to see if pus will come out. A hot compress sometimes helps pus to form more quickly. Soak some pieces of cloth in very hot water and put these on the boil. When they get cold, warm them again in the water. Do this several times, but be careful not to burn the child.**

Never squeeze (press) a boil, because this may spread organisms through the tissues, or into the blood.

Give him a course of penicillin (3.15), if there is spreading cellulitis round a boil, or fever, or if he has many boils. Only use sulphadimidine for septic lesions if they are already open, and pus is coming out.

Give his mother some permanganate crystals to wash him with (11.6). These will help to stop bacteria spreading on his skin and causing more boils.

EXPLANATION. **Tell his mother how to bath him and wash his clothes as described in Section 11.6.**

DON'T SQUEEZE BOILS

Sometimes you have to open a boil or abscess. Wait until the lesion feels fluid and its top is thin. This shows that pus has formed and that it is ready to be opened.

OPENING A BOIL OR ABSCESS

Tell an older child what you are going to do. Say that it will be quickly over, and that it will not hurt so much as cutting healthy skin. Ask a helper to hold him for you. Take a sterile scalpel and quickly cut into the *top* of the abscess only. Then put a pair of forceps into the wound and open them. This will make a way out for the pus without harming anything. *Don't* put the end of the scalpel into the wound, or you may cut an artery or a nerve.

Put a piece of wet gauze into the hole in the abscess. Take it out slowly, a little more every few days, as the abscess heals.

Comfort him, and give him some aspirin or paracetamol (3.42) for the pain.

EXPLANATION. **Tell his mother that the abscess will heal more quickly if you open it. Ask her to bring him back for a clean dressing.**

11.6 Pyoderma

Children often have septic lesions on their skin and scalp for which there is no special name. They may have infected sores, or cuts, or secondarily infected ringworm, scabies, or insect bites. They may have a secondarily infected heat rash. The best name for septic skins like this is 'pyoderma'.

PYODERMA

LOCAL TREATMENT

Soak the child's lesions in hypochlorite (3.48) or permanganate solution (3.48), or saline (3.48) for ten minutes two or three times a day. Make the solution by putting as much permanganate as you can pinch in three fingers into half a bucket of water. Put an infected hand or leg into a bowl of solution. For other parts of the body use a cloth soaked in the solution.

Dry the skin and put on gentian violet or chlortetracycline ointment.

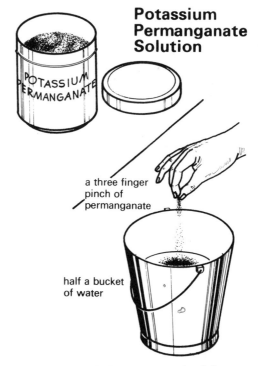

Fig. 11–5 **Making permanganate solution.**

GENERAL TREATMENT

Give him penicillin (3.15) if the lesions are not healed by local treatment, if they are deep or spreading, or if he is 'ill'.

EXPLANATION

Tell his mother that washing is the most important part of the treatment. Ask her to wash him twice a day, and to wash his clothes once a day. Explain that there are organisms on his skin and clothes and that washing removes them. Give her some teaspoonfuls of permanganate crystals or some hypochlorite. Show her how to make permanganate solution, and how to put an infected hand or leg into a bowl of it.

If he has impetigo, show her how to wash away the crusts with wet cotton wool or gauze. Dark healing crusts can be left.

Ask her to bath him for several days after he is well, to prevent the lesions coming back.

If he has head lesions and wears a hat, tell her not to put it on him until they are healed. A clean cotton hat is useful for keeping away flies, but it needs to be boiled often. Infected towels spread infection, so ask her to give him one for himself only and to wash it often.

If you give him gentian violet or chlortetracycline ointment show her how to use them.

A mother may not be able to do all these things, but she will probably be able to do *some* of them. This may be enough to cure his infection. *Before she goes home* from the clinic show her what she can do.

11.7 Skin ulcers

Most cuts and scratches heal easily. Some become infected by bacteria. The edges of an infected cut become inflamed and pus forms under the crust. Sometimes a small cut like this slowly grows larger and forms an ulcer (sore). Children often have several small ulcers on their legs. Sometimes an ulcer grows very large, especially if a child is malnourished. An ulcer may take a long time to heal because skin has to grow in from the edges to cover it. Dust gets into it, and the crust over it is scratched off as it forms. If a big ulcer does not heal for several weeks, the child may need an operation in hospital. A surgeon takes small pieces of skin from another part of the child's body and puts them on the ulcer. Treat small lesions early and carefully, and so prevent ulcers becoming serious.

**PREVENT LARGE ULCERS BY
TREATING SMALL LESIONS EARLY**

SKIN ULCERS

TREATMENT. **This depends on how large they are.**

Small ulcers. **Wash the ulcer in permanganate (3.48), or hypochlorite (3.48). Put gentian violet on it, and cover it with a dry dressing.**

Large ulcers. **Clean the ulcer each day with hypochlorite. Twice a day is better. Put gauze made wet with hypochlorite on it and bandage it. If the child will stay in bed and rest his leg, it will heal quicker.**

Give him penicillin for five days (3.15). If he is anaemic, give him iron (3.33).

PREVENT TETANUS. **If he has not had his DPT injections (4.9), give them to him.**

EXPLANATION. **Teach his mother how to care for his ulcer. If he has many ulcers, tell her to wash them as in Section 11.6. Explain that he should have plenty of protein food.**

A CHRONIC ULCER ON THE SKIN

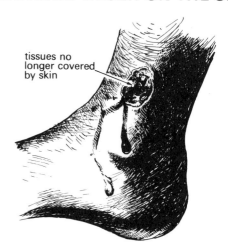

tissues no longer covered by skin

Fig. 11–6 A chronic ulcer on the skin.

Lesions caused by insects

11.9 Insect bites

Children are often bitten by mosquitoes. Bites make them cry, stop them sleeping, and may give them malaria. Sometimes the bites become secondarily infected. Occasionally the bites cause many itchy, red papules to come on parts of the body which have not been bitten. This is called **papular urticaria** (11.24). Let the child sleep under a net. This will prevent bites.

Insects which live in beds and chairs also bite children. The lesions from the bites may be macular, papular, or urticarial. They are often close to one another on the body. They itch, get scratched, and become secondarily infected.

11.10 Scabies

In some villages most children have scabies. Small insects (2–1) which live in holes in the skin cause scabies. Scabies lesions are not dangerous, but they itch, and make a child scratch, especially at night. They may make him so unhappy that he sleeps badly, does not eat, and loses weight. They are often secondarily infected by bacteria, and become septic. Scabies usually infects several people in a family, especially if they sleep in the same bed. A child usually catches it from his mother, who may have only a few lesions. Children become partly immune to scabies, so they have fewer lesions as they grow older.

Scabies causes a symmetrical itchy rash of papules, vesicles, and pustules. If a rash does not itch, it is not scabies. Older children have scabies between their fingers and toes, round their wrists, and on their elbows. They have lesions along the folds of their axillae and on their buttocks, penis, and ankles. There may not be lesions in all these places, but there will probably be lesions in most of them. Babies may have severe scabies, especially on the palms of their hands and on the soles of their feet. Sometimes there are lesions on a mother's breast and on a baby's face.

It is not easy to see the burrows (holes) made by scabies insects. Make the diagnosis from the scratched and often infected lesions in these special places.

**DIAGNOSE SCABIES FROM
THE ITCHING, THE SCRATCHING,
AND THE PLACE OF THE LESIONS**

SCABIES

TREATMENT

Gamma benzene hexachloride. **Mix one part (cup, ml etc) of the lotion concentrate with 19 parts (cup, ml etc) of**

SCABIES IS A DISEASE OF THE WHOLE FAMILY

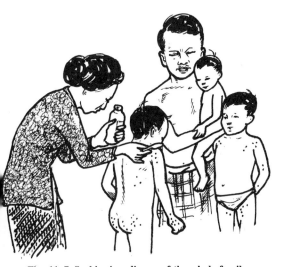

Fig. 11–7 Scabies is a disease of the whole family.

water. Mix well to make a milky solution. DON'T USE UNDILUTED.

OR Benzyl benzoate. **Mix one part of benzyl benzoate with 3 parts of water. Mix to make a milky solution. DON'T USE UNDILUTED.**

OR Sulphur ointment. **Give the child's mother some of this.**

OR Monosulphiram. **This is a good drug to use in districts where people rub their bodies with oil. If rubbing oil is used, ask the child's mother to bring some. Add one part of monosulphiram in spirit to twenty parts of rubbing oil.**

EXPLANATION. **Give the child's mother 75 ml of diluted benzyl benzoate or gamma benzene hexachloride for each child. Give 150 ml for each adult. Tell her to take off all the**

WHERE TO LOOK FOR SCABIES LESIONS

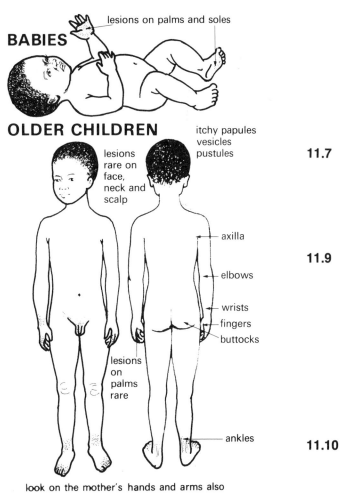

BABIES — lesions on palms and soles

OLDER CHILDREN

lesions rare on face, neck and scalp

itchy papules vesicles pustules

— axilla

— elbows

— wrists

— fingers

— buttocks

lesions on palms rare

— ankles

look on the mother's hands and arms also

Fig. 11–8 Where to look for scabies lesions.

11.7

11.9

11.10

patient's clothes, wash him all over with soap, and dry him. Next, she must cover the whole of his body, except his head with the medicine that you give her. She can use a small piece of cloth to do this. She must not let the medicine get into his eyes. Then she must put him into clean clothes. After this she must wash his dirty clothes, blankets, or mat and put them in the sun. This kills the scabies insects.

Ask her to wash him, and put medicine on him in this way each day for three days. Tell her not to wash him after a treatment, until it is time for the next wash and treatment. If she does, she will wash off the medicine before it can kill all the insects.

Treat anyone else with scabies in the family *at the same time*. Treat anyone who sleeps in the same bed as he does. Treat everyone in the family three times. Ask her to wash their clothes, blankets, and mats also. Treating scabies is hard work! But this is the only way.

**SCABIES IS A DISEASE
OF THE WHOLE FAMILY**

11.11 Head lice

The head louse is a small insect which lives in the hair. It makes a child's head itchy, so that he scratches it. These scratches may become septic. Lice lay small white eggs on the hair called **nits**.

HEAD LICE

TREATMENT. **Kill the lice by putting gamma benzene hex-achloride (3.48), or benzyl benzoate (3.48), on the child's head. Treat everyone in the family. Treat them again a week later when the eggs on the hairs have had time to hatch.**

EXPLANATION. **Show his mother the nits and the lice. Tell her to leave the medicine on his hair until next day, and then to wash and comb it.**

11.12 The tumbu fly (*Cordylobia arthropophaga*)

This fly lays her eggs on clothes while they are drying in the sun. When a child is wearing his clothes, the eggs hatch, and the larvae (young flies) bite their way into his skin. This causes itching. Each larva grows to become a maggot (one of the stages in a fly's life cycle), and a small abscess forms round it. Each maggot breathes through a small hole in the top of its abscess. If you block this hole by putting some ointment or vaseline on the abscess, the maggot cannot breathe. In a few minutes, it comes out for air, and you can pull it out. This is a good test for the tumbu fly, and also good treatment for it. If there are tumbu flies in your district think of them when a child has a boil that itches.

HEAD LICE

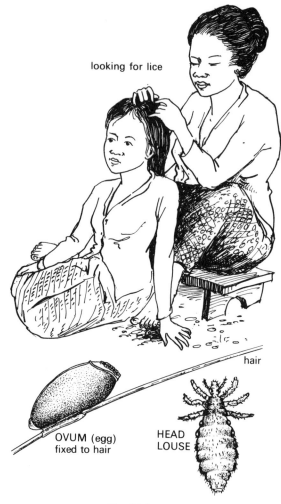

looking for lice

hair

OVUM (egg)
fixed to hair

HEAD
LOUSE

Fig. 11–9 Head lice.

Skin lesions caused by fungi

11.13 Ringworm

Several kinds of fungi (2.2) can grow in a child's skin or scalp, and cause a mild chronic infection called ring-worm. Ringworm lesions heal themselves as a child grows older, but this takes a long time. Soap and water is the best way to prevent them.

Ringworm of the body. The lesion starts as a round papule. This slowly gets larger by growing from its edge, which becomes thicker and redder than the middle of the lesion. The edge is always easy to see. It is raised and may have small vesicles on it. The middle of a lesion is covered with dry white scales. Lesions start as round papules, but because they heal in the middle, they soon become curved lines or rings. This is why they are called 'ringworm'. Sometimes they itch mildly, so they may be scratched and become infected. A child with ringworm usually has a few asymmetrical lesions one or two centimetres across.

Scrape off a small piece of the edge of the lesion and look at it with a microscope (L 11.15). You may be able to see fungi.

Ringworm of the scalp. Several fungi infect the hair and make it so weak that it breaks easily, and forms lesions without hair. One kind of ringworm causes hair to break off above the skin. You can see the short pieces of hair which remain. These lesions are round, pale, and grey.

Another fungus causes the infected hairs to break off at the skin or below it. You can only see the ends of the hairs looking like black dots. In a third kind of ringworm the skin becomes swollen and soft.

Not all scalp lesions are caused by ringworm fungi. The lesions of impetigo (11.4), sometimes look like ringworm, but heal more quickly.

Griseofulvin is the best treatment for ringworm, but it is so expensive that we have not put it in the drug list (3:1).

RINGWORM OF THE BODY AND SCALP

TREATMENT

Uninfected lesions. **Wash the child's skin with soap and water, and put benzoic acid ointment on it twice a day. Do this for ten days. Lesions heal slowly, and you may have to treat him for several months. Never cover more than a quarter of his body with benzoic acid ointment. It is slowly absorbed through his skin. If he absorbs too much, it causes harmful side effects.**

Secondarily infected septic lesions. **First treat them for pyoderma (11.6). Use permanganate, and penicillin if necessary. Only put on benzoic acid ointment after the sepsis has healed.**

EXPLANATION. **Tell his mother how to wash his septic lesions in permanganate, and how to put on his ointment. Explain how useful soap and water are for prevention and treatment.**

11.14 Tinea versicolor (Pityriasis versicolor)

This fungus disease is so common in some districts that about half the children have it. The rash is made of many macules of different sizes, shapes, and colours. Some macules are nearly white and others brown, so 'versicolor' (different colours) is a good name. In a dark-skinned child most of the macules are paler than his normal skin. They seldom itch. They are most common on his chest and back, and are rare on his face. They sometimes spread to the abdomen, and upper arms and

Ringworm

Head—
—chronic
—painless
—round
—bald
—pale

Body—
—chronic
—painless
—round
—thickened edge
—scales in the middle

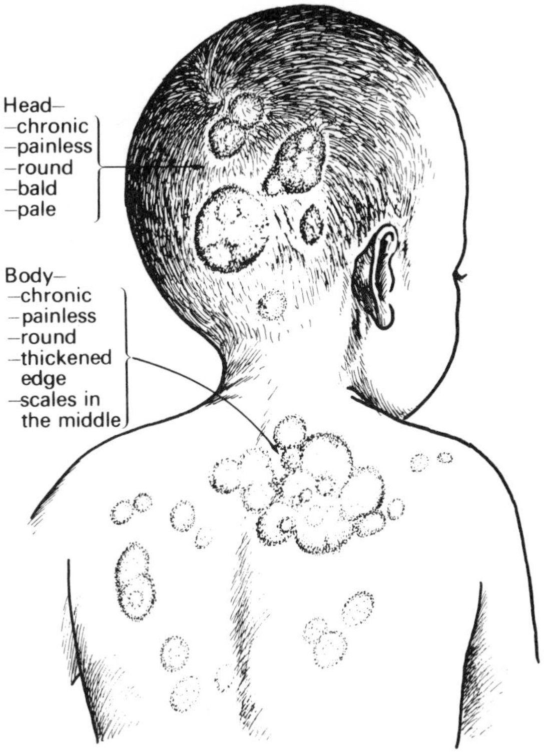

11.11

Ringworm of the head and the body are different diseases. They are shown here on the same child. Both kinds can become secondarily infected

Fig. 11–10 Ringworm is a fungus disease.

legs. The lesions don't look scaly, but scales come off when you scratch them.

The disease is harmless, so you need not treat it. If you want to treat a child, give his mother some 20 per cent sodium thiosulphate solution. Ask her to put it on his skin twice a day for two weeks.

Skin lesions caused by viruses

11.15 'There is a sore on his lip'—herpes simplex

11.12
11.13
11.15

11.14

Herpes means a vesicle. The virus of herpes simplex infects the mouths of young children and gives them **stomatitis** (inflamation of the mouth, 18.6). When this heals the virus stays in the skin of the lips, or around the nose. It causes no harm, except when the child has pneumonia, malaria, or a cold. The fever from these diseases causes the virus to make a painful red macule on the lip—a 'cold sore'. This becomes a vesicle, a pustule, and then a crust. The child's lesion then heals. He stays healthy until he has another fever, and then the lesion starts again, always in the same place. A cold sore is not serious, and many people get one every year. If it becomes septic, put gentian violet on it.

HERPES SIMPLEX OR COLD SORES

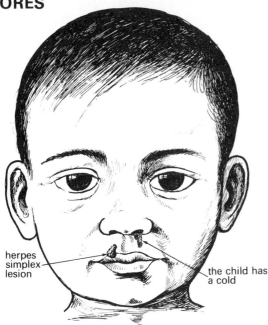

herpes
simplex
lesion

the child has
a cold

Fig. 11–11 Herpes simplex, or cold sores.

ONLY TREAT VIRUS DISEASES
WITH ANTIBIOTICS IF THEY ARE
SECONDARILY INFECTED

11.16 Chickenpox

This is an infectious fever with a skin rash. It is caused by a virus, and it might have been put with the other fevers. But the fever is seldom severe. The rash is usually the presenting symptom. It comes on the day the fever starts.

Chickenpox causes a symmetrical rash, which starts as red macules. These then become papules, vesicles, pustules, crusts, and sometimes scars (11.2). The rash starts on the body, and then comes on the face, arms, and legs. There may be papules and pustules at the same time.

CHICKENPOX

TREATMENT. **Put calamine lotion (3.48) on the lesions that itch, and gentian violet (3.48) on the lesions that become septic. If there is secondary infection, or signs of pneumonia, give the child penicillin (3.15). If his rash is very itchy, and he cannot sleep, give him promethazine (3.45). If necessary, treat his fever (10.3).**

EXPLANATION. **Tell his mother that this is not a serious disease, and that he will recover in one or two weeks. Tell her that there is no need to stop washing him.**

11.17 Herpes zoster

Herpes zoster is caused by the same virus as chickenpox, but is less common. The skin lesions are like the lesions of chickenpox. The lesions of chickenpox are all over the body, but the lesions of herpes zoster are in very special places. They follow a nerve. They are usually close together in a broad line that goes round one half of the body. Sometimes the line goes down part of one arm or leg.

Occasionally, there are lesions on the face and the eye. Corneal lesions are dangerous, so send the child for help. Herpes zoster is easy to diagnose, because of the place of the rash, and also because it is painful. The pain comes first, *before* the rash. The lesions go in about a week. Treat them as if they were chickenpox (11.16).

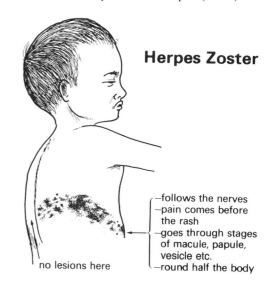

Herpes Zoster

—follows the nerves
—pain comes before
 the rash
—goes through stages
 of macule, papule,
 vesicle etc.
—round half the body

no lesions here

Fig. 11–12 The lesions of herpes zoster follow one of the nerves.

HERPES ZOSTER IS PAINFUL
AND THE PAIN COMES FIRST

11.19 Molluscum contagiosum

This virus disease causes a symmetrical rash of small, hard, smooth, round, solid papules 1–5 mm across. At first there are only a few papules. Later there are many. In the middle of each papule there is a small hole. The lesions are most common on a child's face, neck, lower arms, genital organs, and thighs. They will go by themselves, but they may last 18 months. Treat them by scraping them out with a sterile needle and putting a drop of iodine on them. Be careful not to cause septic infection when you do this.

11.20 Warts

The warts virus causes small chronic thickenings of the skin, usually on the hands and feet. There may be only one wart, or several. They may last for a year or more, but they nearly always go away. There is no easy treatment for them.

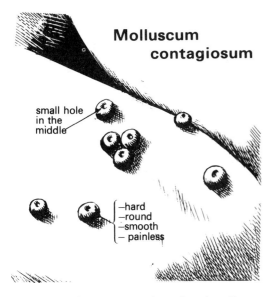

Molluscum contagiosum

small hole in the middle

—hard
—round
—smooth
— painless

Fig. 11–13 Molluscum contagiosum is a virus disease.

Warts

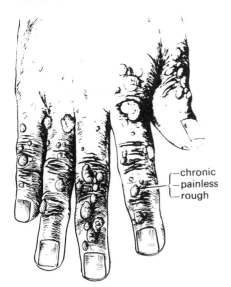

—chronic
—painless
—rough

Fig. 11–14 A hand covered with warts.

Skin lesions caused by worms

11.21 Creeping eruption

To creep is to move slowly, and an eruption is a skin lesion. So creeping eruption is a lesion which moves slowly on the skin. It is not common, but it is easy to diagnose. A child may have a long itchy lesion on his arm, leg, or buttock. The lesion looks like a worm under the skin. If you see him a few days later, you can see that his lesion has moved. Creeping eruption is caused by *Strongyloides* worms (21.6), or several other worms which usually live in animals, such as dogs. Dogs pass the eggs of these worms in their faeces. The eggs hatch into larvae and infect a child when he plays on infected ground. Creeping eruption is not dangerous and the worms die in a few months. They die more quickly if a child is given tiabendazole (3.29). If you have not got this, put plain ointment or vaseline on the lesions and tell his mother that they will go by themselves. Explain that if he wears shoes, he is less likely to become infected again.

Creeping eruption

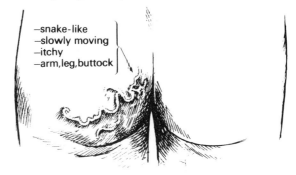

—snake-like
—slowly moving
—itchy
—arm,leg,buttock

Fig. 11–15 Creeping eruption is caused by worms in the skin.

DISEASES WHICH ARE NOT INFECTIONS
Skin lesions caused by malnutrition

11.22 Kwasiorkor

Kwashiorkor sometimes presents as a 'flaking paint rash' (7.10). It is given this name because it looks like old paint which is coming off. The skin of the outer parts of a child's arms and legs becomes dark and comes off in large pieces (7–10). This leaves thin pale skin underneath, which looks as if it has been burnt. He is usually underweight, and has the other signs of kwashiorkor, especially oedema. Treat him for severe malnutrition (7.11).

11.23 Pellagra

This is caused by lack of a vitamin called nicotinic acid. You will see it in adults and *older* children from poor families who eat maize and little other food. Pellagra causes painful symmetrical red lesions. These later become dark, rough, and scaly, with an easily seen edge between normal and diseased skin. The lesions are only on the skin on which the sun shines. This helps diagnosis. There are lesions on the forehead, and on the tops of the

11.17

11.16

11.22

11.19

11.23

11.20
11.21

cheeks. Sometimes there are lesions in a 'V' on the front of a child's neck where his shirt begins. There may also be lesions on the outer parts of his lower arms, and on the backs of his legs. There are no lesions under any clothes.

A child with pellagra is usually underweight (7.8), because he lacks protein, as well as nicotinic acid. If his pellagra is very severe, he may have diarrhoea and mental symptoms.

PELLAGRA

TREATMENT. **Give him two vitamin B tablets, three times a day, until his rash has gone.**

EXPLANATION. **Tell his mother that his rash is caused by lack of the right food. Pellagra can be prevented and cured if a child eats enough protein food. This is because most protein foods contain substances from which the body can make nicotinic acid.**

Other kinds of skin lesion

11.24 Urticaria

An urticarial lesion is a pale itchy papule with erythema around it. It comes and goes in a few hours and does not usually become septic. A rash where all the lesions are like this is called an **urticarial rash**. A mosquito bite is the commonest cause of an urticarial lesion. Occasionally, one insect bite causes urticarial lesions all over the body (papular urticaria). These may be caused by insects in the child's bed. Put DDT powder in his bed.

Urticaria can also be caused by foods, such as fish or shrimps, or by penicillin, or ampicillin (3.15). Most children are not harmed by fish or penicillin. But some children are allergic (3.2) to them. If a child has an urticarial rash, ask his mother if he has had any drugs, or if it has happened before. Ask if he ate any special food the day before. Give him promethazine (3.45).

11.25 Rashes caused by drugs and detergents

Many drugs, especially penicillin, ampicillin, and sulphonamides can cause rashes. Drugs given by mouth and drugs put on the skin can both cause rashes. The rash can spread over the whole body, or only part of it, and may itch. Drug rashes are usually erythematous (red, 11.2), but they can be petechial, or urticarial (11.24). So, if you are not sure what is causing a rash, ask his mother what medicines or injections the child has had. Has she bought any drugs for him from a shop? Most drug rashes go when the drug is stopped. Promethazine (3.45) is good symptomatic treatment for a rash that itches. If a drug causes a rash in a child, he is allergic to it (3.2). Write 'Allergic to . . .' on his weight chart.

Ask the child's mother what detergent she uses to wash his clothes in. These detergents often cause rashes. Ask her not to use a detergent, or to use another kind.

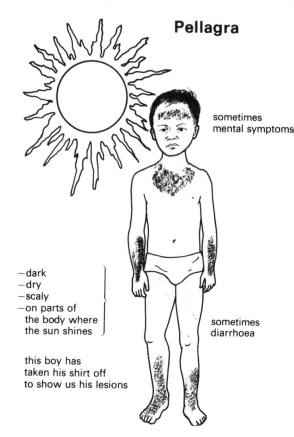

Pellagra

sometimes mental symptoms

—dark
—dry
—scaly
—on parts of the body where the sun shines

sometimes diarrhoea

this boy has taken his shirt off to show us his lesions

Fig. 11–16 Pellagra is a vitamin deficiency.

DRUGS CAN CAUSE RASHES

11.26 Heat rash (Miliaria, prickly heat)

Sometimes, in very hot weather, a child's sweat glands become blocked. This causes a symmetrical itchy rash of many very small macules, papules, and vesicles. These are most common on his chest and neck and forehead. A heat rash looks like the rash of measles, but it itches, and the child is well. Measles does not itch, and the child is ill. In some hot districts children wear too many clothes. Sometimes, so many of them have a heat rash that mothers think this is normal. Teach mothers not to put so many clothes on their children. They should try to keep them cool, and wash them well. If a heat rash needs treatment, wash it with potassium permanganate and put on calamine lotion (3.48). If it becomes secondarily infected, treat it as pyoderma (11.6).

11.26b Intertrigo

This is a wet red lesion in places where the skin is folded. It is common around the neck and under the arms of fat babies. Intertrigo is caused by the skin in the folds being

152

wet all the time. This is usually because mothers do not wash and dry it carefully enough.

INTERTRIGO

EXPLANATION. Tell the baby's mother to wash *and dry* his skin folds. If necessary wash him in permanganate (11.6). Baby powder helps, if she can buy it. Ointments do not help. The fungus which causes thrush sometimes causes intertrigo. If washing and drying does not cure the baby, try gentian violet.

11.27 Eczema

This is a symmetrical, itchy, red, scaly rash. Usually it is chronic and dry. Sometimes it becomes acute and wet. It is worse on the parts of the body which bend. So it is worse on the front of the elbows and behind the knees, around the neck, and under the arms. Acute wet lesions may become secondarily infected. Some children with eczema get asthma when they are older.

Eczema is difficult to treat. Put plain ointment on dry lesions, and calamine lotion on wet lesions. This does not cure them, but it helps a little. If a child scratches himself at night, give him promethazine (3.45), or phenobarbitone in the evening (3.43). Tell his mother to cut his nails very short. She must not put soap on the lesions. If he goes on scratching, ask her to put cotton gloves on his hands. Treat secondarily infected eczema as if it were pyoderma (11.6). Explain that he will recover as he grows older. He may be completely recovered by the time he is an adult.

11.28 Caring for a child with skin disease

If he is newborn go to Section 26.43 and the sections after it.

HISTORY

How long has he had it? (Some diseases, such as cellulitis and lymphangitis are acute. Other diseases, like ringworm, eczema, and scabies, are chronic.)

Is he 'well' or is he 'ill'? (Most skin diseases do not harm the rest of the body. Some, such as measles, chickenpox, or a spreading septic infection, make him 'ill'. If he is 'ill' what other symptoms has he?)

Does anyone else in the family have the same kind of lesion? (Scabies and impetigo spread round a family.)

Has he been having any 'medicine' of any kind, either by mouth, or on his skin (drug rashes)? What detergents does his mother use?

EXAMINATION

Take off all his clothes. Look at the lesions carefully. Try to answer all these ten questions about it.

(1) Where are the lesions?

(2) Are the lesions symmetrical?
(3) How many lesions are there?
(4) How big are the lesions?
(5) What shape are the lesions?
(6) What colour are the lesions?
(7) Are the lesions macules? Papules? Vesicles? Pustules? Or Crusts? Are there lesions of more than one of these kinds?
(8) Are the lesions wet or dry?
(9) What kind of edge has the lesion got?
(10) Does he scratch the lesions?
Pus? (The sepsis may be primary or secondary, 2.6.)
Cellulitis, lymphangitis, lymphadenitis, or fever? (These are signs of a spreading septic infection 2.4; 11.3.)
Ankles swollen (perhaps kwashiorkor, 19.8)?

11.27

SPECIAL TESTS

If he might have ringworm, look for fungi (L 11.15).

If he might have leprosy, look for bacilli in a skin scraping (L 11.11b).

DIAGNOSIS

It is useful to group diseases together for diagnosis, as we have done below. But, although diseases usually present like this, they do not always do so. Drug rashes, for example, may present in other ways than with many small lesions.

11.24

The septic lesions. Boils (11.5)? Impetigo (11.4)? Secondarily infected heat rash (11.26)? Pyoderma (11.6)? Secondarily infected ringworm (11.13)? Secondarily infected scabies (11.10)? Spreading septic infection (11.3)?

The chronic patch, or patches. Ringworm (11.13)? Leprosy (12.5)?

11.28

Many small lesions all over the body. Heat rash (11.26)? Measles (10.6)? Drug rash (11.25)? Scabies (11.10)? Urticaria (11.24)? Tinea versicolor (11.14)?

11.26

Vesicles. Impetigo (11.4)? Herpes zoster (11.17)? Herpes simplex (11.15)? Chickenpox (11.16)?

11.25

Large symmetrical lesions in an underweight child. Kwashiorkor (7.10)? Pellagra (11.23)?

'The others.' Insect bites (11.9)? Ulcers (11.7)? Head lice (11.11)? Detergent rashes (11.25)? Chickenpox (11.16)? Herpes zoster (11.17)? Herpes simplex (11.15)? Warts (11.20)? Molluscum contagiosum (11.19)? Tumbu fly (11.12)? Eczema (11.27)? Creeping eruption (11.21)?

MANAGEMENT IF DIAGNOSIS IS DIFFICULT

Try to decide if the lesion is septic or not. Is there pus on it? If it is septic, treat it as pyoderma (11.6). If it is not septic, treat it symptomatically with plain ointment or calamine lotion. If it is a 'patch', are you sure it is not leprosy?

11.26b

12 The child who might have leprosy

12.1 'Could this be leprosy?'

Leprosy is serious, but you can treat it easily. If you treat it early you can cure it completely. Whenever you see a chronic skin lesion in an older child, ask yourself—'Is this leprosy?' Bacilli which grow in the skin and nerves cause leprosy. The injured nerves are more important than the skin lesions. So leprosy has a chapter to itself and is not with the other skin diseases. Young children can be infected and show signs of early leprosy. But it is a slow, chronic disease, so you will not see serious signs until children are older.

If leprosy harms a nerve, the nerve swells and becomes tender and painful. If the nerve goes to a child's skin, he loses the feeling in that part of his skin. He cannot feel cotton wool touching it, or pain from a needle. Skin with no feeling is **anaesthetic**. A child with anaesthetic lesions may injure or burn himself without knowing because he cannot feel pain. These injuries can become infected, so that ulcers form, especially on his feet. Leprosy lesions can become anaesthetic, so can skin that looks normal.

Nerves also go to muscles and make them move. If leprosy destroys the nerve to a muscle, the muscle becomes wasted and weak. Then other normal muscles can pull the patient's arms or legs into an abnormal shape, and cause a **deformity**. He cannot use a deformed or anaesthetic hand normally, or walk on a deformed leg, so he has a **disability**. Treatment stops lesions getting worse, but it cannot make an injured nerve grow again. So a patient's disability lasts for the rest of his life. So nerve lesions are more important than skin lesions, and are why we must diagnose and treat leprosy *early*.

DIAGNOSE AND TREAT LEPROSY EARLY

Leprosy probably spreads by contact and droplets. It is only *mildly* infectious. A child must be close to an infectious leprosy patient for a long time before he is infected. The best way to prevent it is to treat all the infectious leprosy patients in a community.

12.2 The different kinds of leprosy

If leprosy bacilli go into a child, his body fights them. If his body can fight them strongly, he does not become sick. Most children have much immunity (2.3), so that the bacilli cannot multiply and cause disease. These are the healthy children in Picture A, Figure 12–1. They can live with an infectious leprosy patient for many years. They are never infected.

Sometimes a child has very little immunity. The bacilli multiply into many millions, they spread through his body, and cause **lepromatous leprosy**. This is the most severe and infectious kind of leprosy (Picture D). Lepromatous lesions swell and you cannot easily see the edge between the lesion and the healthy skin around them. The lesions are not usually anaesthetic, and the nerves are only harmed late in the disease. Often, there are nodules (small swellings) on a child's face, or on his ears. This is the most infectious kind of leprosy.

Some children have a moderate immunity, but not enough to win the fight completely. The bacilli grow slowly, and cause **tuberculoid leprosy**. This causes anaesthetic skin lesions and harms the nerves early. Tuberculoid leprosy is not infectious, and bacilli are difficult to find.

If a child has a little less immunity he may get **borderline leprosy**. This is half way between tuberculoid and lepromatous leprosy.

Early in the disease we often cannot diagnose if a child's leprosy is lepromatous, tuberculoid, or borderline. He has leprosy, but it is not yet one of these three kinds. This early kind of leprosy is called **indeterminate leprosy**. You will most often see this kind of leprosy in children. The child has a pale or red macule (11–3) on the upper parts of his arms or legs, or on his chest or abdomen. You cannot find any bacilli, or only a few bacilli. It is mildly anaesthetic, and his nerves are normal. Most *early* leprosy lesions heal themselves in a few months. Sometimes they stay the same for a long time. Sometimes lesions change into one of the other kinds of leprosy, as shown in Figure 12–1. This usually happens in older children. We don't know which lesions

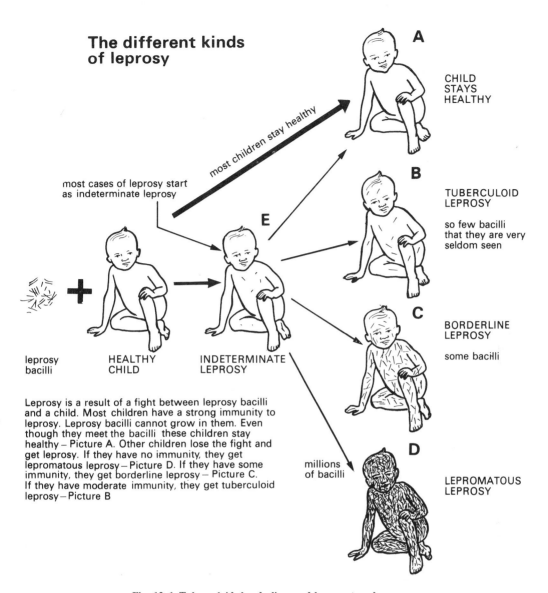

The different kinds of leprosy

most children stay healthy

most cases of leprosy start as indeterminate leprosy

A CHILD STAYS HEALTHY

B TUBERCULOID LEPROSY

so few bacilli that they are very seldom seen

C BORDERLINE LEPROSY

some bacilli

D LEPROMATOUS LEPROSY

millions of bacilli

leprosy bacilli

HEALTHY CHILD

INDETERMINATE LEPROSY

E

Leprosy is a result of a fight between leprosy bacilli and a child. Most children have a strong immunity to leprosy. Leprosy bacilli cannot grow in them. Even though they meet the bacilli these children stay healthy – Picture A. Other children lose the fight and get leprosy. If they have no immunity, they get lepromatous leprosy – Picture D. If they have some immunity, they get borderline leprosy – Picture C. If they have moderate immunity, they get tuberculoid leprosy – Picture B

Fig. 12–1 Tuberculoid, borderline, and lepromatous leprosy.

are going to heal themselves, so we must treat *all* children with leprosy.

12.3 'Has Ketut got leprosy?'—diagnosing leprosy

There are many kinds of leprosy lesion, but the important question is this—is it leprosy, or is it not? Here is some help in diagnosis.

Age. Leprosy is a disease of older children. It is very rare in children under two years old. Lepromatous leprosy is rare in children under fifteen.

The look of the lesion. Leprosy usually causes one large (1 cm or more), chronic, round or egg-shaped, painless, skin lesion. Sometimes there is more than one lesion. These large lesions are called **patches**. They may be macules (flat) or papules (raised). Leprosy lesions are never tender, they are never itchy, and they never have vesicles or pus. Sometimes they heal in the middle. Lesions can be anywhere. But they are most common on the legs, especially the thighs and buttocks.

In dark-skinned children leprosy lesions are often paler than the rest of the skin. They have less than the normal amount of pigment (coloured substance)—they are mildly **hypopigmented**. But not all hypopigmented lesions are leprosy. If a lesion has been pale since birth, it is congenital (2.1) and it is *not* leprosy. *Completely* white lesions without any pigment are not leprosy either.

In pale-skinned children lesions are often mildly erythematous or brown.

A PALE LESION MIGHT BE LEPROSY

Anaesthesia. If a child's skin lesions are anaesthetic, we can be sure he has leprosy. No other disease causes anaesthetic skin lesions. You must test for anaesthesia in the right way, because it is difficult in children. If a child is frightened, or you are busy, ask him to come back another time. If you are careful, you can test for anaesthesia in a child who is three years old. Examine carefully, because the anaesthesia may be mild. It may be in part of a lesion only.

TESTING FOR ANAESTHESIA

Take the child into a place where you can examine him quietly. Make friends with him for a few minutes. Play with him. Make testing a game.

Sit him down and touch a healthy part of his skin with a pointed piece of cotton wool, a feather, or a thread. Touch

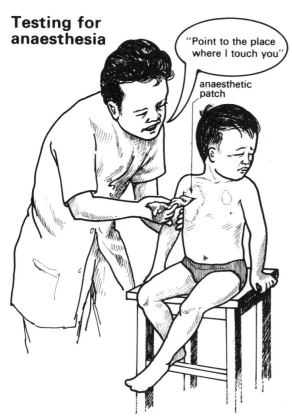

Testing for anaesthesia

"Point to the place where I touch you"

anaesthetic patch

Fig. 12–2 Testing a child's skin lesions to see if they are anaesthetic.

his skin with the cotton wool. Don't brush him with it. Ask him to point to the place which you touched. Touch him in several places until he knows what to do.

Then, ask him to shut his eyes. Touch him on healthy skin on the other side of his body. Then touch him on the lesion. Test each part of the lesion carefully. If he can tell when you touch healthy skin, but not when you touch his lesions, they are anaesthetic. He has leprosy.

AN ANAESTHETIC LESION IS LEPROSY

Thickened nerves. The small nerves in the skin round a leprosy lesion may be thickened. The larger nerves, especially those near a lesion, may also be thickened (12–3). Diseased nerves are sometimes so thick that you can see them. Most often, you can see the nerves at the sides of the neck going up towards the ears. Thickened nerves are a difficult sign to be sure of.

EXAMINING FOR THICKENED NERVES

Feel the nerves on both sides of the body. First touch the skin over the nerve. Then press slowly more and more. Look at the child's face to see if he feels pain. If a nerve is thicker, or harder, or more tender on one side than the other, it is abnormal. Nodules (lumps) on a nerve are also abnormal.

Around the lesions. Use the edge of the nail of your first finger to feel for small thickened nerves in the skin round the lesions.

Ulnar nerves. Take the child's right hand in your left hand. Bend his elbow. Place your right first finger on the bone of the inner side of his elbow (medial epicondyle). Feel for the ulnar nerve in the groove behind this bone. Feel the nerve with two fingers and follow it upwards. Do the same on the left side.

Peroneal nerve. Sit the child down in front of you with his knees bent. Put your finger on the bone at the upper outer part of his lower leg (head of the fibula). Move your finger backwards. First you will feel a tendon, then you will feel the peroneal nerve. Feel this nerve upwards and downwards with two fingers.

Great auricular (ear) nerve. Turn the child's head away from you. This nerve crosses the middle of the (sternomastoid, 19–1b) muscle that goes from the mastoid to the top of the sternum.

Bacilli in the skin. You can do a special test called a **skin scraping** to find leprosy bacilli (L. 11.11b). Take some tissue from the edge of the lesion and put it on a slide (piece of glass). Stain it (colour it), and look at it with a microscope. In the laboratory, the stained bacilli are washed with acid and alcohol. Most bacteria lose their colour when we do this. Leprosy bacilli and TB bacilli keep their colour. We call them 'AAFB' or 'acid-and alcohol-fast bacilli'. AAFB in the *skin* show that a patient has leprosy. We can stain sputum for TB bacilli in the same way. AAFB in the *sputum* show that he has TB.

Lepromatous lesions have millions of bacilli, but they are not always anaesthetic. Tuberculoid lesions are always anaesthetic, but you cannot find bacilli. So, in leprosy, you will usually find *either* anaesthesia, *or* bacilli. A few patients have both. Some patients have neither.

12.4 Management and treatment

If you diagnose leprosy, be sure to treat it. Treatment takes a long time. Treat children with tuberculoid leprosy for at least two years. Treat children with lepromatous and some kinds of borderline leprosy with many bacilli, for at least ten years. *Treat them even if they seem to be well.* They may need treatment all their lives.

If a mother has leprosy, she *must* breast-feed her baby (26.66). If she does not do this, he may get marasmus (7.9) and die.

You can help to protect anaesthetic hands and feet, and prevent deformities. But this does not usually happen until a child is older, so we will not describe it here.

LEPROSY

MANAGEMENT. **If possible send the child for help. If you have to treat him yourself, see him every month. Treat him like this.**

TREATMENT. **What kind of leprosy has he got?**

Indeterminate and tuberculoid leprosy. **Give him dapsone (3.24) for at least two years.**

Lepromatous leprosy, and borderline leprosy where there are many bacilli. **Give him dapsone for at least ten years. He may need it all his life. AND, give him clofazimine (3.24b) for six months.**

EXPLANATION. **Explain to his mother that leprosy is an ordinary curable disease. He is the same as any other sick child. Tell her that you can treat him with tablets. He must take them for at least two years, or 10 years, or longer, if he has lepromatus leprosy. Explain that the drugs take a long time to kill all the organisms in his nerves. He must take the tablets even if he seems to be well. If he does not take his tablets, he may get lesions again and become severely disabled when he is older.**

HEALTH EDUCATION LESSONS. **Teach families these things. (1) Healthy-looking well-nourished children can get leprosy. (2) Children can get leprosy even if they are not in contact with a leprosy patient. (3) We can cure almost all early leprosy lesions completely — *if we give the right treatment for the right time.* (4) We must examine other people in the house of a patient with leprosy.**

RECORDING AND REPORTING. **Put him in the special care register and don't forget him. Make sure you have his**

Tuberculoid leprosy

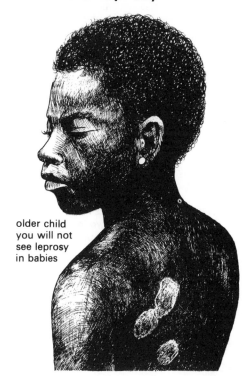

older child
you will not
see leprosy
in babies

ALWAYS	SOMETIMES
—chronic	—pale
—more than 1 cm	—anaesthetic
—painless	—bacilli ++
—not itchy	
—no pus	

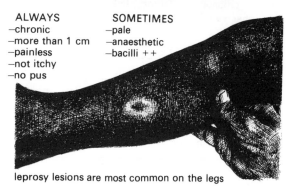

leprosy lesions are most common on the legs

Fig. 12–2b Tuberculoid leprosy.

right address, so you can find him if he does not come for treatment.

12.5 Caring for a child who might have leprosy

A child may have one lesion or several. We write this section as if the child you are looking at has several lesions.

HISTORY. **How old is he? (Leprosy is a disease of older children.)**

How long has he had the lesions? (All leprosy lesions

are chronic. A lesion which has only lasted a few days, or is quickly getting worse, is not leprosy).

Who did he catch leprosy from? Who has he infected?

EXAMINATION. Take off all his clothes, and examine him in a good light. Look carefully for pale or red macules.

How large are the lesions? (Lesions less than a centimetre across are not usually leprosy.)

Feel the lesion. Is it raised above the skin around it (perhaps leprosy)?

Are the lesions painful, or itchy, so that they are scratched? Is there pus on them? (If they are any of these things, they are *not* leprosy.)

Are his lesions anaesthetic (12.3)? (If they are anaesthetic, he has leprosy.)

Is any skin that looks normal anaesthetic (probably leprosy)?

Can you feel any thickened nerves in the skin round the lesions? Examine the nerves shown in Figure 12–3. Are any nerves thickened, tender, or harder than normal? (These are signs of leprosy.)

Muscle wasting? Contractures? (Probably leprosy, if there are other signs also.)

SPECIAL TESTS. Look for **AAFB** in a scraping from the edge of the lesion and from the lobes of his ears (L11.11b).

DIAGNOSIS. **Leprosy (12.4)? Or something else?**

MANAGEMENT IF THE DIAGNOSIS IS DIFFICULT. If you think he probably has leprosy, treat him. If you are less sure, observe him carefully, and put him on the special care register. Most patches of indeterminate leprosy heal themselves. If his lesions don't heal, if they become anaesthetic, or if other lesions come, treat him for leprosy.

Where to look for thickened nerves

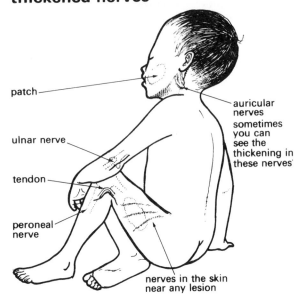

Fig. 12–3 Nerves that are sometimes thickened in leprosy.

Table 12:1   The signs of leprosy

Always	Sometimes
The child is more than two years old The skin lesion is – — chronic, it has lasted for more than a month — more than one centimetre across — painless, and not tender — not itchy — without pus — not cured by other treatment, such as benzoic acid ointment	The skin lesion is — pale — anaesthetic – DIAGNOSTIC — full of leprosy bacilli (AAFB) as shown by a skin scraping – DIAGNOSTIC **The child sometimes has –** — thickened nerves – DIAGNOSTIC (if you are sure about them) — other signs of leprosy, such as weakness, deformity, ulcers, or nodules on his face and ears — a leprosy patient living in the same house

13 The child who might have TB

13.1 How TB presents

TB is an infectious disease caused by TB bacilli. These bacilli take weeks or months to make a child ill, or kill him. So TB is usually a *chronic* disease, except in babies who can die from TB very quickly. When we treat a child, he recovers slowly.

TB usually spreads from adults to children. Sometimes, cows are infected with TB which spreads to children in unboiled milk.

TB can cause disease in any part of the body. TB most often harms the lungs. Sometimes it harms the lymph nodes and the meninges (coverings of the brain, 15.2), the bones, and the kidneys.

TB has four common presenting symptoms. It can also present in several less common ways. These are shown in Table 13:1. *Many other diseases can also cause these symptoms.* TB causes few *signs* until a child is very ill. So TB is difficult to diagnose.

13.2 How TB harms a child

When an adult with infectious TB coughs, droplets of his sputum go into the air. These contain living TB bacilli. If a child inhales TB bacilli they multiply slowly, and cause a lesion in his lungs. Some bacilli spread through the lymph vessels to the lymph nodes next to the main bronchi. Here the bacilli grow and make the nodes enlarge (TB lymphadenitis). A small lesion in a lung, with enlarged lymph nodes is called a primary TB lesion. The child has a **primary TB infection**. If a child drinks unboiled milk from TB cows, his primary infection is in the lymph nodes of his gut. Many children have a primary TB infection at some time. In towns most children have a primary TB infection before they go to school. In rural areas they are usually infected later. A child's immunity (how good he is at fighting TB bacilli) decides if he becomes ill or stays healthy—

The child with strong immunity. Most children have a strong immunity, and soon kill the TB bacilli which infect them. They have a mild TB *infection without symptons. They are not ill.* Their primary lesion soon heals. A few children have a short illness with fever and loss of weight, and then they recover by themselves. We do not usually diagnose these illnesses (10.10).

The child with weak immunity. TB bacilli spread in his body. The lesions in his lungs and lymph nodes become bigger and he becomes ill. *When TB spreads like*

Table 13:1	Ten ways in which TB presents
Common	**Four common presenting symptoms**

These symptoms last several weeks and there are usually several of them.

1. *Losing weight (7.13).* A child with TB does not grow normally. Usually he loses weight, so that his growth curve falls. Sometimes he is so severely malnourished that he presents with marasmus (7.9), or kwashiorkor (7.10).

2. *The 'ill' child (5.15).* He is irritable and 'not well'. He does not eat, or run about and play normally.

3. *Cough (8.1), or wheezing (8.13).* Coughs are common, and there is no need to think a child might have TB until he has been coughing for a month or more.

4. *Fever (10.10).* This is usually mild, and comes and goes.

Six less common ways TB presents

1. Pneumonia which is not cured by sulphadimidine or antibiotics (8.16).

2. The child who does not recover after measles (10.6) or whooping cough (8.17).

3. Painless (not tender) enlarged lymph nodes usually in the neck (19.3).

4. As phlyctenular conjunctivitis (16.11).

5. With meningeal signs (TB meningitis 15.6).

Uncommon 6. Pain in the back or hip (24.6).

Less common

HOW TB SPREADS

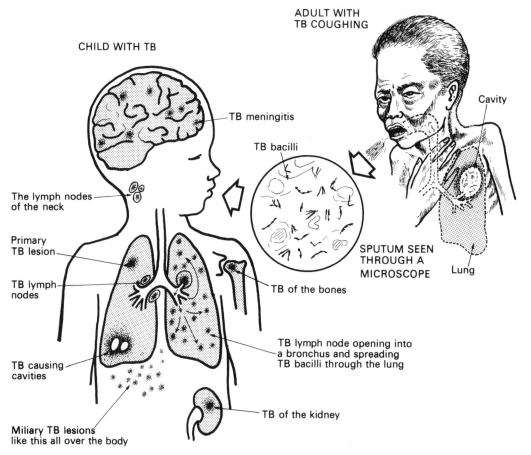

ADULT WITH
TB COUGHING

CHILD WITH TB

TB meningitis

TB bacilli

Cavity

The lymph nodes
of the neck

Primary
TB lesion

TB lymph
nodes

SPUTUM SEEN
THROUGH A
MICROSCOPE

Lung

TB of the bones

TB causing
cavities

TB lymph node opening into
a bronchus and spreading
TB bacilli through the lung

TB of the kidney

Miliary TB lesions
like this all over the body

Fig. 13–1 How TB spreads.

this it causes symptoms and the child becomes sick. Sometimes, an enlarged lymph node presses on a bronchus and obstructs it. This prevents air going to part of a lung (8–4). Occasionally, an infected lymph node opens into a bronchus, and TB bacilli spread from it all through a child's lungs. This is very serious.

Sometimes, TB bacilli spread to all parts of a child's body and cause millions of small lesions. This makes him very ill, and is called **miliary TB**. Or the bacilli may spread to part of his body only, and cause TB lymphadenitis (19.3), or TB meningitis (15.6), or TB of the kidneys, or TB of the bones or joints (24.6).

children have less immunity to TB than older children. Another reason is malnutrition. TB is *more* common in malnourished children. Whenever we see a malnourished child, we must ask ourselves—has he also got TB? TB makes a child's nutrition worse, and is one cause of the 'vicious circles of malnutrition and infection' (7.5).

TB bacilli spread more easily in a child when his body has been weakened by whooping cough (8.17), or measles (10.6) or some other infection such as malaria or chronic diarrhoea. If a child does not recover from any of these diseases, he may have TB.

MANY CHILDREN ARE INFECTED WITH TB, BUT FEW BECOME ILL

Why are some children so good at fighting TB bacilli that they never become ill? Why do other children get severe TB? We do not always know. Age is one reason. Young

---

MALNOURISHED CHILDREN GET TB MORE OFTEN

13.3 How adults infect children

A child with TB rarely infects other children, because

TB bacilli are rarely able to get out of his body. An adult with TB is different. He can be very dangerous and easily infect children. He becomes infectious by coughing out the middle of his lung lesion. This makes a hole in his lung, called a **cavity**. TB bacilli grow in the walls of this cavity, and are coughed out in the sputum. A cavity sometimes bleeds, so blood in the sputum is an important sign of TB in an adult. An adult with TB is usually only mildly ill until he is dying. He can walk about coughing out bacilli. When you find an adult with infectious TB, look for the children he might have infected. These children are his **contacts**. When you see a child with TB, look for the adult with a chronic cough who probably infected him. Look also for other children the adult might have infected.

Infectious adults cough up sputum containing millions of TB bacilli. We can see these bacilli if we examine their sputum with a microscope (L 11.1). This is useful, because, if we can see TB bacilli, we can be sure the patient has TB. Laboratories don't usually report 'TB bacilli seen'. Instead, they report 'AAFB' seen (12.3). Usually, we cannot examine children's sputum, because they swallow it.

BLOOD STAINED SPUTUM IS USUALLY CAUSED BY TB

Preventing TB

13.4 BCG vaccine

We can prevent TB in children in two ways.

(1) We can diagnose and treat TB in adults. We must examine the sputum of all adults who have had *a cough for more than a month*. We must then treat all infectious adults we diagnose, so that living bacilli do not get out of them. An adult soon stops being infectious when he is treated. *But he must finish his treatment, and take his drugs regularly.* If he does not finish it, the bacilli may start growing, so that he becomes infectious again. We must teach infectious adults to cover their mouths when they cough. They should swallow their sputum and not spit onto the floor. This is important because bacilli can get from the floor into the air, and into children.

(2) We can make a child better at fighting TB. Making his nutrition better makes his immunity stronger. Even better, we can give him an artificial active immunity (4.2) with BCG vaccine (4.6). This contains living harmless organisms called BCG bacilli and gives a child a safe, mild infection. BCG does not make a child completely immune to TB. But, it is useful, because he is much less likely to become ill than a child who has not had BCG. He is most unlikely to get miliary TB or TB meningitis.

13.6 Treating TB

There are four older TB drugs—isoniazid (INH 3.20), streptomycin (3.21), Thiacetazone (3.22) and amino-

salicylate (PAS, 3.23). There is also a newer drug called ethambutol (3.23b).

Never treat a child for less than one year. TB bacilli can become resistant, (1) if you give one drug only, (2) if you give too little, (3) if the child takes it irregularly, or (4) if treatment stops too soon. Help to prevent resistance by giving two or three drugs at the same time (3.12) but always give isoniazid. Make sure his mother gives them to him regularly. *If isoniazid is the only drug you have, you can give it to him alone.* Even if the TB bacilli inside a child become resistant to isoniazid, they are unlikely to infect other children. Never give adults isoniazid alone. Isoniazid resistant TB bacilli can more easily get out of an adult and infect another person.

NEVER GIVE ADULT PATIENTS ISONIAZID ALONE

There are several other TB drugs—rifampicin, pyrazinamide. They cure TB more quickly—in six months, instead of a year or more. But they are more expensive and are not yet so widely used as the older drugs.

TB

CONTACT WITH SYMPTOMS
Treat them for TB.

CONTACT WITHOUT SYMPTOMS
If they have not had BCG, give it to them. If they have had BCG, observe them carefully.

THE CHILD WITH TB SYMPTOMS—CURATIVE TREATMENT

DRUGS. Give him daily streptomycin for three months. This is a long time. So if a mother cannot bring her child for as long as this, try hard to make her bring him for at least one month.

Give him these drugs for one year. Give him isoniazid once a day. If you are working in a country where thiacetazone can be used, give isoniazid and thiacetazone compound tablets. If his mother has to buy his drugs, ask her to buy enough for a whole year. Ask her to buy them now while he has symptoms.

If you cannot use thiacetazone, give him aminosalicylate (3.23) or ethambutol with his isoniazid.

OTHER TREATMENT. Don't forget these—
Nutrition. Tell his mother she must feed him well, especially if he is underweight (7.8).
Malaria. If he is under five years, suppress his malaria (3.25).
Anaemia. If he is anaemic, examine his stools. If he has hookworms, treat them (22.5).

RECORDING AND REPORTING. Put him in the 'special care register' with the other TB children (6.3). Be sure you know where to find him if he does not come to the clinic. Write TB in large letters on his weight chart.

EXPLANATION. **Explain to** *both* **his parents and perhaps his grandmother about TB. Tell them you can cure it. Explain that this will take one year. Explain that he must take his drugs regularly for all this time, even if he seems well. If he stops taking them the disease may come back again. If he has another disease, such as measles, he** *must* **go on taking his TB drugs.**

EXAMINE HIS FAMILY. *Try to see as many of his family as possible. Look for the person with the chronic cough who infected him. Test this person's sputum. If the child is less than two years old he was probably infected at home. This person probably lives in his home. Older children may have been infected outside, or at school.*

FOLLOW UP. *If he has got TB, he should start to recover in three or four weeks. He may gain weight quickly when he is given TB drugs. This helps you to be sure of the diagnosis.*

LOOK FOR TB IN HIS FAMILY. DON'T GIVE TREATMENT FOR LESS THAN A YEAR

13.7 Caring for a child who might have TB

TB is a difficult disease to diagnose. Think of it whenever a child presents in one of the ten ways in Table 13:1. Ask about the four common symptoms. Ask how long a child has had them. *If he has had two or more symptoms for 4 or more weeks, he may have TB.* When you examine him, *you may find no signs.* You may have to make your diagnosis from the symptoms alone. If you think a child might have TB, and are not sure, don't be afraid to treat him. If possible give him the full TB treatment. If necessary don't be afraid to give him isoniazid alone. Isoniazid is easy, cheap and safe, but he needs treatment for a year.

Don't diagnose TB too often. Don't diagnose it in every child who has had a cough for a few days only. Only diagnose it if a child has had several TB symptoms for several weeks.

If he is newborn and his mother might have TB go to Section 26.66.

HISTORY. **How many of the four common symptoms of TB has he got (13:1)? (1) Loss of weight? Look at his weight chart. (2) 'Ill'? (3) Coughing or wheezing? (4) Fever? How long has he had these symptoms?**

Has anyone in the family got TB or a chronic cough (possibly TB)? Are they coughing up blood (almost certainly TB)?

EXAMINATION. **Are his respiratory rate and chest movements normal? (These are usually normal in TB, except when it is very severe. If they are** *abnormal,* **he probably has a septic lower respiratory infection.)**

Has he any signs of severe malnutrition (7.10)? (TB is common in malnourished children.)

Has he any enlarged painless lymph nodes which might be TB lymphadenitis? Look for them in his neck, under his arms, and in his groins.

BCG scar on his right upper arm? (If he has a scar, he is more likely to be immune, and less likely to have serious TB.

SPECIAL TESTS. **If an older child can cough up some sputum, examine it for AAFB.**

Try to get his chest X-rayed.

DIAGNOSIS. **TB (13.6)? Or something else? Who infected him?**

MANAGEMENT IF DIAGNOSIS IS DIFFICULT. **Think about any other diseases he might have such as malaria (10.7), whooping cough (8.17), or typhoid (10.8), or a pyogenic infection, especially in his urinary system (23.4) or malnutrition (7.13). Do any tests for these that you can. Weigh him.**

If he might have a pyogenic infection, give him an antibiotic for two weeks. Weigh him again. If he does not gain weight, and his symptoms don't go, and you cannot find another diagnosis, give him isoniazid and thiacetazone. Give him streptomycin too if possible. If he now gains weight and his symptoms go in a few weeks, he probably has TB. So continue full TB treatment for a year. If he does not improve, send him for help. He has probably not got TB.

IF HE MIGHT HAVE TB START HIM ON ISONIAZID

---

14 Injuries and poisoning

14.1 We can prevent accidents

An accident causes death or injury by mistake. Children have accidents because they are finding out about the world around them. They touch things, pull things, or try to eat or drink them. They have not yet learnt which things are dangerous. Many accidents happen because a child's home, and especially his mother's kitchen, are very dangerous places. A baby can crawl into a fire, or turn over a lighted lamp. He can fall off a bed or a chair, or his older sister may drop him. When he starts to walk he can pull a pot of hot food over himself, or fall into water, or into a latrine. He can drink harmful fluids, especially kerosine, and eat dangerous tablets. When he is older he can fall from trees and break his bones, or hit his head so that he becomes unconscious. He can be hurt by a buffalo, or bitten by a dog, a snake, or a scorpion. He can also drown, or injure himself on the road, or harm himself with fireworks.

HOME CAN BE A DANGEROUS PLACE

Accidents to a young child happen in or near his home. Accidents to older children happen further away. We can prevent accidents. We can take danger away, or teach children to prevent themselves being harmed. Both ways are important. We must take dangers from very young children. For example, when you give a mother some tablets, tell her to lock them up, so that her children cannot find them. As children grow older they must learn how to cross a road safely. They must learn how to swim so that they do not drown. They must learn that fire and fireworks are dangerous.

Before we can prevent accidents we must find out what kinds of accident happen in our community. Many communities have accidents of the same kind. Kerosine, for example, is a danger wherever it is used for cooking. Children may be burnt with hot water anywhere in the world. But each community also has its own special kinds of accident. For example, in districts where sugar cane is grown, small boys ride on the trains which carry it. They fall off and are injured. We must tell parents in these districts that this is dangerous.

So we need to think carefully about how accidents happen in our community and how we can prevent them. This is part of the community diagnosis (2.10). If we see a child who has an accident, we must try to prevent the same kind of accident happening to another child.

14.1

13.7

TRY NOT TO LET THE SAME ACCIDENTS HAPPEN AGAIN

When you visit a child's home, look for the things in the list below. When you find something, show his mother how dangerous it is. Help her to find some way to prevent it hurting her child.

IS A CHILD'S HOME SAFE?

Has his mother made her stove as safe as she can?
   Can he reach the lamps?
   Are there any disinfectants (3.11), detergents, or bottles of kerosine in places where he can reach them?
   Are there any pills or medicines which he could eat or drink?

CHILDREN ARE OFTEN IN DANGER

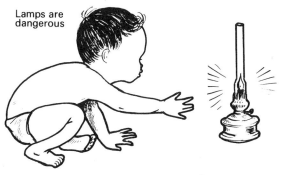

Lamps are dangerous

Fig. 14–1 Children are often in danger.

Are there any medicines in the kind of bottles usually used for drinks (14–9)?

Is the hole in the latrine so large that he might fall through?

Is there any broken glass on the ground?

Is there a cover on the well?

Are there any other signs of danger?

SHOCK

14.2 'My son has become cold and pale'—shock, fainting

Sometimes a child suddenly becomes white and cold, and his skin becomes damp (wet). This can happen either because he has **fainted**, which is not serious, or because he is **shocked**, which is very serious. Diagnosis is easy.

Fainting. An abnormality in the way in which blood is pumped round the body causes fainting. A child only faints when he is old enough to stand. He feels 'dizzy', but as soon as he lies down, he feels better.

Shock. Any serious harm to the body can cause shock. It can last for many hours, and can cause death. A severely shocked child has a fast weak pulse, and does not move. Sometimes he breathes deeply. If he is severely shocked he becomes unconscious. Any serious accident can cause shock, especially if there is much bleeding. Any severe disease, such as pneumonia, diarrhoea (9.18), or cerebral malaria (10.7), can also cause shock.

CARING FOR A CHILD WITH SHOCK

TREATMENT. **Lie him flat without a pillow in a quiet place. Put a blanket over him.**

If he has bled a lot, give him an intravenous drip with Darrow's solution (9.27). Give him a drip if he might be bleeding from an injury inside his body.

Treat the disease which is causing the shock, such as a burn, or an injury.

EXPLANATION. **Explain to his mother what has happened to him. He will be very frightened, so make sure that someone is with him to comfort him.**

BURNS

14.3 'My baby fell into the fire'—burns

Burns differ in three important ways. How big they are, how deep they are, and where they are.

How big is the burn? A large burn is much more dangerous than a small burn. A large burn causes more pain, and more shock, and more easily becomes

WHAT PERCENTAGE OF HIM IS BURNT?

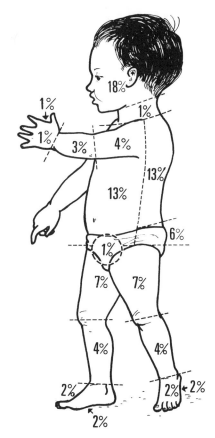

Fig. 14–2 What percentage of him is burnt?

infected. A burn becomes wet with fluid containing protein. So a child with a large burn loses much protein and fluid. Children with large burns become very ill and die from infection and loss of fluid.

The size of a burn is important, so measuring the size of a burn is useful—if a burn is the size of the palm of a child's hand, it covers about 1 per cent of his body. If a burn covers 5 per cent of a child's body, he has a 5 per cent burn.

How deep is the burn? The skin has two layers (parts). The thin outer layer is the **epidermis**. The thicker inner layer is the **dermis**. The parts of the epidermis which make hair (hair follicles) and sweat (sweat glands) are deep in the dermis. Full thickness burns destroy all the epidermis and the hair follicles and sweat glands. Less severe burns harm or destroy part of the epidermis only.

Superficial burns. Superficial means outer or on the surface. These burns are the least serious. The epidermis

164

is harmed but it is still alive. The burnt skin is red (erythema) but it soon heals. Scales form as the epidermis heals, but there are no blisters.

Superficial partial thickness burns. These burns destroy only the outer part of the epidermis. The part which is still alive quickly grows to replace the dead part. These burns also heal quickly and usually leave no scar. Vesicles (blisters) form a day or two after the burn. These vesicles are a good sign because they show that the skin is not seriously burnt.

SUPERFICIAL PARTIAL THICKNESS BURNS HAVE VESICLES

Deep partial thickness burns. These burns destroy the epidermis but the hair follicles and sweat glands are still alive. These burns heal easily because cells from the hair follicles grow and form new epidermis.

Full thickness burns. These burns are the most serious. They completely destroy the epidermis, the hair follicles, and the sweat glands. Healthy epidermis from the edge of the burn grows slowly over the burn to heal it. This takes a long time if the burn is big, and it leaves a bad scar. If the burn is bigger than the size of a child's hand, he will probably need a skin graft. In this operation small pieces of healthy skin are cut from some other part of his body and put on the burn.

Burns are not always of the same kind all over. For example, part of a child's burn may be deep partial

HOW DEEP IS HIS BURN?

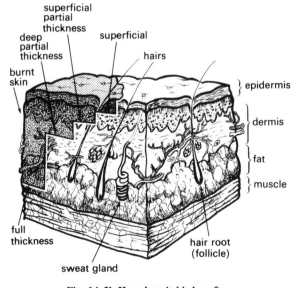

Fig. 14–2b How deep is his burn?

thickness, and the rest superficial. Burns with hot cooking oil are usually full thickness.

Where is the burn? Burns on a child's face are serious because they leave scars and deformities. If his eyes are burnt, he may become blind. If his hands are burnt, he may get contractures (1–9), so that he cannot straighten his fingers. If he has inhaled hot smoke, his respiratory tract may be burnt, and he may get pneumonia.

BURNS   14.2

IMMEDIATE TREATMENT. **If you see a child within 30 minutes of a burn, put the burnt part in cold water. This prevents the burn going deeper. After 30 minutes, cold water does not help.**

If he is shocked, treat him for shock (14.2).

EXAMINATION. **If he has a large burn, leave his clothes on until he reaches hospital.**

What percentage of his body has been burnt?

Look at Figure 14–2b. Try to find out what kind of burn he has. Have blisters started to form (superficial partial thickness)? Often we cannot diagnose how deep a burn is. We have to wait and see how it heals.

MANAGEMENT. **Decide early whether or not to send a child to hospital. Don't wait for him to get complications. Superficial burns of any size cure themselves. A child with a partial thickness burn of less than 5 per cent seldom needs intravenous fluid. If he has 5–15 per cent partial thickness burns he may need fluid. If he has more than 15 per cent partial thickness burns, he certainly needs fluid.**

If possible send him to hospital when he has—
—2 per cent or more full thickness burns.
—more than 15 per cent partial thickness burns (or less if care at home is not good, and you have few dressings).
—severe burns of his hands and face, or he is very young.
—inhaled hot smoke.

TREATMENT. **If the burn is dirty or there is ointment or local medicine on it, wash the burn. Use soap and clean water. If there is hair round the burn, cut it short.**

If there are vesicles on the burn, don't break them. They help to protect the burn from infection.

Dress the burn with sterile vaseline gauze, ordinary gauze, cotton wool, and a bandage. The vaseline gauze will stop the dressing sticking to the burn, and the cotton wool will absorb the fluid. Put on these dressings very carefully, so that the child does not become infected in the clinic. Don't put on the dressings too tight. If the burn is over a joint put on a splint. This keeps the joint straight and prevents contractures.   14.3

Change the dressings every two or three days.

Give him penicillin (3.15) for several days. If his burn becomes severely infected, he may need chloramphenicol or tetracycline. Prevent tetanus—see Section 18.16.

SEVERE BURNS AT HOME. **If you cannot send a severely burnt child to hospital, care for him at home. If possible let him sleep under a mosquito net. This will keep flies away. Treat any infection with antibiotics. Leave his burn open without a dressing. Give him plenty of food and fluids.**

EXPLANATION. **Teach mothers that if a child is burnt they must put the burnt part into cold water** *immediately.* **If his clothes are burning, they must put his whole body into water.**

If his mother has to look after him at home, tell her what she can do for him.

HEALTH EDUCATION LESSONS. **Think carefully about how to prevent burns in your district. Can mothers make fires safer? Can fireplaces be raised, so that children do not fall into them so easily? Can you teach mothers to turn the handles of their cooking pots away from the edge of the stove, so that children cannot pull the pots off the fire? Tell them not to put butter, or sauce, or anything else onto a burn.**

CUTS

14.4 'Yoyo has cut himself'

Children often cut themselves. Small cuts usually heal well if we clean them carefully, and cover them with iodine and a dry dressing. Sometimes the edges of a cut are pulled apart. There is a space beneath the edges of the skin and the skin no longer covers the tissues underneath. These cuts heal slowly because new skin takes time to grow in from the edges. Cuts heal more quickly if their edges are held together, so that skin covers the deeper tissues. You can do this with stitches, or with adhesive strapping. Before you decide to stitch up a cut, see if you can pull its edges together with strapping. This often works and is much less painful.

Usually, only the skin is cut. Sometimes nerves or tendons (the 'cords' which join muscles to bones) are cut also. These only heal if you sew them up. This is difficult in a health centre, so send these injuries to hospital.

Sometimes, a foreign body, such as a piece of bamboo, goes into a child's skin. If you do not take it out, it becomes infected and pus forms. Try to take it out. If you cannot take it out, send the child for help.

CARING FOR A CHILD WITH A CUT

HISTORY. **When was he cut? (If he was cut yesterday or earlier, his cut is probably infected, so don't stitch it.)**

EXAMINATION. **How big is the cut and where is it? (Send large cuts and cuts on the face to hospital.)**

Are any nerves or tendons cut? (This is especially important in the hand.) Ask him to touch the end of each of his fingers with his thumb. If he can do this his tendons have not been seriously cut.

Ask him to shut his eyes. Touch the skin below the cut with a piece of cloth. Can he feel it? (If he can feel when you

TESTING TO SEE IF NERVES OR TENDONS HAVE BEEN CUT

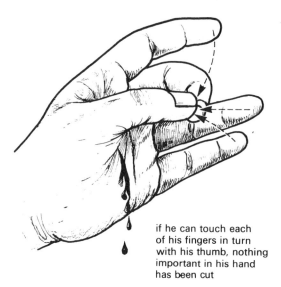

if he can touch each of his fingers in turn with his thumb, nothing important in his hand has been cut

Fig. 14–3 **Testing to see if nerves or tendons have been cut.**

touch him, his nerves are not cut. If there is any part which has no feeling, a nerve probably is cut.)

Is there dirt or any other foreign body in the wound? (If you stitch up a dirty cut it will probably become septic.)

Is there pus in the cut? (If a cut is already septic, don't stitch it, because it will not heal. Leave these cuts open and treat them as ulcers, 11.7.)

MANAGEMENT. **Send children to hospital if they have a large cut, or a cut on the face, and especially if they have a cut nerve or tendon.**

TREATMENT. **Ask a helper to hold the child. First try to clean all the dirt out. Hold the cut under a tap, or soak it in clean saline (3.48). If necessary take out larger pieces of dirt with forceps, or scrub the wound with gauze.**

Closing a cut with adhesive tape. **Cut the tape into pieces as shown in Figure 14–4. These easily stick to the skin and they do not stop fluid draining from the cut. Pull the edges of the skin together with them.**

Stitching. **Don't make the stitches too tight. Just bring the edges of the skin together. If you cannot get surgical nylon, use sewing thread or nylon fishing line. Sterilize this. Boil it.**

Put gauze on the wound and cover it with adhesive tape.

Antibiotics are not needed for every cut. Give a child penicillin if his cut is deep, or dirty, or if it has already become septic when you see it.

Prevent tetanus—see Section 18.16.

EXPLANATION. **Teach mothers how to care for cuts. Cuts easily become septic and cause ulcers or cellulitis.**

CLEAN THE DIRT OUT OF WOUNDS

OTHER INJURIES

14.5 'Tosin has hurt his leg and cannot walk' —bruises, sprains, and fractures.

A **bruise** is caused by bleeding into the tissues, such as the skin. A **sprain** is a tear in a joint or muscle. A **fracture** is a broken bone. Bruises and sprains heal well. Fractures heal if there is no deformity (abnormal shape) of the bones. But a fracture will not heal well if a child's arm or leg is deformed (bent) into the wrong shape. A fracture is also serious if a wound in the skin goes down to a broken bone. Bacteria can go in through the skin wound and infect the bone. Fractures like this are called **compound fractures.**

BRUISES, SPRAINS, AND FRACTURES

DIAGNOSIS. **Was he able to walk after the accident? (If he was able to walk, and the pain and swelling came later, he has probably not got a fracture.)**

Is there a cut in the skin over the injury? (If there is, he may have a compound fracture.)

EXAMINATION. **Don't move his injured arm or leg if this hurts him. Move his healthy arm or leg into the same position as the injured leg. Do they look the same? (A bruise or a sprain may cause a swelling, but the bone will be the same shape underneath it. If the fracture has caused a deformity, the bone will be a different shape.)**

MANAGEMENT. **If there is no deformity, treat him in the health centre. If there is deformity, or if the fracture is compound, send him for help.**

TREATMENT. **If necessary, treat the child for shock (14.2). Rest an injured arm until he wants to use it again. Tie a piece of cloth loosely around his neck and his wrist. We call this a 'collar and cuff'. If one leg is fractured, tie it to the other before you move him.**

Give him paracetamol (3.42) or aspirin (3.41) for his pain. Prevent tetanus—see Section 18.16.

POISONING

14.6 'Hannah has eaten her brother's tablets' —poisoning

Children swallow poisons of many kinds. These may be things in the house, such as kerosine, petrol, detergents, or bleaches. They may be poisonous leaves or berries. They may be drugs that the family have left lying about, such as aspirin, iron, pyrimethamine, or dapsone tablets.

HOW TO STITCH UP A CUT

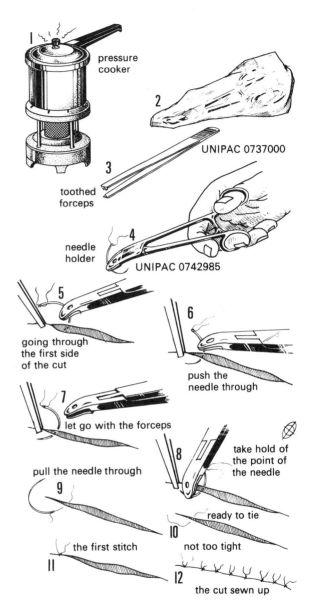

14.5

1 pressure cooker

2

UNIPAC 0737000

3 toothed forceps

needle holder

4 UNIPAC 0742985

14.4

5 going through the first side of the cut

6 push the needle through

7 let go with the forceps

8 take hold of the point of the needle

pull the needle through

9

10 ready to tie

the first stitch

not too tight

11

12 the cut sewn up

CLOSING A CUT WITH ADHESIVE TAPE

14.6

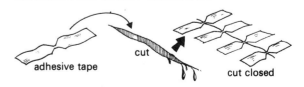

adhesive tape

cut

cut closed

Fig. 14–4 How to stitch up a cut.

Tablets are especially dangerous if they are covered with sugar and look like sweets. Any of these things may make a child very 'ill'. They can also cause coma, fits, and death. Fortunately, we can usually help him. We can find out what poison he has swallowed. If necessary we can remove it. We can also treat the symptoms it has caused.

What poison has the child taken? Some poisons need special treatment. So we must find out what poison a child has taken. We can wash some poisons out of a child's stomach. But washing out kerosene is dangerous. If even a little kerosine gets into his lungs by mistake, it may cause serious pneumonia. A corrosive ('burning') chemical, such as a strong acid or alkali, may injure his oesophagus. If you make him vomit, his oesophagus may tear.

When did the child eat the poison? If he took the poison only a few minutes ago, we can remove it before it causes much harm. If he took the poison many hours ago, and he has no symptoms, we need not worry about him. If he has no symptoms 36 hours after he ate the poison, he is probably safe.

RESTING A CHILD'S ARM IN A COLLAR AND CUFF

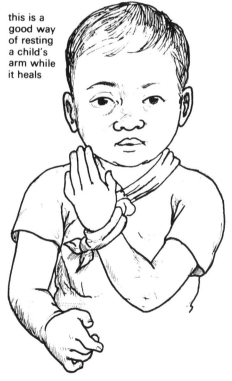

this is a good way of resting a child's arm while it heals

Fig. 14–5 Resting a child's arm in a 'collar and cuff'.

Remove the poison—empty his stomach. Some poisons cause diarrhoea and vomiting which helps to remove them from the body. If this does not happen, we can give the child ipecacuanha (3.47). This will make him vomit the poison. If you have not got ipecacuanha—put a spatula down his throat. Do this as soon as possible. But don't try to make him vomit if he has swallowed a corrosive poison or kerosine. Don't make him vomit if he is comatose or half comatose, because vomit may go into his lungs and kill him.

MAKING A CHILD VOMIT BY PUTTING A SPATULA DOWN HIS THROAT

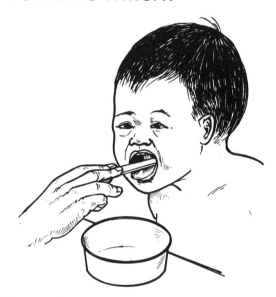

Fig. 14–6 Making a child vomit by putting a spatula down his throat.

MAKING A CHILD VOMIT

USING IPECACUANHA. **Go to Section 3.47.**

USING A RUBBER TUBE OR A SPATULA. **If the child has not eaten or drunk for more than an hour, his stomach will be almost empty. Give him a drink so that he has something to vomit the poison with. Lay him across a couch or bed. If necessary get several helpers to hold him. Rub the back of his throat with the tube from a stethoscope, or a spatula, or your finger, until he vomits.**

MAKE A CONSCIOUS CHILD VOMIT HIS POISON SOON, BUT NOT WHEN HE HAS SWALLOWED KEROSINE OR CORROSIVES

14.7 Caring for a poisoned child

HISTORY

What has he swallowed? (Some poisons, such as kerosine, need special treatment.) How much has he swallowed? When did he swallow it? (If a poison has not caused any symptoms in 36 hours, it probably won't harm him.) Has he vomited? (This may have removed some of the poison.)

MAKING A CHILD VOMIT THE POISON HE HAS SWALLOWED

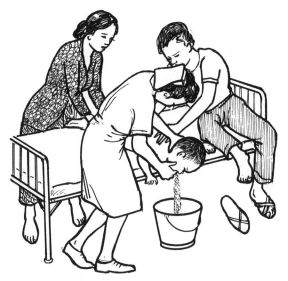

Fig. 14–7 Making a child vomit the poison he has swallowed.

EXAMINATION   14.7

Is he 'well' or is he 'ill'? (Don't worry about a well child who swallowed poison more than 36 hours ago.)

Is he shocked? (Severe poisoning may cause shock.) Is he drowsy or comatose? (Some drugs, such as phenobarbitone, may cause drowsiness or coma.) Has he any signs of pneumonia? (Some poisons cause penumonia after a few hours.)

MANAGEMENT AND TREATMENT

ALL POISONS, EXCEPT KEROSINE, CORROSIVES, AND THE UNCONSCIOUS CHILD

It is less than four hours since he swallowed poison. **Make him vomit (14.6), if he has not already vomited a lot. Observe him carefully.**

It is between 4 and 36 hours since he swallowed poison. **If he has any symptoms, send him for help. If he has no symptoms, observe him carefully until 36 hours have passed.**

It is more than 36 hours since he swallowed poisons. **If he is well, he needs no treatment. If he has any symptoms, send him for help. If you cannot do this, treat any symptoms you can.**

KEROSINE OR CORROSIVE POISONING (STRONG ACIDS AND ALKALIS)
Don't make him vomit, and don't wash out his stomach. If he swallowed kerosine, give him procaine penicillin for five days. If he has any symptoms send him for help.

TREATING SYMPTOMS (ALL POISONS)
Treat any dehydration (9.17), fits (15.9), pneumonia (8.15), or coma (14.8) which the poison has caused.

Don't put kerosene in 'Coke' bottles!

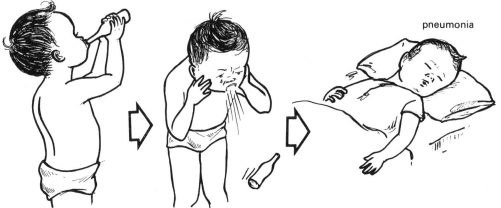

Fig. 14–8 Kerosine (paraffin) is a very common poison.

169

EXPLANATION AND EDUCATION

Explain to his mother what you are doing for him. Teach families to keep their kerosine where children cannot get it. Teach them not to store poisons with food. Teach them not to leave medicine, especially sugar-covered tablets, in places where children can get them.

DROWSINESS OR COMA

14.8 'Siti seems to be asleep, but I cannot wake her up'—coma

Any severe illness can make a child drowsy (abnormally sleepy). As the disease becomes worse he goes into coma (5:2). If a healthy child is sleepy, or asleep, we can easily wake him up. But we cannot wake a child who is drowsy or in coma. A child in coma is in great danger and may easily die.

Drowsiness and coma can be caused by any very severe illness especially cerebral malaria, meningitis, dehydration, a head injury, or poisons. Most fits (15.1) cause coma for a short time after the fit. Head injuries and fits are easy to diagnose. But we can easily forget that a child might have cerebral malaria. So, if this might be the cause of his drowsiness or coma, give him chloroquine or quinine by injection—now.

DON'T FORGET CEREBRAL MALARIA WHEN A CHILD IS IN COMA

An unconscious child cannot cough, so if vomit or saliva goes into his lungs, he cannot cough it up. If it stays in his lungs, he may drown or it may cause pneumonia. We can prevent this. Lie him on his side, so that vomit and saliva fall out of his mouth, and do not go into his lungs. Also, if an unconscious child lies on his back, his tongue may fall back into his throat and obstruct his breathing. Prevent this. Lie him on his side.

ABNORMAL DROWSINESS AND COMA

HISTORY. **Has he had an accident? A fit? Does he live in a malarious area? Has he taken any poisons? What symptoms did he have before his drowsiness or coma began?**

EXAMINATION. **How deep is his coma? Can you wake him a little? Meningeal signs (15.6)? Signs of dehydration (9.18)? Large spleen (malaria)? Other signs of severe illness?**

SPECIAL TESTS. **Examine a blood slide for malaria parasites (L 7.31). If he has not had a head injury, or swallowed poison, he needs a lumbar puncture (15.3).**

DIAGNOSIS. **Any very severe illness? Cerebral malaria (10.7)? Head injury? Poisoning (14.7)? Meningitis (15.6)? Hypoglycaemia from severe malnutrition (7.10)?**

MANAGEMENT. **Send a child in coma to hospital quickly. While he is waiting to go, or if you have to treat him yourself, treat him like this.**

KEEP MEDICINES AWAY FROM CHILDREN

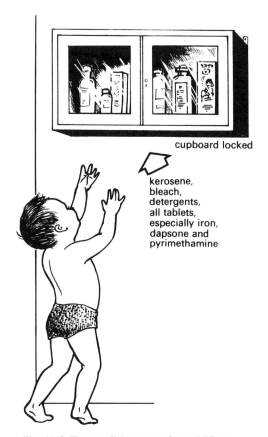

cupboard locked

kerosene,
bleach,
detergents,
all tablets,
especially iron,
dapsone and
pyrimethamine

Fig. 14–9 Keep medicines away from children.

Coma

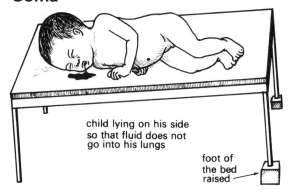

child lying on his side
so that fluid does not
go into his lungs

foot of
the bed
raised

Fig. 14–10 Lie a comatose child on his side.

SYMPTOMATIC TREATMENT. **Lie the child on one side or on his front with his head on one side. Put his feet higher than his head, so that if he vomits, his vomit comes out of his lungs more easily. If you have a sucker, suck out his throat.**

Look at his breathing carefully and listen to it. If he has difficult breathing, move his head into the position where he breathes most easily. Try gently pulling his tongue and jaw upwards and forwards. If possible, put in an airway. This is a short curved tube. Put it into a patient's mouth to keep his tongue forward and so help him to breathe more easily.

If his eyelids are not shut, close them.
Give him penicillin if he has signs of pneumonia.
Give him intravenous fluid. He needs 120 ml/kg/day.

TREAT THE CAUSE OF HIS COMA. **If he might have cerebral malaria, give him chloroquine or quinine (3.25).**

**DON'T LEAVE A COMATOSE CHILD
ON HIS BACK**

14.8

15 Fits

15.1 Fits are serious

When an older child has a fit, he suddenly becomes unconscious and falls to the ground. All his muscles contract at the same time so that his body becomes stiff (unable to bend). He stops breathing, and he becomes cyanosed (blue). His eyes move around, and turn upwards, but he does not seem to see anything. Sometimes he vomits, passes urine or faeces, or bites his tongue. After about half a minute, he starts to breathe again. His arms and legs make strong movements. These movements stop after two or three minutes and then he sleeps deeply.

Fits are not so easily recognized in a baby. His mother probably sees he is having a fit, only if she is holding him. A baby moves his eyes in the same way as an older child. He becomes blue and stiff for a minute or two, and then he goes to sleep.

Learn to diagnose fits from the history. For example, if a mother says that her baby became blue and stiff, ask her if his eyes moved. Mothers usually know about fits, and there is usually a local word for them. Fits are different from the spasms (contractions) of tetanus (18.16). A child with tetanus has spasms of his muscles, especially his back muscles. These spasms make him bend over backwards. He does not lose consciousness, and he cries with pain.

**A CHILD WITH FITS LOSES CONSCIOUSNESS
A CHILD WITH THE SPASMS OF TETANUS
IS CONSCIOUS**

15.2 The meninges and the CSF

Fits are caused by lesions of the brain. Before you can treat a child with a fit, you must know about the fluid round the brain.

At the bottom of the brain there is a big nerve called the **spinal cord**. It is about as thick as your little finger and goes down inside the **vertebral column** (spine). The brain and the spinal cord are soft and easily injured, so they are protected by several coverings called **meninges**. There is a narrow space between the meninges, filled with a clear fluid called the **cerebrospinal fluid** or **CSF**. The CSF goes all round the brain and spinal cord. Normal CSF looks like clean water and contains a little protein (less than 40 mg/dl) and a few white cells (less than 5 in a microlitre). We can count these cells with a microscope. There is also an easy test to see if there is more protein than normal in the CSF (Pandy's test, 15–6).

15.3 Lumbar puncture

Healthy CSF is sterile. If organisms grow in a child's meninges and CSF, he has **meningitis**, and is seriously ill. The best way to diagnose meningitis is to take some CSF from a child and examine it. We take CSF by lumbar puncture. 'Lumbar' means the lower part of the back. To puncture something is to make a hole in it. When a child has a lumbar puncture, we push a needle between the bones of his spine into the space containing CSF.

We can easily do a lumbar puncture in a health centre. The child need not go to hospital. Lumbar puncture must be done with a completely sterile needle. If you put an infected needle into a child's CSF, the organisms on the needle may cause meningitis. So only people who have been carefully taught should do lumbar puncture.

**ONLY DO A LUMBAR PUNCTURE
IF YOU HAVE BEEN TAUGHT HOW**

The best needle for a child is a sterile disposable 0·9 × 40 mm short bevel intramuscular needle (3–8). These needles are very useful, because they are already sterilized. If you have not got a sterile disposable needle, use an ordinary intramuscular needle. It should be new and it must be sharp. Intramuscular needles are useful for children less than five years old. Older children and adults need special lumbar puncture needles.

Make lumbar puncture safer by using iodine as an antiseptic. Iodine kills organisms on the child's skin, and on your fingers. If you use an ordinary needle, sterilize it in a pressure cooker or boil it carefully. Don't let microorganisms get onto it after it has been boiled, and before it goes into the child. Don't touch its point with your

HOW WE TAKE CSF FROM A CHILD BY LUMBAR PUNCTURE

the needle in the child

A

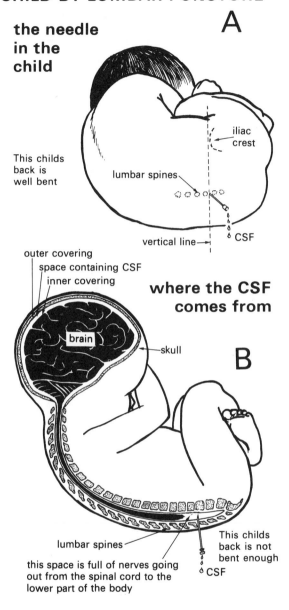

This childs back is well bent

iliac crest

lumbar spines

vertical line

CSF

outer covering
space containing CSF
inner covering

where the CSF comes from

brain

skull

B

lumbar spines

this space is full of nerves going out from the spinal cord to the lower part of the body

This childs back is not bent enough

CSF

Fig. 15–1 How we take CSF from a child by lumbar puncture.

fingers—if organisms got into the CSF, they grow very easily. So there must be *no* live organisms on a lumbar puncture needle.

A DIRTY LUMBAR PUNCTURE CAN CAUSE MENINGITIS

NEEDLES FOR LUMBAR PUNCTURE

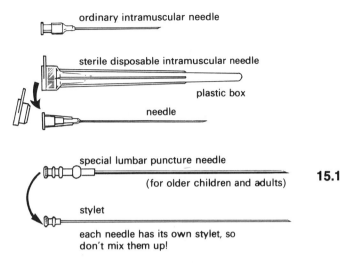

ordinary intramuscular needle

sterile disposable intramuscular needle

plastic box

needle

special lumbar puncture needle

(for older children and adults)

stylet

each needle has its own stylet, so don't mix them up!

Fig. 15–2 Needles for lumbar puncture.

15.1

15.3

LUMBAR PUNCTURE

Give the child some paraldehyde (3.44) to make him sleepy.

A HELPER AND THE EQUIPMENT. **Find someone to help you. Put some tincture of iodine into a small bowl—no other antiseptic is so good. Get a syringe, some cotton wool or gauze, and two small clean bottles (or tubes) for the CSF. Take two disposable 0·9 × 40 mm intramuscular needles. If you have not got these, get two ordinary intramuscular needles. Blow water through them with a syringe to make sure they are not blocked. Use a pressure cooker for sterilizing. If you have not got this, get a pan with a lid, and a stove which will boil water fast. Two needles are better than one, because one of them may touch something unsterile by mistake, or fall on the floor.**

STERILIZING IN A PRESSURE COOKER—**see Section 6.13**

STERILIZING BY BOILING
1. Put the needles into the pan. Cover them with about 3 cm of water. Put the lid on the pan and boil the water. After it has started boiling, keep it boiling for 15 minutes.

2. Hold the lid on the pan and carefully pour out all the water. Don't let the needles fall out. Practise this before you boil the needles.

3. The needles are now nearly dry inside the sterile pan. Leave them there until you are ready. Never put the needles anywhere else. Keep them on the sterile bottom of this pan.

GETTING THE CHILD READY
Before you wash, show your helper how to hold the child.

15.2

STERILISING LUMBAR PUNCTURE NEEDLES

1 Sterilising

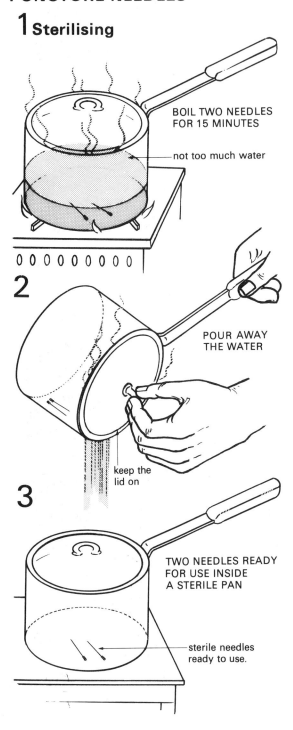

BOIL TWO NEEDLES FOR 15 MINUTES

not too much water

2

POUR AWAY THE WATER

keep the lid on

3

TWO NEEDLES READY FOR USE INSIDE A STERILE PAN

sterile needles ready to use.

Fig. 15–3 Sterilizing lumbar puncture needles.

The way the child is held is very important. His back must be well curved.

Put him on the side of a table or hard couch. Ask your helper to put one hand behind his head, and the other hand behind his knees. Tell him to bend the child's back as much as possible. This opens up the spaces between the vertebrae (bones of the spine). Make sure that his back is straight up and down, like the wall, not sloping. The child in Picture A, Figure 15–1 is held very well, but the child in Picture B is not bent enough.

PUTTING IN THE NEEDLE

Wash your hands. If possible use a scrubbing brush and running water.

Make a piece of cotton wool or gauze wet with iodine. Swab the lower part of the child's back and iliac crest with iodine. The iliac crest is the top part of the pelvic bone. Start cleaning over the place where you are going to make the hole and move outwards in circles. Do this three times using three iodine swabs. *Leave the iodine on the skin.*

Dip the fingers of both your hands into the bowl of iodine.

Use your left little finger to feel for his iliac crest. Follow a line from the iliac crest down across the child. This is the line shown in Picture A Figure 15–1. It will cross the fourth lumbar spine, or the space between the third and fourth spines. You can easily feel the lumbar spines and the

DOING A LUMBAR PUNCTURE

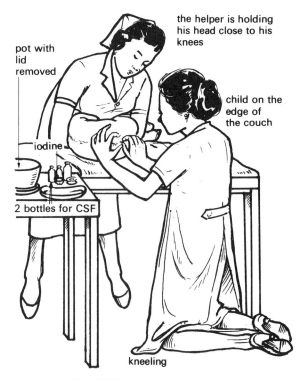

the helper is holding his head close to his knees

pot with lid removed

iodine

2 bottles for CSF

child on the edge of the couch

kneeling

Fig. 15–4 Doing a lumbar puncture.

174

spaces between them through the skin. Put your needle into the middle of any space below the second lumbar spine. If you put it into a higher space, you may harm the spinal cord.

Do not touch the point of the needle with your finger. Don't let the needle touch anything that has not been covered with iodine.

Push the needle into the child between two of his lumbar spines. Push it straight in and point it towards his umbilicus. It must go in parallel to (in the same direction as) the top of the table. It must not point up or down. It will suddenly go in more easily when it gets into the space containing CSF. CSF will come out as soon as it is in this space. If no CSF comes out, turn the needle round, and push it a little further in.

If you feel the needle hit bone, pull it out, and push it in again. If still no CSF comes, take the needle out. Put the second needle into the next space. If no CSF comes, stop—see Section 5.23.

If the neeedle touches anything before it goes into the child don't use it. Use the second needle or boil it up again.

As soon as CSF comes out, hold each of the two small bottles underneath. Allow about 2 ml to drip into each.

Sometimes the needle cuts a small blood vessel, so that there is blood in the CSF. This does not harm the child, but it spoils the CSF for testing. Stop and try again later, if necessary. If the child might have purulent meningitis, treat him for it.

**LUMBAR PUNCTURE IS EASIER IF
A CHILD IS HELD PROPERLY**

---

the needle in horizontally

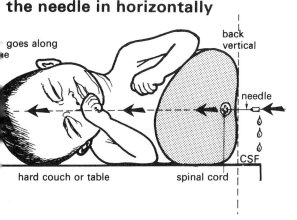

goes along ¦e

back
vertical

needle

CSF

hard couch or table   spinal cord

Fig. 15–5 Hold the child's back vertical and put in the needle horizontally.

15.3b Examining the CSF

A health centre should have a small laboratory which can examine CSF. If there is no laboratory, here are two easy ways you can examine CSF.

Is the CSF clear or turbid (cloudy, milky)? White cells from the blood can get into the CSF and make it into pus (2.4). This makes the CSF turbid. If CSF is even a little turbid, it is abnormal, and has at least 100 cells per microlitre. In severe purulent meningitis the CSF looks like pus. If lumbar puncture has been difficult, blood may get into the CSF and make it red. But, if lumbar puncture has been easy, and the CSF is even slightly cloudy, the child probably has meningitis.

EXAMINING THE CSF FOR TURBIDITY

Get a small test tube or bottle, like the bottle the CSF is in. Fill it with clean water. Hold the tubes of CSF and the water up to the light. If the CSF is as clear as the water it has got less than 100 white cells per microlitre. It is probably normal. The bottles or tubes must be clean and clear (not scratched).

Pandy's test for protein in the CSF. Pandy's solution is a mixture of phenol in water. When you add a few drops of normal CSF to it, nothing happens. But, if the CSF contains too much protein, it becomes cloudy. Most diseases of the meninges, and some diseases of the brain, cause more protein to come into CSF. They give a positive Pandy's test. This shows that a child has a disease of his brain or meninges. But it does not show what kind of disease he has. A positive Pandy's test usually means that he has meningitis. If Pandy's test is negative, and his CSF is clear, he has probably not got meningitis.

Pandy's test is useful because it becomes positive when there is between 25 and 35 mg/dl of protein in the CSF. But a normal child may have a CSF protein up to 40 mg/dl. So occasionally a very mildly positive (trace positive) Pandy's test is normal, especially in newborn babies. A strongly positive Pandy's test is always abnormal. It usually means that the child has meningitis.

Occasionally, there are bacteria in the CSF when Pandy's test is negative, and there are a normal number of cells. So, if possible, stain (colour) the CSF and examine it with a microscope (L 11.5).

PANDY'S TEST

Fill a bottle (about 100 ml) a quarter full of phenol. Fill it to the top with water. Shake it, and leave it until the next day. There will be liquid phenol at the bottom of the bottle, and a mixture of phenol in water on top of it. This is Pandy's solution.

Carefully pour some Pandy's solution into a test tube. Don't let the liquid phenol come with it. Let a few drops of CSF fall into it. Look at it against something dark. If it is cloudy, Pandy's test is positive.

These are the easiest ways of examining the CSF. A health centre laboratory should also be able to count the cells in it (L 9.9). The laboratory should be able to say what kind of cells they are and look for bacteria (L 9.11).

These special tests make the diagnosis of meningitis more exact—always do them if you can.

Diseases which cause fits

15.4 'Ismail has had a fit'—febrile convulsions, cerebral malaria, dehydration, meningitis, epilepsy, poisoning

Often, we cannot easily diagnose if a child has meningitis or a febrile convulsion. But the diagnosis is important. Meningitis is serious and rare. Febrile convulsions are not serious and are common.

15.5 Febrile convulsions

A convulsion is a fit. Acute infections cause a high fever. This fever can cause convulsions. So these fits are called febrile convulsions. The acute infection can be otitis media, malaria, or something else. The best way to treat a febrile convulsion is to cool a child's fever. When his temperature is lowered, his fit stops. A child who has had a febrile convulsion may have another convulsion when he has a fever again. Febrile convulsions are most common in children between six months and four years old. As a child grows older he is less likely to have convulsions.

THE COMMONEST FITS ARE FEBRILE CONVULSIONS

FEBRILE CONVULSIONS

TREATMENT. **Treat him for hyperpyrexia (10.4). Cool him immediately, and then treat the cause of his fever, such as**

PANDY'S TEST AND EXAMINING THE CSF FOR TURBIDITY

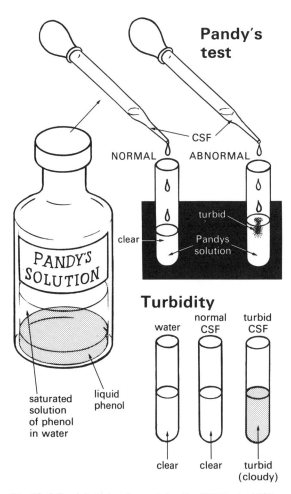

Fig. 15–6 Pandy's test and examining the CSF for turbidity.

DIAGNOSE MENINGITIS BEFORE THIS HAPPENS

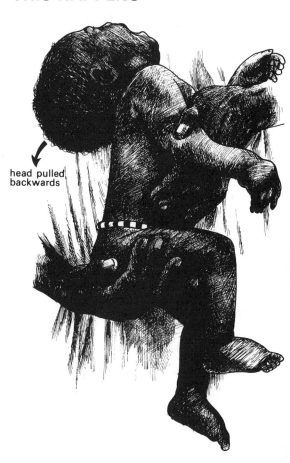

head pulled backwards

Fig. 15–6b Diagnose meningitis before this happens.

otitis media (17.9). Give him paracetamol (3.42) or aspirin. Phenobarbitone helps to stop fits, so give this for three days (3.43).

PREVENTION. If he has had several convulsions with fever, malaria has probably caused them. So suppress his malaria with pyrimethamine or chloroquine (3.25).

EXPLANATION. Ask his mother what she thinks caused his fits. Explain how you think they were caused. Tell her to keep him cool, both in this illness, and when he has a fever again. Tell her to put very few clothes on him when he has a fever (10.4). If she feels him getting hot, tell her to cool him with water (10–4), and give him aspirin. Explain the dose carefully. If his malaria is not being suppressed, she must give him chloroquine when he has a fever again.

15.6 Meningitis

Organisms can grow in a child's meninges and CSF, and harm his brain. This causes meningitis. Organisms get into his CSF from the top of his nose, which is very close to his brain, or from his middle ear (17.2). They can come through his blood from some other part of his body, such as his gut. They can also get into his CSF on a dirty lumbar puncture needle (15.3). Pyogenic bacteria cause purulent meningitis. Viruses, and TB bacilli also cause meningitis. Purulent meningitis and TB meningitis always kill a child if you don't diagnose him early and treat him carefully. TB usually causes symptoms (13:1) for several months before it causes meningitis. Prevent TB meningitis by diagnosing and treating TB early. Viruses meningitis is less serious. Most children recover by themselves.

PREVENT TB MENINGITIS—DIAGNOSE AND TREAT TB EARLY

The meningeal signs. These signs are caused by the muscles of a child's back contracting, but there are no muscle spasms. (Tetanus causes abnormal muscle contractions *and* sudden spasms.) Meningitis which has lasted several days makes a child's head bend backwards, like the child in Figure 15–6b. You must diagnose meningitis before it does this. You will see meningeal signs most easily in adults and older children. Sometimes, you will see them in a one-year-old child. You will seldom see them in babies.

THREE MENINGEAL SIGNS IN OLDER CHILDREN

NECK STIFFNESS, PICTURE A (15–7).
Lie an older child on his back. Put your hand behind his head and lift it forwards, so that his chin touches his chest. A normal child can easily touch his chest with his chin. A

Neck stiffness

OLDER CHILDREN **A**
a healthy child can touch his chest with his chin, this child with meningitis cannot

PAIN!

15.4

15.5

15.6

YOUNGER CHILDREN **B**
a healthy child cannot be made to sit up, but meningitis makes a child's neck stiff so that he can be raised to the sitting position

PAIN!

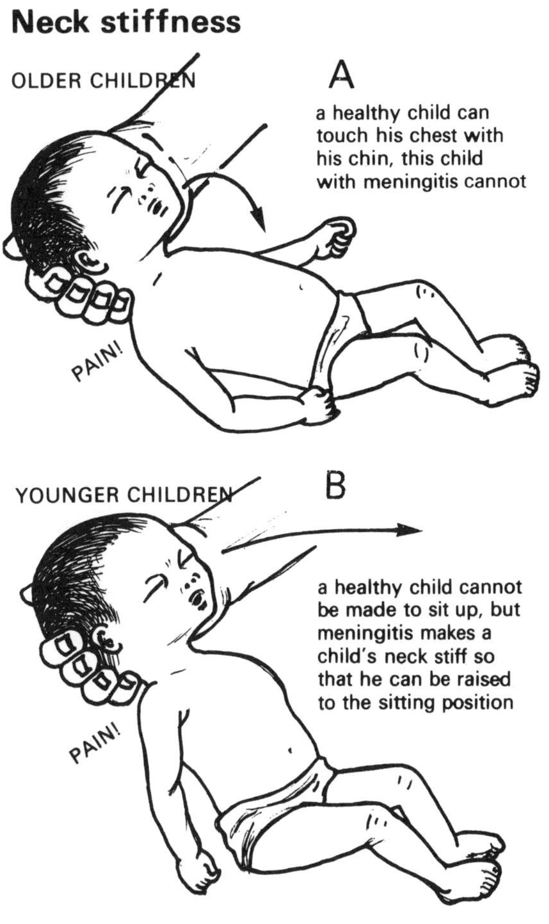

Fig. 15–7 Examining child for neck stiffness.

child with meningitis cannot do this. Bending his head forwards hurts him.

If he is only about a year old, lie him on his back—Picture B (15–7). Put your hand behind his head, and try to lift him, so that he sits up. A healthy child bends his neck and back, and you cannot make him sit up. If he has meningitis his back muscles contract, so that you can easily lift him up by his head.

KERNIG'S SIGN, PICTURE C (15–8)
Lie him on his back with his knees bent. Bend one of his thighs upwards as shown in the figure. Try to straighten his knee. You can easily do this in a healthy child, and it does not hurt. But if a child has meningitis you cannot straighten his knee. The muscles at the back of his leg contract and hurt him as they are pulled. A child like this has a positive Kernig's sign.

'HEAD BETWEEN THE KNEES SIGN' PICTURE D (15–8)
Try to put his head between his knees. A normal child can do this easily. A child with meningitis cannot do this, because his back is too stiff.

KERNIG'S SIGN AND THE HEAD BETWEEN THE KNEES SIGN

Kernig's sign

You can straighten a healthy child's leg without hurting him, You cannot do this if he has meningitis

C

PAIN!

The head between the knees sign

D

You can easily put a healthy child's head between the knees. You cannot do this if he has meningitis

PAIN!

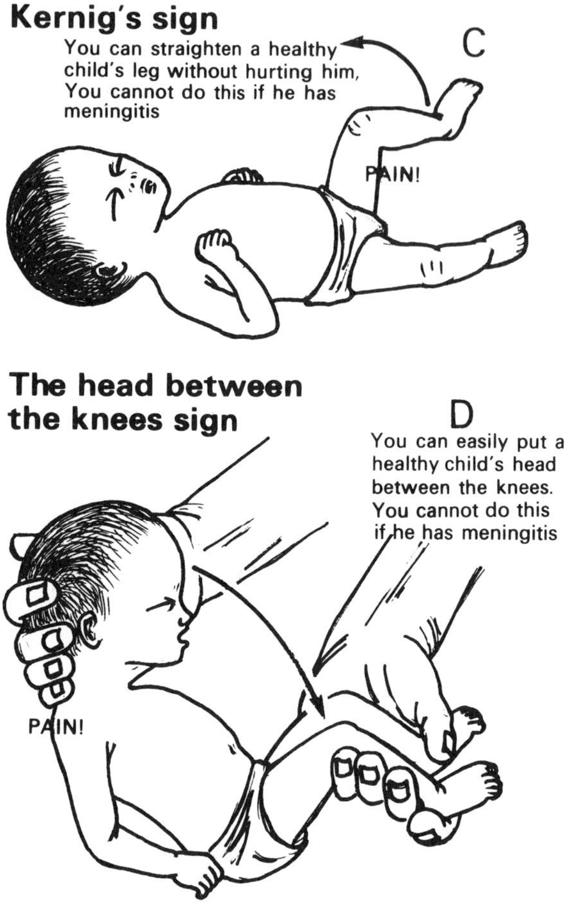

Fig. 15–8 Kernig's sign and the head between the knees sign.

Babies have a meningeal sign of their own—the swollen fontanelle. A child's fontanelle closes as he grows older. So you can only diagnose meningitis (or dehydration 9.17) by this sign, when a child is less than about a year old. Meningitis often causes vomiting, and vomiting causes dehydration. This reduces the swelling caused by the meningitis. So you may not find a swollen fontanelle if a baby with meningitis has been vomiting. Swelling of the fontanelle is a *late* sign. Try to diagnose meningitis before the fontanelle swells.

A SWOLLEN FONTANELLE—BABIES IN WHOM THE FONTANELLE HAS NOT CLOSED FIGURE 15–9
The fontanelle of a healthy baby is soft and almost flat. Meningitis makes it swell and stops it pulsating (moving). Feel his fontanelle to see if it is swollen. Crying makes a

Signs in the fontanelle

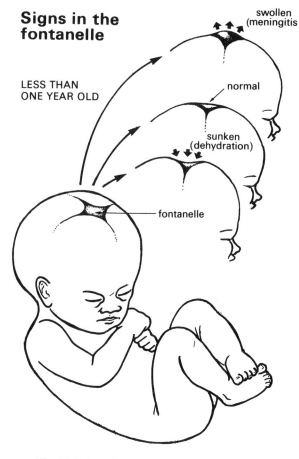

LESS THAN ONE YEAR OLD

swollen (meningitis

normal

sunken (dehydration)

fontanelle

Fig. 15–9 A swollen fontanelle is a sign of meningitis.

normal fontanelle swell a little, so try to feel it at the beginning of the examination, before he starts to cry.

DIAGNOSE MENINGITIS EARLY

Occasionally, some other disease, such as pneumonia, malaria, tonsillitis, or otitis media, causes meningeal signs. But the child's CSF is normal and he does not have meningitis. He has **meningism** which is harmless. Lumbar puncture is the only way to find out if a child has meningism or meningitis.

Signs at any age. In children of *any* age meningitis causes fever, not eating (or sucking), vomiting, fits, and drowsiness. Children who are not treated go into coma. You *must* diagnose them and send them for treatment *before* they become drowsy and go into coma. Occasionally, there is a petechial rash (11.2). Usually, the other signs come before the fits. Sometimes, the fits come first.

Signs in older child. He is old enough to say that he has a severe headache. Usually he has meningeal signs.

Signs in a child between one and two. He has a high sharp 'meningeal cry'. He may have meningeal signs, or he may not.

Signs in a baby under one year. He has small movements of parts of his body ('twitches') and a meningeal cry. He usually has no meningeal signs. Sometimes he has a swollen fontanelle.

Meningitis is difficult to diagnose in a child under two. If he has several signs, such as fever, drowsiness, not sucking, or fits, he may have meningitis. The only way to be sure he has not got meningitis is to do a lumbar puncture.

What kind of meningitis is it? This is often difficult to decide. Virus meningitis and purulent meningitis come quickly, usually in a few hours, or one or two days. TB meningitis comes more slowly. A child has usually been ill for more than ten days before he comes to see you. But a mother may not tell you this if you do not ask her. Often the first sign she notices is a fit or vomiting. TB meningitis is difficult to diagnose from purulent meningitis in a health centre. If you are not sure, treat a child for purulent meningitis. If he is not much recovered in two days he may have TB meningitis.

All kinds of meningitis cause more protein and white cells to come in the CSF, so that it looks turbid. If a child's CSF is turbid, he needs treatment immediately. If his CSF is not turbid, examine it for cells, protein and bacteria (L 9.12). This is the only way to be sure he has not got meningitis.

A CHILD WITH A TURBID CSF NEEDS IMMEDIATE TREATMENT

A primary care worker must diagnose meningitis and send the children who have it to hospital. But you may have to treat a child yourself. Treat him for purulent meningitis in the way described below. Penicillin is the most important part of the treatment. Start IMMEDIATELY and give him a complete course. If he is treated late or if he is not treated carefully, his brain may be harmed. He may become backward (24.12), blind, or deaf.

PURULENT MENINGITIS

MANAGEMENT
If you have done a lumbar puncture, send the child to hospital with his specimen of CSF. Give him his first penicillin injection before he goes. If possible, give him *benzyl* penicillin (*not* procaine penicillin) slowly intravenously.

EARLY TREATMENT

INTRAVENOUS DRIP
Put up a drip of half strength Darrow's solution and give him—
— 50 ml per hour if he is over 20 kg
— 25 ml per hour if he is between 5 and 20 kg
— 10 ml per hour if he is under 5 kg
If you cannot give him an intravenous drip, give him intragastric fluid. Each day he needs 120/ml/kg.

ANTIMICROBIAL DRUGS
Give him all these drugs at the same time. If he cannot take his oral drugs by mouth, give them down a tube.

Penicillin. If he is over 5 kg give him 600 mg (one mega-unit) of benzyl penicillin into his drip every three hours.
If he is under 5 kg give him 150 mg ($\frac{1}{4}$ mega-unit) of benzyl penicillin into his drip every six hours.

Chloramphenicol. Give him 100 mg/kg/day. If he is less than two months old, don't give him chloramphenicol. Give him 30 mg/kg/day of intramuscular streptomycin.

Chloroquine. If he comes from a malarious area, give him one dose of chloroquine by subcutaneous injection immediately (3–17).

FITS
Give him phenobarbitone by mouth to prevent fits. If necessary you can double the dose in Figure 3–16.
If he has fits before this treatment has had time to work, or if it does not work, give him phenobarbitone or paraldehyde (3.44) by injection.

COMA
Keep his airway clear and nurse him on his front (14.8).

LATER TREATMENT
Each day see how 'well' or 'ill' he is (5.15). Take his temperature, feel his fontanelle, look for signs of dehydration. Ask how much urine he has passed, or if he has had fits.
If, in two or three days, he is getting better, change the penicillin to 300 mg by intramuscular injection four times a day. Go on with penicillin and chloramphenicol treatment for fourteen days.
If he was treated early and is not much better in 48 hours, he probably has TB meningitis.

EXPLANATION
Tell his mother that treatment takes a long time, but that he must have it all. Explain that he must have plenty of fluids.

15.7 Cerebral malaria

Malaria causes fever. If this is severe it may cause febrile convulsions. The parasites of falciparum malaria (10.7) can also cause fits. The parasites block the capillaries of the brain. So a child with cerebral malaria can have fits for two reasons—fever, and malaria of his brain. Often, we cannot be sure which of these two is causing his fits. In febrile convulsions the CSF is always normal. But cerebral malaria occasionally gives a positive Pandy's test with up to 100 mg/dl of protein, and up to 100 cells per microlitre. Cerebral malaria rarely makes the CSF turbid. It often kills children. So, where *P. falciparum* is common, the only safe rule is to give subcutaneous chloroquine (3.25, 10.7) or intravenous quinine to every child with a fit.

IN A MALARIOUS AREA A CHILD WITH A FIT NEEDS SUBCUTANEOUS CHLOROQUINE IMMEDIATELY

15.8 Epilepsy

This is a brain disease which causes fits. It usually starts between the ages of five and twenty-five years. If a child has a fit without a fever, and then gets well, he probably has epilepsy. If he has several fits like this with days or weeks between them, he almost certainly has epilepsy. Epilepsy can also make a child backward (24.9). Phenobarbitone (3.43) may prevent his fits, but don't give him so much that he becomes drowsy. Send him for help.

15.9 Caring for a child with a fit

If a child is still having a fit when you see him, treat him quickly. If it goes on too long it will harm his brain and may make him backward. When his fit has stopped, you can start to diagnose what caused it.

If the baby is newborn go to Section 26.42

IF HE IS STILL HAVING A FIT. **Turn the child onto his front, so that if he vomits, the vomit will come out of his mouth, and not go down into his lungs (14.8). Make sure his tongue is forward, so that he can breath easily.**

If you have oxygen, and he is cyanosed, give it to him.

Don't stop him moving, but stop him hurting himself. He may bite his tongue, so put something between his teeth, such as a piece of cloth wrapped round a spatula.

Give him paraldehyde (3.44) or phenobarbitone (3.43), intramuscularly, to stop the fits before they harm his brain. If his fit has still not stopped ten minutes later, give him one more **dose.**

If he feels hot, don't wait to take his temperature. Take off all his clothes and cool him with water (10.4).

In a malarious area give all children with a fit subcutaneous chloroquine immediately (3.25, 10.7), and also any other treatment they may need.

HISTORY. **Did he have sudden high fever for a few hours before the fits (febrile convulsions)?**

Did his illness come on quickly (febrile convulsions, purulent meningitis)? Was he mildly ill (stage C, and los-

ing weight 5:2) for several weeks, or months before the fit (TB meningitis)?

Has he had fits before with other fevers (febrile convulsions)?

Has he swallowed any poison (some poisons cause fits)?

Milestones normal (several diseases which cause fits also make a child backward)?

EXAMINATION. **What is his temperature? (If he is hotter than 39°C, his fever may have caused his fits.)**

Has he got severe diarrhoea? Is he dehydrated? (If he has severe diarrhoea he probably has hypernatraemic dehydration 9.18. He needs intravenous fluids 9.27, 9.29).

Examine his ears (otitis media).

Examine his throat (tonsillitis).
Look for the signs of a lower respiratory infection (8.9) (pneumonia).

Severely malnourished (hypoglycaemia)?

LUMBAR PUNCTURE. **Most children who have had a fit during the last few hours** should **have a lumbar puncture. There is no other way to be sure they have not got meningitis. A child does not need a lumbar puncture if—**

—you know he has epilepsy, and he has no fever.

—his fit was more than six hours ago and he is now completely normal.

He has probably had a FEBRILE CONVULSION so that lumbar puncture is less important if—

—he is one to five years old

—AND he has only had one fit

—AND there was a sudden rise in temperature before the fit

—AND the fit lasted less than 15 minutes

—AND he is completely conscious after it

—AND he has some other infection outside his brain, such as tonsillitis.

HE MUST have a lumbar puncture if—

—he is under one year old

—OR his fontanelle is swollen or not pulsating

—OR he has no signs of dehydration, or of an infection such as otitis media (17.9) which is causing his fever

—OR he has had more than one fit during this illness

—OR he has had a fit which lasted more than 15 minutes

—OR the movements of his fit were in one part of his body only, such as his arm (focal fits)

—OR he was paralysed or unconscious for more than half an hour after the fit

—OR he has any meningeal signs, such as neck stiffness, or a positive Kernig's sign.

In a malarious area, he should have a lumbar puncture, even if there are malaria parasites in his blood. He may have malaria and meningitis.

SPECIAL TESTS. **Examine his CSF for turbidity and protein (Pandy's test, 15–6). Count the cells in it, and stain it for bacteria (L 9.11).**

If he comes from a malarious area, look for malaria parasites in his blood film (L 7.31) (cerebral malaria).

DIAGNOSIS. **Febrile convulsions because of otitis media,**

tonsillitis, or pneumonia (15.5)? Whooping cough (8.17)? Cerebral malaria (10.7)? Dehydration (9.18)? Meningitis (15.6)? Typhoid (10.8)? Epilepsy (15.8)? Poisoning (14.6)? Hypoglycaemia from severe malnutrition (7.10)?

MANAGEMENT WHEN DIAGNOSIS IS DIFFICULT. **If you cannot do a lumbar puncture, and he might have menin-** gitis, send him for help. **If you cannot send him for help, and he might have meningitis, treat him for it.**

IF A CHILD HAS A FIT TURN HIM ONTO HIS FRONT

15.8

15.9

16 Eyes

16.1 Preventing blindness

Eye diseases are important because they can make a child blind, so we must prevent them, and treat them early. Bacteria, viruses, lack of vitamin A, injuries, and foreign bodies can all cause eye disease.

16.2 Examining the eye

Look carefully at a healthy eye with a magnifying glass. The white part is the **sclera**. Thin smooth wet mucosa called the **conjunctiva** covers the sclera. The conjunctiva folds round inside the eyelids. It forms a pocket called the **conjunctival sac**. This sac is wet with tears, which are made in a gland at the side of the nose. Look at the small blood vessels on the conjunctiva. These dilate and you can see them more easily when the conjunctiva is inflamed (conjunctivitis).

The **cornea** is the shining glass-like 'window' at the front of the eye. Corneal scars are very serious, because they often make the cornea milky white. Light cannot get through a white cornea into the eye. So a child cannot see normally. A special thin mucosa covers the cornea. There are no blood vessels in a healthy cornea. If you see any, they are a sign of disease. Look carefully at the place where the healthy cornea joins the sclera. Lesions form here when a child has trachoma. Behind the cornea is a circle of brown or blue tissue called the **iris**. The black hole in the iris is the **pupil**. Smooth muscle in the iris can make the pupil larger or smaller. So more or less light goes into the eye. The **anterior chamber** is a space filled with clear fluid behind the cornea and in front of the iris. When the eye is infected this sometimes fills with pus. Behind the iris is the **lens**. This is like one of the lenses of a pair of spectacles, except that it is smaller and

HOW THE EYE IS MADE

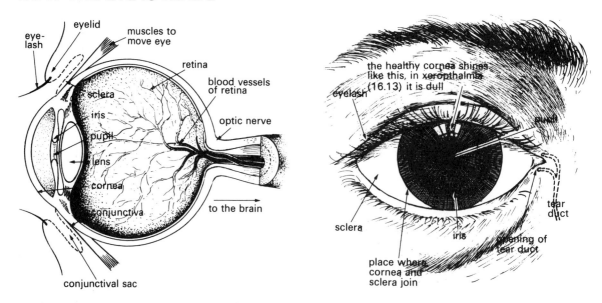

Fig. 16–1 How the eye is made.

182

thicker. Special cells at the back of the eye form the **retina**. When light shines on the retina these cells send messages down the optic (eye) nerve to the brain.

EXAMINING THE EYE

AN OLDER CHILD. **Take him into a good light. Sit him on his mother's knee, and ask her to hold his head.**

Ask him to look up and down, right and left, so that you can look at his cornea and sclera. Gently pull down his lower lid and examine the conjunctiva covering it.

If he will not do what you say, you may have to pull his upper eyelid upwards, and his lower eyelid downwards. Do this quickly and gently, before he can shut his eyes and make them even more difficult to examine.

Lastly, look at the conjunctivae inside his upper eyelids. Ask him to look at his toes.

1. Take hold of his upper eyelashes with your thumb and first finger. Pull his upper eyelids gently forwards and downwards away from his eyes.

2. Put a matchstick on the top of the back of his upper eyelids.

3. Turn his eyelid upwards and slightly outwards over the matchstick, so that its inside turns outwards.

4. Keep his eyelid like this while you examine it with a magnifying glass. Ask him to keep looking at his toes while you hold his eyelashes against his eyebrow.

This does not hurt. Practise on an adult. Turning over the eyelids is useful when you examine a child for trachoma, or foreign bodies.

A YOUNG CHILD. **Try to see as much as you can before touching him.** Look at his eyes while he is sucking from the breast. He usually opens his eyes then. If you cannot

EXAMINING A BABY'S EYES

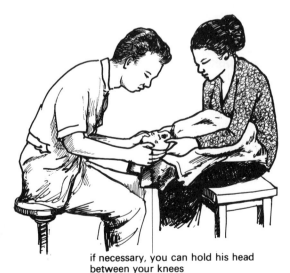

if necessary, you can hold his head between your knees

Fig. 16–2 Examining a baby's eyes.

EXAMINING THE UNDERNEATH OF THE UPPER EYELID

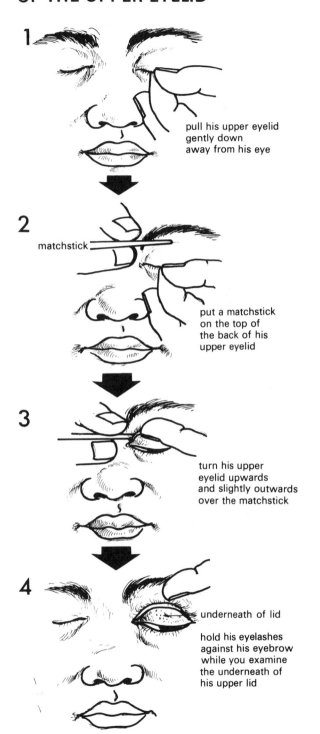

1

pull his upper eyelid gently down away from his eye

16.1

2

matchstick

put a matchstick on the top of the back of his upper eyelid

16.2

3

turn his upper eyelid upwards and slightly outwards over the matchstick

4

underneath of lid

hold his eyelashes against his eyebrow while you examine the underneath of his upper lid

Fig. 16–3 Examining the underneath of the upper eyelid.

see enough, put a blanket round him and put him across his mother's knees. Ask her to pull down his lower lids, while you pull up his upper lids:

We can put some drugs, such as chlortetracycline, into the conjunctival sac. This is made into a special eye ointment in small tubes. If you give a mother a tube, show her how to use it like this.

PUTTING OINTMENT INTO A CHILD'S EYE
Pull down the child's lower lid. Squeeze a 1 cm length of ointment onto his conjunctiva from the tube.

EXAMINE A CHILD'S EYES WITH A MAGNIFYING GLASS

16.3 'There is a red swelling on Pablo's eyelid'—a stye

Children sometimes get small red swellings on their eyelids. These are caused by bacteria infecting one of the small glands round the eyelashes. They cause a small abscess called a **stye**. If a stye becomes very large and swollen there may be lymphadenitis of the lymph nodes in front of the child's ear.

PUTTING OINTMENT IN THE EYE

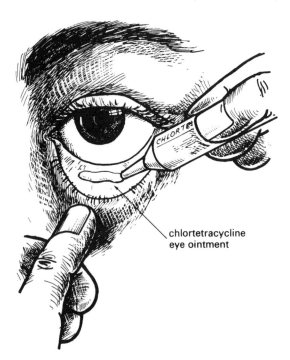

chlortetracycline eye ointment

Fig. 16–4 Putting ointment in the eye.

STYES

TREATMENT. **Put chlortetracycline eye ointment in the child's eye three times a day. If his whole eyelid is swollen and painful, give him penicillin injections (3.15).**

EXPLANATION. **Sometimes a child has several styes, one after the other. His mother may be able to prevent them by washing his eyes with clean water and a clean cloth. Explain that she must not squeeze a stye, because this spreads the infection.**

A STYE IS A SEPTIC INFECTION ROUND ONE OF THE EYELASHES

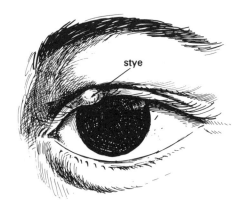

stye

Fig. 16–5 A stye is a septic infection round one of the eyelashes.

Red painful eyes

16.4 'Ade's eyes are red and painful and watery'—acute conjunctivitis, measles, foreign body, burns, harmful liquids, corneal ulcer, trachoma, phlyctenular conjunctivitis

These are the most common eye diseases. Most of them are easy to diagnose. The red eyes of measles are helpful for diagnosing the cause of a fever (10.6).

16.5 Foreign body

Foreign bodies often get into the eyes of older children. One of a child's eyes suddenly becomes red and watery, and he knows that he has something in it.

Usually, a foreign body only goes into the conjunctival sac. Occasionally, a foreign body goes through the sclera deep inside his eye. If you think this has happened, look carefully. There may be only a small hole, or sometimes no hole that you can see. A foreign body inside the eye is very serious, because it easily becomes infected and causes blindness.

184

A FOREIGN BODY IN THE EYE

MANAGEMENT. **If a foreign body might have gone inside a child's eye, try to send him to hospital immediately. But, if it is only in the conjunctival sac, you can probably take it out.**

EXAMINATION. **Look at his eye carefully (16.2).**

TREATMENT. **An older child can usually tell you where he can feel a foreign body. It may be high up under the top lid, under the bottom lid, or deep in one of the corners of the conjunctival sac. So, ask him to look up and down, right and left. Turn over his upper eyelid and see if the foreign body is there. When you have found it, gently brush it away. Use a piece of clean cloth, or some cotton wool on the end of a match stick.**

If there are many foreign bodies, wash them away with saline (3.48). Fill a small glass to the top with saline. Bend his head forwards. Put his eye into the saline in the glass. Tell him to open and close his eye several times.

Look for an ulcer on the cornea. If the foreign body might have scratched the cornea, use fluorescein paper (16.7). If you find an ulcer, treat it (16.7).

When a foreign body is removed, a child usually feels better immediately. Sometimes, he still feels that there is something in his eye. If his eye is very inflamed, give his mother some chlortetracycline eye ointment (3.17) to put in it.

16.6 Burns or harmful liquids in the eye

If a child's eyes have been burnt, look carefully for foreign bodies and remove them. Put chlortetracycline ointment into his eyes and put pads over them. A severe burn may cause a corneal scar which makes him blind.

If a harmful liquid gets into a child's eyes, wash it out quickly with plenty of water.

16.7 Corneal ulcer

The thin mucosa over the cornea of a child's eye is easily injured, so that a corneal ulcer is formed. Harmful organisms can get in and cause an infection which destroys his eye. Corneal ulcers need careful treatment.

A child with a corneal ulcer usually has one red painful watery eye. He keeps his eye shut and does not like looking into the light. The redness is most severe near the cornea. In conjunctivitis the redness is most severe at the sides of the sclera and *away* from the cornea. Examine his cornea by letting a bright light, such as that from a window, shine onto it. Look at the reflection (as in a mirror) of the light on his cornea. You may see that part of his cornea is not as smooth and shining as it should be. Ulcers are difficult to see. Staining them with fluorescein (a yellow substance) helps you to see them more easily. Fluorescein colours a corneal ulcer green and a conjunctival ulcer yellow. Touch one corner of the child's eye with a small piece of fluorescein stained

HYPOPYON-PUS BEHIND THE CORNEA

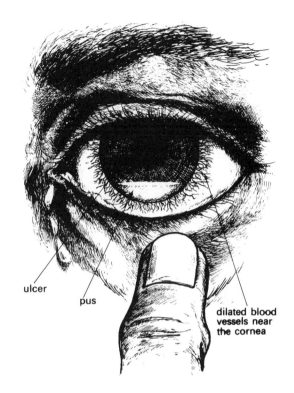

16.3

16.6

Fig. 16–5b Hypopyon—pus behind the cornea.

paper. The fluorescein dissolves in the tears, and colours the ulcer.

Bacteria sometimes spread through a corneal ulcer into the eye and cause pus to form in the anterior chamber—**hypopyon**. The pus falls to the bottom of the anterior chamber and has a straight upper edge, like liquid in a glass. This is a serious sign of infection inside the eye.

16.4
16.7

Conjunctivitis sometimes causes a corneal ulcer. So, if a child has severe conjunctivitis, look carefully at his cornea to see if he has an ulcer. Vitamin A deficiency can also cause a corneal ulcer—it is one of the first signs of keratomalacia (16.13).

16.5

CORNEAL ULCERS

MANAGEMENT. **See the child every day. Send him for help quickly if he is not much better in two days, or if pus starts to form behind his cornea (hypopyon).**

TREATMENT. **Put chlortetracycline eye ointment into his eye three times a day. Give him penicillin (3.15). If vitamin A deficiency is common in the district, give him vitamin A.**

EXPLANATION. **Explain to his mother that a corneal ulcer**

**can be very serious. Be sure she brings him to see you
every day.**

16.8 Acute conjunctivitis

This is common, and very infectious. It can quickly
spread through a family or a school, especially if several
people use the same towel. Bacteria or viruses can cause
conjunctivitis. It is more common where there is a lack of
soap and water, and where many people live close
together.

Conjunctivitis usually attacks both eyes, but one eye
may be inflamed more than the other, or before the
other. A child's conjunctivae become red and painful. If
his disease is severe, his conjunctivae swell in folds that
push out his eyelids. Sticky pus forms which dries and
makes crusts. Pus sticks his eyelids together while he
sleeps. When he wakes, he may not be able to open his
eyes until the crusted pus has been washed away.

The measles virus also makes a child's eyes red. Usually, pus does not form, and no treatment is needed.
Sometimes there is a secondary bacterial infection (2.6)
and pus does form. This bacterial conjunctivitis is much
more serious and can harm the cornea, so treat it.

Acute conjunctivitis

OPEN

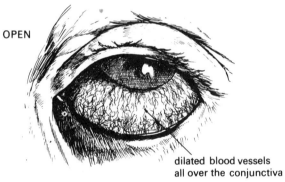

dilated blood vessels
all over the conjunctiva

CLOSED

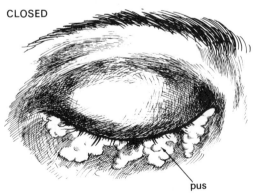

pus

Fig. 16–6 Acute conjunctivitis.

Newborn babies sometimes get a serious conjunctivitis from their mothers. The bacteria (gonococci)
which cause gonorrhoea in adults, can cause conjunctivitis in babies (26.40). Gonococci from infected
parents can also spread to the eyes of older children.
Gonococcal conjunctivitis is very severe with much
swelling of the eylids. It quickly causes blindness. So
treat any very severe conjunctivitis as if it were gonococcal.

Teaching a child's mother how to clean pus from his
eyes is very important. Antibiotics do not work unless an
eye is cleaned first.

ACUTE CONJUNCTIVITIS

MANAGEMENT. **If a child's conjunctivitis is severe, ask his
mother to bring him to see you every day. If he is not much
recovered in two days send him for help.**

TREATMENT. **If his conjunctivitis is very severe with much
swelling of the eyelids, treat it as if it were gonococcal
conjunctivitis (26.40). If it is less severe, put chlortetracycline eye ointment into his eye four times a day. Do
this after his eyes have been cleaned. If you put ointment
in at night, his eyes will not be stuck together in the morning.**

**If his eyelids are swollen, give him penicillin (3.15). Don't
cover his eyes with a pad and bandage. This keeps the pus
in, and it should come out.**

EXPLANATION AND EDUCATION—CLEANING THE EYES.
**If a child's eyes are very sticky with pus, show his mother
how to clean them. She can use soft clean toilet paper
which she can throw away. Or she can use several small
pieces of cloth. Ask her to wet one of these cloths with
clean water and to wipe her child's eyes from the middle
outwards.**

**Tell her not to use the same cloth more than once. Ask
her to wash, or, better, boil the cloth and dry it before she
uses it again. Tell her to clean his eyes like this three times
a day, and then put antibiotic ointment into them. Tell her
not to put any local medicines into his eyes.**

**ANY VERY SEVERE CONJUNCTIVITIS
MAY BE GONOCOCCAL**

16.9 Trachoma

Trachoma is a chronic infection. The organisms causing
it are half-way between viruses and bacteria. Trachoma
spreads by contact from the eyes of one person to the
eyes of another person. Flies also spread it. Trachoma is
common in districts where people are poor, and where
there is much dust, little water, and many flies. The
trachoma organism causes chronic inflammation of the
conjunctiva which heals after some months or years. But
it causes much scarring and deformity of the eyelids.
Eyes which have been deformed by trachoma easily
become secondarily infected by bacteria. Even if a

child's trachoma infection has stopped, bacterial conjunctivitis can make him blind.

Trachoma is much more serious in some countries than others. In some countries trachoma makes many people blind. These countries have *blinding trachoma*. In other countries there is trachoma but few people go blind. These countries have *non-blinding trachoma*.

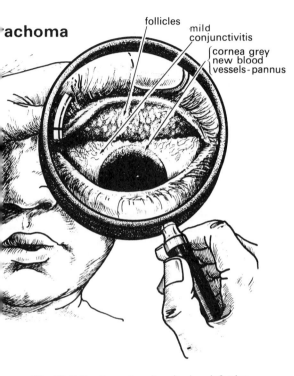

Fig. 16–7 Trachoma is a chronic virus infection.

Trachoma goes through four stages. By the time a child reaches the last stage he may have become an adult. You can treat the first two stages and kill the organism. But when scarring has deformed the eye in the third and fourth stages, treatment will not make it normal again. There is no strong immunity to trachoma, so a child often has several infections. You may see signs from several stages at the same time.

First stage—early trachoma. The child has mildly red watery eyes for a month or two. There are other signs, but these are not easy to see. So trachoma is difficult to diagnose at this stage. Many children recover completely, but some go on to the second stage. If trachoma is common in your community, and you see a child who might have early trachoma, treat him.

Second stage—later trachoma. Turn over the child's upper eyelid (16.2) and look at the conjunctiva underneath it. You will see many small blood vessels, and also some small pinkish grey swellings called **follicles**.

Use a magnifying glass to look at the place where his cornea joins his sclera. The edge of his cornea looks mildly grey, and small blood vessels go beyond the grey part into the cornea. This greyness of the cornea with new blood vessels in it is called **pannus**. It slowly grows over the cornea. Think of the eye as being like a clock. Pannus starts at the place where 12 o'clock would be, so look for it there first. If you see pannus and follicles, the child has trachoma.

Allergic conjunctivitis (16.10) causes follicles, but only trachoma causes follicles *and* pannus.

Third stage—healing trachoma. After several years, the follicles slowly go, and a scar forms, but the pannus remains.

Fourth stage—the stage of healing and scarring. This happens after several more years. By this time the child is probably an adult. The pannus slowly goes. His corneae are grey and scarred, so he cannot see through them normally. His eyelids are now so deformed that they don't close normally over his eyes. Tears fall from his eyes. Scarring and deformity turn his eyelashes inwards, so that they scratch his corneae. His eyelids no longer protect his eyes, so bacteria can infect them and cause more conjunctivitis. This makes his blindness worse.

Remember that cleaning the eyes of a child with trachoma is as important as putting antibiotics into them.

TRACHOMA

MANAGEMENT. **Try to see the child at least once a month until his trachoma is healed.**

TREATMENT. **Put chlortetracycline eye ointment into his eye twice a day for five days, each month for six months.**

EXPLANATION. **Show his mother how to put ointment into his eyes. Explain that he has a slow disease, which will take six months to cure. If it is not cured, he may become blind. Show his mother how to clean his eyes as explained in Section 16.8. Show her how to put the ointment into them. Tell her to come and fetch more ointment when the first tube is finished.**

Teach mothers to prevent trachoma by washing their children's eyes every day.

FACE-WASHING PREVENTS TRACHOMA

16.10 Allergic conjunctivitis

These children have a mild chronic conjunctivitis. Their eyes sometimes become allergic to substances in dust, or to substances from some kinds of plants. Allergic conjunctivitis comes and goes. Usually it is severe at the same time each year. It is not serious and rarely causes blindness, but it makes the sclerae look brown. It may cause follicles in the conjunctiva or the upper lid, but it never causes pannus.

ALLERGIC CONJUNCTIVITIS

MANAGEMENT. **Observe him carefully to make sure he has not got trachoma.**

TREATMENT. **Give him promethazine tablets (3.45).**

EXPLANATION. **Explain that his disease is not dangerous. Tell his mother that he will recover, but he may get the disease again. Explain that you would like to see him again in a month, so you can be sure he has not got any more serious disease (trachoma). Explain that the brown colour in his eyes will slowly go as he grows older.**

16.11 Phlyctenular conjunctivitis

A **phlycten** is a small (1 or 2 mm) painful yellow swelling on the sclera, close to the cornea. The conjunctiva is red near the phlycten, but further away it is normal. The child's eye is acutely red and full of tears. Looking at a light hurts him. Phlyctens are usually caused by TB. They are one of the special ways in which TB presents (13:1). They are common in malnourished children.

PHLYCTENULAR CONJUNCTIVITIS

DIAGNOSIS. **Ask about TB symptoms (13:1).**

TB TREATMENT. **Go to Section 13.6 and treat him for TB.**

EYE TREATMENT. **Put a pad and bandage over his eye.**

A phlycten

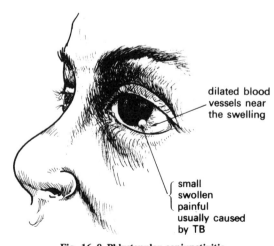

dilated blood vessels near the swelling

small swollen painful usually caused by TB

Fig. 16–8 Phlyctenular conjunctivitis.

EXPLANATION. **Tell his mother that his sore eye will slowly recover during several weeks, and that he must have TB treatment. Help her with his nutrition (7.13).**

16.12 Caring for a child with red painful eyes

Acute conjunctivitis is the most common cause of a red painful eye.

HISTORY. **Has anything gone into his eye (foreign body)?**

Did the redness start a few days ago (acute conjunctivitis) or a few weeks ago (trachoma or allergic conjunctivitis)?

EXAMINATION. **Is one eye red (corneal ulcer, foreign body, or phlycten) or both of them (acute conjunctivitis, trachoma, allergic conjunctivitis)?**

Examine his eye (16.2). There is no need to turn over his upper eyelid if he has acute conjunctivitis.

Where is the redness? All over his sclera (conjunctivitis)? In part of it only (phlycten)? Is there a yellow swelling in the middle of the redness (phlycten)?

If he has chronic conjunctivitis, look for follicles underneath his upper eyelids (trachoma or allergic conjunctivitis).

Use a magnifying glass to look at the place where his cornea and sclera join. Is the edge of his cornea grey with new blood vessels in it? (This is pannus—Stage two and three trachoma.) Scarred eyelids (stage three and four trachoma)? Deformed eyelids (stage four trachoma)?

SPECIAL TESTS. **If he might have a corneal ulcer, put a piece of fluorescein paper into the side of his eye. Let the fluorescein dissolve. Look carefully all over his cornea. Is there any dull green lesion which might be a corneal ulcer?**

If there is much swelling and pus, look for gonococci (L 11.5).

DIAGNOSIS. **Acute 'ordinary' conjunctivitis (16.8)? Foreign body (16.5)? Corneal ulcers (16.7)? Trachoma (16.9)? Allergic conjunctivitis (16.10)? Phlyctenular conjunctivitis (16.11)? Gonococcal conjunctivitis (26.40)?**

Vitamin A deficiency

16.13 A disease we can easily prevent

There is vitamin A (retinol) in animal foods such as liver. The body can make vitamin A from yellow substances called carotenes. There are carotenes in yellow or orange fruit and vegetables, and in dark green leaves. Many children do not get enough Vitamin A or carotene in their food, so they have signs of vitamin A deficiency. Lack of vitamin A harms the retinae, the conjunctivae and the glands which make tears. Vitamin A deficiency is especially common in children between six months and five years old. It has three stages—(1) nightblindness, (2) xerophthalmia, and (3) keratomalacia.

Vitamin A deficiency is common in some districts only. There may be much in your district, or none.

***First stage. 'He falls over things in the dark'
—night-blindness.*** When a child's retinae lack vitamin
A he cannot see in the dark—he has **night-blindness**.
Mothers sometimes call it 'Chicken blindness' (chickens
cannot see in the dark). Night-blindness is more often
noticed in an older child. His mother may say he falls
over things in the dark, or he loses his toys in the evening. Occasionally, the mother of a younger child says
that in the evening he cannot see to put his hand into a
pot of food. This is usually worse after a very bright day.
But few mothers notice this. So in a young child vitamin
A deficiency usually becomes xerophthalmia or keratomalacia before his mother brings him to see you.

Night-blindness is not serious, and is easily treated. In
some communities it is so common that most school-
children are blind at night. Test for it like this.

NIGHT-BLINDNESS

OLDER CHILDREN. **Take the child into a darkened room.
Stand beside him and hold out your hand. Hold up some
fingers and ask him to count them. If he cannot count, ask
him to hold up the same number of fingers as you do. Shut
the door a little, and ask him to count them again. Go on
doing this until the room becomes dark and you cannot
see your own fingers. If the child has night-blindness, he
stops being able to count fingers while you can still see
them.**

YOUNGER CHILDREN. **If a child can feed himself, see how
much light he needs to do it. Put him and his porridge in a
darkened room or slowly bring a lamp nearer to him. If you
can see his porridge before he starts eating, he probably
has night-blindness. Another way is to put the child and
his mother in the dark and to see if he can find her.**

Second stage. Xerophthalmia—'dry eyes'. The
conjunctivae and the tear glands need vitamin A. If a
child lacks it his conjunctivae do not shine or look normally shining and wet. Instead, they become dry and he
has *xerophthalmia*. His whole conjunctiva may be dry, or
it may only be dry in parts. Dryness usually comes first in
the place where Bitot's spots form later. As his xerophthalmia becomes worse small folds form in his conjunctiva round the edge of his cornea. His cornea
becomes dull, instead of shining like a mirror, and his
sclera becomes grey.

Lesions called **Bitot's spots** form on the outer sides of
the conjunctiva close to the cornea. These are frothy
(bubbly) grey or white lesions with sharp edges. Usually
they are in both eyes. You can remove Bitot's spots from
the eyes with a cloth. Mothers sometimes have a name
for them, and they may be a presenting symptom. Bitot's
spots are sometimes caused by other diseases. If the
conjunctiva underneath a Bitot's spot is dry, it is probably caused by vitamin A deficiency.

We can cure early xerophthalmia with large doses of
vitamin A. But, if there are any ulcers on the cornea, it
may *quickly* become keratomalacia, and the child

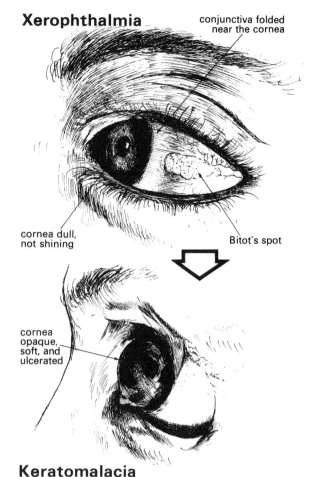

Xerophthalmia

conjunctiva folded near the cornea

16.12

cornea dull, not shining

Bitot's spot

16.11

cornea opaque, soft, and ulcerated

Keratomalacia

Fig. 16–9 Xerophthalmia and keratomalacia.

becomes blind. So a child with *dull dry corneae and any
other corneal lesions is an emergency*. His disease is
especially serious if he is between six months and five
years and is malnourished. He needs vitamin A *now*.

**THE BLINDNESS OF VITAMIN A DEFICIENCY
IS SUDDEN**

16.13

Third stage. Keratomalacia—'soft eye'. As a child's
vitamin A deficiency becomes worse his scleras become
more grey and his conjunctivae become more folded.
His corneae become opaque (cloudy). They become soft
and ulcerated so that a hole forms, and his eye becomes
infected. This makes him completely blind. Although his
eyes are being destroyed he has no pain. Often, the
disease is so acute that he becomes blind in both eyes in a
few hours or days. If he has only been blind for a few
days treat him. As the scar in his eye heals some sight

might come back. When he has been blind for longer than this, vitamin A does not help.

Many of these children die, either soon after they become blind, or later. Put all the blind children in your special care register (6.3).

16.14 Prevention and treatment

Vitamin A deficiency can be prevented by eating plenty of yellow fruit and vegetables, or dark green leafy foods such as cassava leaves, or papaya leaves, or animal foods, such as eggs, liver, or milk. All village families can get leafy foods, so vitamin A deficiency could easily be prevented. In some districts, very poor people never get vitamin A deficiency. They must eat leafy foods, because they have nothing else. The rich people who can eat anything they want do not get it. The moderately poor people have vitamin A deficiency most often. They don't want to eat leaves, because these are the poorest people's food.

VITAMIN A PREVENTS KERATOMALACIA

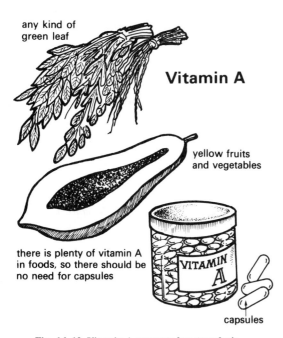

any kind of green leaf

Vitamin A

yellow fruits and vegetables

there is plenty of vitamin A in foods, so there should be no need for capsules

VITAMIN A

capsules

Fig. 16–10 Vitamin A prevents keratomalacia.

GREEN LEAVES PREVENT BLINDNESS

Vitamin A is stored in the body and used slowly. So we can also prevent vitamin A deficiency by giving a child a capsule of vitamin A every six months. Don't give more vitamin A than the dose you see here. Too much vitamin

A causes vomiting, headache, swelling of the fontanelle, and peeling of the skin.

WE CAN PREVENT VITAMIN A DEFICIENCY

16.15 Caring for a child who might have vitamin A deficiency

Sometimes, children present with signs of vitamin A deficiency. More often you find it when you examine a child for malnutrition or an infection. Think of it whenever you see an underweight child, or a child with any kind of eye disease.

HISTORY. **Has he been falling over things in the dark (night-blindness)?**

Has he been eating any foods containing vitamin A?

A FEW GREEN LEAVES WOULD HAVE PREVENTED HIS BLINDNESS

A child blind from keratomalacia

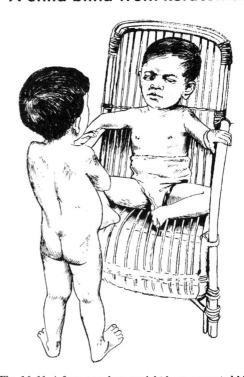

Fig. 16–11 A few green leaves might have prevented his blindness.

EXAMINATION. **Conjunctiva dry, all over, or in parts? Conjunctivae folded near the edge of the corneae? Bitot's spots (xerophthalmia)?**

Have his corneae started to become opaque, soft and ulcerated (keratomalacia)?

SPECIAL TESTS. **Test for night-blindness (16.13).**

DIAGNOSIS. **Are his signs of vitamin A deficiency negative? Doubtful? Mild? Moderate? Or severe? (16.14).**

PREVENTION

CHILDREN UNDER ONE YEAR. **Give a capsule of 100 000 units of vitamin A every six months.**

CHILDREN 1–6 YEARS. **Give two capsules of 100 000 units of vitamin A every six months.**

CHILDREN WITH MALNUTRITION AND INFECTION. **Children who lack vitamin A may suddenly get keratomalacia when they get an infection or severe malnutrition. So, if vitamin A deficiency is common, give a capsule of vitamin A to all children with malnutrition or a severe infection.**

TREATMENT

MILD. **Night-blindness, Bitot's spots, and dry folded conjunctivae with *normal* corneae.**

Give the child one capsule (100 000 units) of vitamin A by mouth. If his eyes are not normal in a week, give him another capsule.

SEVERE VITAMIN A DEFICIENCY. *Any corneal lesion* caused by vitamin a deficiency, such as dryness, greyness, or softness of the corneae.

Inject 100 000 units of water-miscible vitamin A (retinyl palmitate). This is special vitamin A for injection. *Don't* inject ordinary oily vitamin A. (If you have not got vitamin A for injection, give him a capsule of 100 000 units by mouth.) Next day give him a capsule of 100 000 units by mouth. Two weeks later give him one more capsule. (If he is over two years old, give him two capsules each time.)

If you have no vitamin A be sure he has plenty of food containing vitamin A.

Put a pad and bandage over his eye.

EXPLANATION. **Tell his mother why he became ill, and how she can help him by giving him plenty of green vegetables.**

17 Ears

17.1 A discharging ear is not normal

Many children have discharging ears, so mothers sometimes think this is normal. But a child with a discharging ear can become deaf, and sometimes dies. In some districts many adults are deaf. In a health education lesson they cannot hear what the teacher says. You can prevent this deafness and these deaths. Examine children carefully and treat them early.

17.2 The ear

Figure 17–1 shows the three parts of the ear—the outer, middle, and inner ear. **The outer ear** is the part of the ear on the outside of the head, and also the 'ear hole' or **meatus**. The meatus of an adult is about 2·5 cm long. The opening of the meatus is wide, and the next part is narrower. Further in the meatus becomes wide again. At the end of the meatus is the **ear drum**. This is like an

THE PARTS OF THE EAR

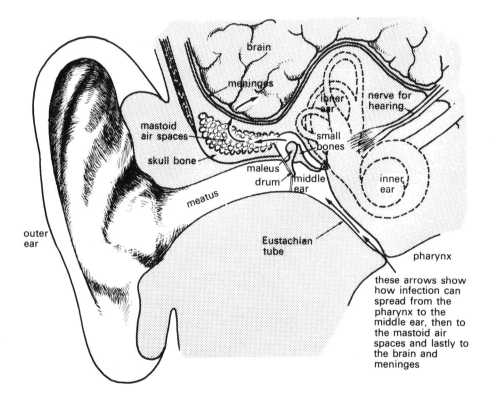

Fig. 17–1 The parts of the ear.

rdinary drum because it is made of tight skin with air on both sides. The air in the meatus is outside the drum, and the air in the middle ear is on the inside of the drum. Inflammation of the outer ear is called **otitis externa**.

The **middle ear** is a small space filled with air in the bone of the skull. The walls of the middle ear are covered with thin mucosa. Inflammation of the middle ear is called **otitis media**. The **inner ear** is deeper inside the skull. It is seldom diseased in children.

There is a small bone in the drum called the **malleus**. Sound causes very small movements in the air. These move the drum, and the malleus. Two other small bones take the movements to the inner ear. A nerve then takes the sound from the inner ear to the brain.

A tube called the **Eustachian tube** takes air from the pharynx to the middle ear. It also drains (removes) fluid from the middle ear. When a child swallows, his Eustachian tubes open and let air go to his middle ears. When you swallow, you can hear your own Eustachian tubes opening.

As a child grows, small spaces filled with air grow into the bone from the back of his middle ears. These are the **mastoid air spaces**. They are in the **mastoids** which are bony swellings behind the ears.

On the outside of each middle ear is the ear drum and the meatus. On the inside of the middle ear is the bone which contains the inner ear. The roof of the middle ear is made of thin bone, and on top of this is the brain. The Eustachian tube comes into the front of the middle ear. The mastoid air spaces join onto the middle ear from behind.

THE EAR DRUM IS BETWEEN THE OUTER AND MIDDLE EAR

17.3 Examining the ear

For this we need an **auriscope**. This is an electric torch with a small bulb, which shines light down on a **speculum** into the ear. There are speculae of different sizes. The big speculae are for the big meatus of an adult, and the small speculae are for children. The light must be bright, so keep spare batteries and a spare bulb. Don't leave the auriscope on when you are not using it.

EVERY CLINIC MUST HAVE AN AURISCOPE WHICH WORKS

EXAMINING A CHILD'S EAR

Do this at the end of the examination. The child may not like it and he may fight. If he fights, examining him will be difficult. Make sure that the auriscope is working before you start. If possible, examine him in a dark place. Choose the largest speculum that will go into his ear and not hurt him.

Sit the child sideways on his mother's knees, with his head against her body. If he sits like this, he cannot move his ear away when you examine it. Put one of his hands behind her back. Ask her to hold his head firmly with one hand. Ask her to put her other hand round his body and other arm (17–1b). If he is older, stand him in front of his mother. If he will not hold his head still, wrap him in a blanket. Ask a helper to hold him as shown in Figure 5–9.

Sit down in front of him. Before you put in the speculum, examine his outer ear, the skin behind it, and the outer part of his meatus. Look for signs of inflammation and discharge.

Hold the auriscope with one hand and his ear with the other. Pull the ear of a young child gently backwards. Pull the ear of an older child or an adult gently upwards and backwards. The meatus is slightly bent and this straightens it out, so that you can see the drum better. **17.1**
Gently pull the ear a little more or a little less. Change the **17.2**
way the speculum is pointing until you see something smooth and pink–grey beyond the hairy skin of the meatus—this is the drum.

HOLDING A CHILD TO EXAMINE HIS EAR

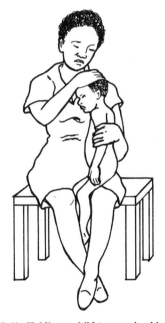

17.3

Fig. 17–1b Holding a child to examine his ear.

17.4 The normal ear drum   **17.4**

When you look into a normal meatus you see hairs, skin, and brown wax. At first you will not see the drum, especially in young children. So practise on adults and look at the ears of your friends. The bottom of the drum shines brightly in the light of the auriscope. A broad yellow–grey line comes down and slightly backwards from the top of the drum. This is the **handle of the malleus**. A small piece of bone sticks out from the top of the malleus. This is the **short process** of the malleus. Look for this if an ear has been deformed by disease. It helps you to know what you are seeing. Ask an adult to blow up his cheeks, while holding his nose. You will see his ear drum move outwards slightly. He is blowing air through his Eustachian tubes into his middle ears.

THE UNICEF AURISCOPE

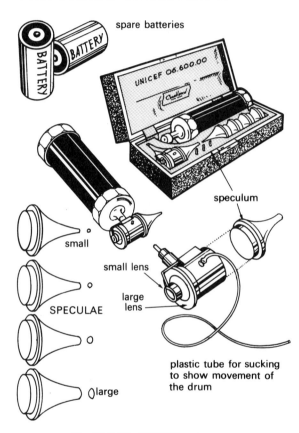

Fig. 17–2 The UNICEF auriscope.

17.5 Dry-swabbing

Wax and pus often stop us seeing the drum well, so we must clean them away. If there is pus or only a little wax, you can remove it by dry-swabbing. But if there is much wax and pus, remove it by syringing. Dry-swabbing means cleaning the ears with cotton wool on the end of a stick. It is useful for diagnosis and treatment, so learn how to do it well and teach mothers how to do it cleanly. Dirty swabbing may put harmful organisms into a child's ears, especially the bacteria which cause tetanus (18.16). *Never leave cotton wool in a child's ear.* It stops pus coming out and helps bacteria and fungi to grow.

DRY-SWABBING A CHILD'S EAR

Wash your hands. Sit the child on his mother's knees.
  First make a swab like this—
  1. If possible, use a special metal wool-carrier. One end of this is rough and has a screw for holding the wool. The other end has a loop for taking wax out of ears. Sterilize it each time you use it, or you may infect one child from another. If you have not got a wool-carrier, use wooden applicator sticks.
  2. Take a piece of cotton wool and pull it out flat.
  3. Put the end of the wool-carrier into the wool and turn it round. The wool wraps round tightly and stays in place.
  4. The biggest part of the wool should make a strong point about half a centimetre beyond the end of the wool carrier. Make sure that part of the wool goes back along the wool carrier. You can hold this part of the wool and stop it falling off into the ear.

THE NORMAL EAR DRUM

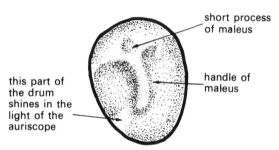

Fig. 17–3 The normal ear drum.

Don't make the swab too long (5), too fat (6), or too loose (7).
  8. Sterilize it. Light it with a spirit lamp, or a match and then quickly put the flame out.
  Put the sterilized swab gently into the child's ear and turn in round. Take it out and throw the dirty swab away. Take some more cotton wool and make another swab. Go on swabbing out the ear a little deeper each time until the wool comes out clean. This shows that there is no more wax.

EXPLANATION. **Show the child's mother how to swab her child's ear. Let her do it in the clinic, and watch how she does it. She will not have a spirit lamp at home, but she may have a candle or a lamp. Give her some cotton wool and some applicator sticks. Explain that she *must* do it cleanly.**

17.6 Syringing

This means 'injecting' water into the ear fast. When the water comes out of the ear it carries wax and pus with it. You can use a metal ear-syringe, or a rubber bulb. Whatever you use, don't block the meatus with it. If water cannot easily get out of the meatus, it may burst

CLEANING THE EAR WITH A SWAB OF COTTON WOOL

1 metal applicator stick UNIPAC 0703000

screwed end for wool

2

pull out a thin flat piece of cotton

3

roll it round an applicator stick

just right   GOOD **4**

too long   BAD **5**

too fat   BAD **6**

too loose   BAD **7**

light it quickly and blow at the flame

8

gently clean the pus from the ear **9**

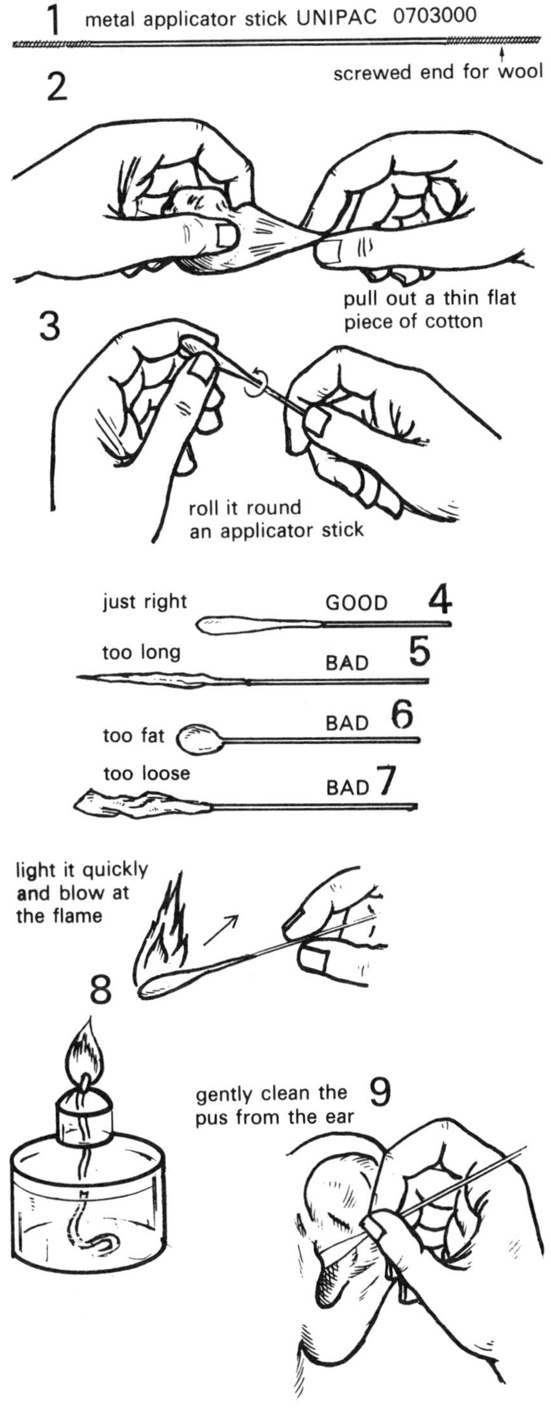

Fig. 17–4 Cleaning the ear with a swab of cotton wool.

the ear drum. Or it may spread infection to the mastoid air spaces.

There are two ways of syringing ears. One way is for removing wax or foreign bodies. The other way gently washes pus from the ear. If a drum might be perforated, syringe *very gently*, or you may spread the infection and cause vertigo (a feeling that the world is going round).

SYRINGING AWAY PUS FROM THE EAR

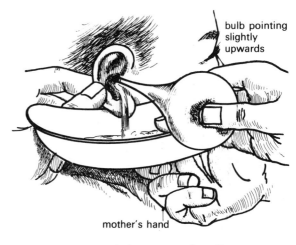

bulb pointing slightly upwards

mother's hand

Fig. 17–5 Syringing away pus from the ear.

SYRINGING

Take a cup of clean warm water, as near to the temperature of the body as possible (37°C). This is specially important if there is a perforation. When you put your finger into the water, it should not feel either hot or cold.

Sit the child on his mother's knee. Put a towel over his shoulder and another towel on her knees. Ask her to hold his head and to hold a kidney-dish under his ear. Fill the syringe with the warm water that you have made. Hold his ear and pull it gently backwards. Put the end of the syringe into the meatus pointing slightly upwards and forwards.

TO REMOVE WAX, OR A FOREIGN BODY. If there is wax in the ear, inject the water fast and slightly upwards. Make the water go along the roof of the meatus so that it pushes out the wax as it comes out (17–6). Fill the syringe and 'inject' more water. Do this several times until all the wax comes out into the kidney-dish. When the wax has come out, look into the meatus with an auriscope. This is the only way to be sure the ear is clean. Dry the child's ear with a swab.

17.5

17.6

GENTLY WASHING AWAY PUS. Syringe *much more gently* than when removing wax. Then dry the child's ear and look at it.

You can also clean wax and pus from an ear with drops of 2 per cent hydrogen peroxide four times a day. This bubbles and makes a noise in the ear, but it does not hurt.

IF THE DRUM MIGHT BE PERFORATED, SYRINGE GENTLY

SYRINGING THE EAR TO REMOVE WAX

squirt water along the roof of the meatus so that it gets behind the wax and pushes it out

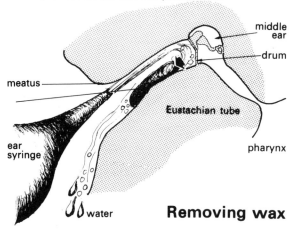

Removing wax

Fig. 17–6 Syringing the ear to remove wax.

17.7 Is he deaf?

Sometimes we need to find out if a child is deaf (24.16).

TESTING FOR DEAFNESS

AN OLDER CHILD. Turn his head away from you, so that he cannot see from your lips what you are saying. Put your finger over the meatus of the ear you are not going to test. Move your finger about so as to make a small noise. This will stop him hearing with that ear. Say a few words into the ear you are testing, and ask him to say the words back to you. Do this several times, speaking more quietly, and further away each time. When you have tested a few normal children, you will be able to diagnose if a child is deaf. A normal child should be able to hear a quiet whisper (speaking) a metre away from his ear.

A BABY. Ask a helper to show the baby something interesting to make him look to the front. Crumple (squeeze into a ball) some paper, or hit a cup with a spoon. Do this behind him on his right where he cannot see it. Then do it on his left. If he can hear, he will turn his head or eyes towards the noise.

17.8 'Dolores has discharge (or pain) in her ear'—acute or chronic otitis media, otitis externa, foreign body, caries (pain only)

Discharge and pain are the two most common presenting symptoms of ear disease in children. If a child has a sudden ear pain and fever, he probably has acute otitis media. A child who is too young to say he has a pain, pulls at his ear. But this does not always mean that he has ear disease. His ears may only be itching. Sometimes caries causes ear pain. There is no fever and the ear is normal.

17.9 Acute otitis media

This is an acute septic infection in the middle ear. Organisms go up the Eustachian tube to the middle ear. Otitis media is thus a common complication of all upper respiratory infections ('URI', 8.6). The mucosa of the middle ear becomes inflamed and thickened, and the space inside fills with pus. If pus cannot get out down the Eustachian tubes, the drum swells and softens. A hole forms, and the pus comes out. The hole is called a **perforation**.

Otitis media usually starts suddenly. A child wakes up in the night crying with pain, or pulling his ear. He has fever, and he may have a cough and a nasal discharge. His ear drum and the deeper part of the meatus near it

THE SIGNS OF ACUTE OTITIS MEDIA

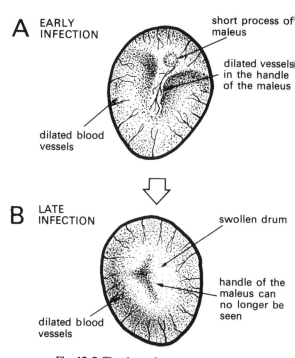

Fig. 17–7 The signs of acute otitis media.

are red. Dilated blood vessels go into the drum from its edge. There are also blood vessels along the handle of the malleus (17–7). Moving his ear does not hurt—unlike external otitis (17.12). Occasionally, when a child has a bad pain in his ear, his drum looks normal. Some of these children get otitis media during the next few days and some do not.

A RED DRUM IS THE FIRST SIGN OF OTITIS MEDIA

If you do not treat a child with an acutely red drum, his middle ear fills with pus and he becomes deaf. His drum becomes dull and opaque, instead of shining and transparent. The drum begins to swell. It soon covers the handle and short process of the malleus, so that you cannot see them. Then the drum perforates, pus discharges from his ear, and his pain and fever get less. Try to diagnose and treat otitis media before a child's drum perforates. You may prevent his otitis becoming chronic. Small perforations usually heal, but larger ones don't. If his ear is still discharging in three weeks, he has chronic otitis media (17.10).

Acute otitis media can also present as fever without ear pain (10.10), fits (15.9), or vomiting (20.15).

TREAT OTITIS MEDIA BEFORE THE DRUM PERFORATES

ACUTE OTITIS MEDIA

TREAT HIS INFECTIONS. **If he has a fever, give him ampicillin (3.16), or penicillin (3.15) *and* sulphadimidine (3.14) or tetracycline (3.17) or chloramphenicol (3.18) for five days. If possible give him depot penicillin (3.15). Don't give antibiotics for more than ten days, because they will not do any more good.**

TREAT HIS PAIN. **Give him paracetamol (3.42), or, if he is over two years, aspirin (3.41). If he is very restless, give him promethazine (3.45).**

If he has severe pain, and his drum is normal, one or two drops of warm oil in his ear may help. Cooking oil, or liquid paraffin can be used. Make sure the oil is not too hot. Test it first. Put a few drops on the back of your hand.

EXPLANATION. **If his drum has already perforated, show his mother how to swab out his ears (17–4).**

17.10 Chronic otitis media

Sometimes a child comes to see you more than three weeks after his ear drum has perforated. There is pus and dirt, and sometimes flies in his meatus. Syringe these away, and look at his drum. You will see a perforation. Look through the perforation. You may see the shining inner wall of his middle ear (17–10).

Chronic otitis media is difficult to treat. Antibiotics sometimes help a child. But, if his discharge has not stopped in ten days, more antibiotics will not cure him. The best way to help him is to show his mother how to swab his ears clean. The infection in his middle ear will get less. The discharge will stop for a time, and the perforation may heal. A clean ear is also less likely to be infected with tetanus (18.16).

17.8

PUS DISCHARGING FROM THE MIDDLE EAR

17.9

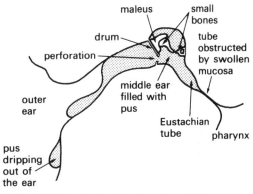

Fig. 17–8 Pus discharging from the middle ear.

CHRONIC OTITIS MEDIA

MANAGEMENT. **Ask the child's mother to bring him back to the clinic once a week. Swab, or syringe and dry his ear each time he comes. Record how much discharge there is (+ to ++++, 1–8), and what you find in his ear. It should heal slowly during a few weeks.**

17.7

TREATMENT. **Give him an antibiotic for ten days as for acute otitis media, if he has one or more of these four things—**
(1) Discharge for less than a month.
(2) Redness of the drum or the meatus near it.
(3) Pain in or near the ear.
(4) Fever.
If he has *none* of these things, antibiotics will probably not help. But his mother will want treatment for him. So, if you have enough antibiotics, give them. If necessary, give him DPT, or tetanus toxoid also (4.9).

EXPLANATION. **If you think that his mother can swab out his ear safely, show her how to do it (17.5). If you think she cannot do it safely, show her how to clean out the outer part only. Explain that careful swabbing is the best way to help him. Tell her to bring him often until his ear has healed.**

17.10

Tell her not to put any local medicine, safety pins, or chicken feathers into his ear. If he is older, tell her that he must not go swimming. This is dangerous for a person with a perforated ear drum.

LOOKING THROUGH A PERFORATED EAR DRUM

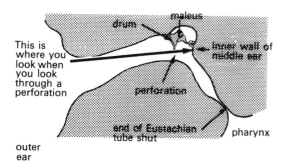

Fig. 17–10 Looking through a perforated ear drum.

17.11 The complications of otitis media—mastoiditis, meningitis, and brain abscess

These sometimes complicate acute otitis media. They are more common in children with chronically discharging ears.

Mastoiditis. Infection sometimes spreads from a child's middle ear to the air spaces in his mastoid. He has fever and pain in his ear, and is deaf. The bone behind his ear (mastoid) becomes swollen and tender. The swelling is fixed to the bone of his skull. Its edges are difficult to feel. Sometimes it pushes his ear forward.

MASTOIDITIS
Send him to hospital quickly. His mastoid spaces must be opened to let out the pus. Give him penicillin (3.15) before he goes. If you cannot send him to hospital, treat him for osteomyelitis (24.5).

Meningitis and brain abscess. Bacteria which are infecting the middle ear sometimes go into the brain through small holes in the skull. They can cause meningitis, or an abscess in the brain. A child with this kind of brain abscess has a discharging ear, and a high fever (10.4). He may also have vomiting (20.14), fits (15.9), and vertigo, and he may keep falling over. Sometimes there are meningeal signs (15.6). For management and treatment, go to Section 15.6.

17.12 Otitis externa

Otitis externa is an acute septic infection of the skin of the meatus and outer ear. The child has ear pain and discharge. But his drum is normal, if you can see it. Moving his ear hurts him, because it moves his inflamed meatus. This is a useful sign, because moving the ear of a child with otitis media does not hurt. His disease is too deep inside his head. Otitis media makes a child deaf (17.7), otitis externa does not usually make him deaf.

This is another useful difference between these two diseases.

Occasionally, a child has a boil in his ear which blocks it. Sometimes, a child's outer ear and his meatus become inflamed, swollen, and wet with pus. This is cellulitis (2.4) of the outer ear.

Lymph from the scalp and outer ear goes to a small lymph node behind the ear. This becomes larger and tender (lymphadenitis) when the outer ear or scalp are infected. Swelling of this node causes a lump which is easily felt and moved. It is different from the swollen bone of a mastoid infection.

TWO CHRONIC PERFORATIONS IN THE EAR DRUM

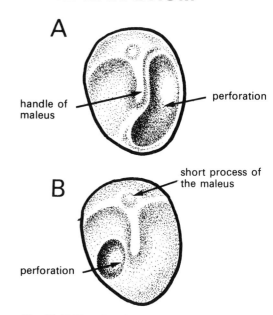

Fig. 17–11 Two chronic perforations in the ear drum.

OTITIS EXTERNA
TREATMENT. **Swab away any discharge (17.5).**
   If there is little swelling, put gentian violet on the lesion.
   If there is much swelling, give the child penicillin (3.15).

EXPLANATION. **Show his mother how to keep his ear clean.**

17.13 Foreign body

Children sometimes put foreign bodies such as beads or peas into their ears. These cause pain, secondary infection, and discharge. Don't try to take them out with forceps. This will push them further in, and you may harm the drum—DON'T HARM THE DRUM.

FOREIGN BODY

Sit him on his mother's knee, and ask her to hold him. Syringe his ear (17.6). This removes most foreign bodies. If syringing does not remove the foreign body, *try to send the child for help.* If you cannot send a child for help, remove the foreign body like this:

Wrap the child in a blanket, so that he cannot move his hands. Ask a helper to hold his head firmly. Sit in a good light.

1. Take a paper clip, or any other kind of *thin*, strong wire.
2. Straighten it out.
3. Bend one end downwards so as to make a very small hook about 3 mm long.
4. Carefully put the hook into the ear flat against the wall of the meatus.
5. Gently push the hook past the foreign body. Don't push it far in, or you may harm the drum.
6. Turn the hook back into the meatus.
7. Gently pull the foreign body out of the ear.

DON'T USE FORCEPS TO TAKE FOREIGN BODIES OUT OF THE EAR

17.14 Caring for a child with pain or discharge from his ear

To make a diagnosis you must be able to see the drum easily.

HISTORY. **How long has the child had a discharge? (If it has lasted more than three weeks, it is chronic.)**

How long has he had pain? (Sudden acute ear pain, with or without discharge, is probably otitis media.)

EXAMINATION. **Look at his outer ear and the opening of the meatus. Pus? Foreign body? Inflammation? Is the ear pushed forward by a swelling behind it (mastoiditis)?**

Look and feel behind his ear. Is there a swelling? If there is, is it a bean-shaped moveable lump (septic lymphadenitis)? Or is it a large tender swelling fixed to the mastoid bone (mastoiditis)?

Press both mastoid processes at the same time. If he moves quickly, away from one of them, it is tender (mastoiditis).

Does moving his ear hurt (otitis externa)?

Is he deaf (17.7 blocked meatus, otitis media, foreign body)?

Take his temperature. Fever (otitis media, mastoiditis)? Examine both his ears with an auriscope (17.3). If necessary swab (17.5) or syringe (17.6) them so that you can see his drums.

Foreign body? Pus? Wax?

Abnormally red drum? Dilated vessels round the edge of the drum, or over the handle of the maleus? Opaque drum? Swollen drum hiding the handle and short process of the malleus? (All these are signs of otitis media.)

Perforation of the drum (otitis media, acute or chronic)?

Look at his teeth (caries).

REMOVING A FOREIGN BODY FROM THE EAR

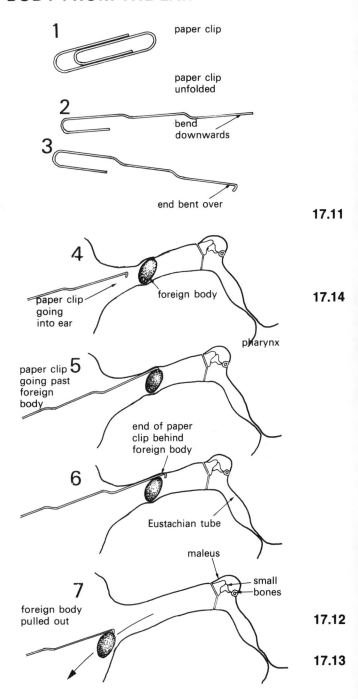

1 paper clip

paper clip unfolded

2 bend downwards

3 end bent over

17.11

4 paper clip going into ear foreign body

pharynx

17.14

paper clip 5 going past foreign body

end of paper clip behind foreign body

6 Eustachian tube

maleus

small bones

7 foreign body pulled out

17.12

17.13

Fig. 17–12 Removing a foreign body from the ear.

DIAGNOSIS. **Acute otitis media (17.9)? Chronic otitis media (17.10)? Otitis externa (17.12)? Foreign body (17.13)? Caries (19.5)? Mastoiditis (17.11)?**

MANAGEMENT IF DIAGNOSIS IS DIFFICULT. **If you cannot see the drum you cannot diagnose if he has otitis media or externa. Fortunately the early treatment of both diseases is the same—penicillin. Swab out his ears carefully. If he is 'ill', give him penicillin. Observe him carefully and examine him again in a few days.**

18 The mouth and throat

18.1 Don't forget to examine the throat

A child can have lesions in his mouth or throat. This makes them sore, so that eating hurts. An older child can say that his mouth or throat feels sore. But a younger child cannot tell us anything. When his mouth or throat are sore he stops eating. He presents as the child who has stopped eating. Often his mother can see lesions in the front of his mouth, and tell us about them. But she cannot see into the back of his throat. So a young child can have throat lesions, and his mother does not know.

So sore mouths and sore throats in older children are usually easy to diagnose. But sore throats in young children are more difficult. They often present as fever (10.10), coughing (8.20), vomiting (20.15), fits (15.9), or abdominal pain (20.13). Sore throats present in many ways, so we must examine the throat of every 'ill' child.

18.2 Examining a child's mouth and throat

Sit him up, he may vomit. If he vomits lying down, the vomit may go into his lungs. Use a sterilized spatula (tongue depressor 3.18). If a spatula is not sterilized, but only washed, it may carry harmful organisms from one child to another. A few 'ordinary' organisms on a spatula do not cause harm. But we must kill the harmful organisms from other sick children. Some health workers sterilize spatulae by washing them in antiseptic, but this is not safe. A clinic needs at least 20 spatulae. You must sterilize them every time you use them. If you cannot get wooden spatulae, ask a carpenter to make some. The best size is 15 × 2 × 0·3 cm with rounded ends.

There are two special organs called the tonsils at each side of the throat. Lymph from the tonsils goes to the tonsillar lymph nodes under the angles of the jaw. Remember to examine these for tenderness and swelling whenever you examine a child's throat. Large tender tonsilar lymph nodes show he has an infection in his throat.

EXAMINING THE MOUTH AND THROAT

LYMPHADENITIS. **Feel for enlarged or tender lymph nodes under the angles of his jaw. The nodes for his mouth are** under the front of the jaw (19–1), so feel for them also. Use both hands and feel both sides together.

HIS MOUTH AND THROAT. **Do this at the end of the examination, because the child may fight. Use a torch, and keep a spare bulb and batteries for it.**

Sit him on his mother's knee with his back against her body. Ask her to put one hand round his head. Tell her to try to stop him turning his face away. Ask her to put her other arm round his body and hold both his arms. If he fights, she may be able to hold his feet between her knees. Sometimes, you need a helper to hold his arms.

Sit in front of him with your head low, so you can see into his mouth when he opens it.

Examining the throat

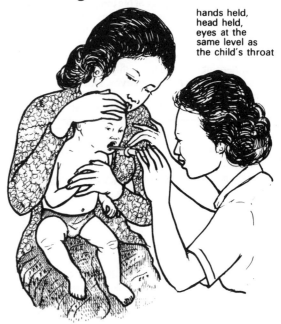

hands held,
head held,
eyes at the
same level as
the child's throat

Fig. 18–1 Examining a child's mouth and throat.

201

The normal throat

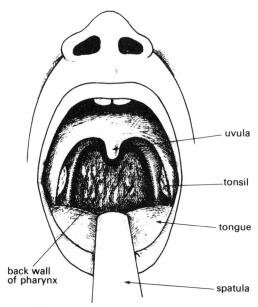

Fig. 18–2 Get a good look at his throat.

Light the torch, and shine it towards his mouth. Ask him to open it. Some children can open it for you without the need for a spatula. First look at his tongue, teeth and gums. Now put the spatula sideways and look inside his cheeks. Are there any Koplik's spots (10–7)? Even if he closes his teeth, you can still examine his cheeks.

Next press down the back of his tongue with the spatula. This makes him open his pharynx, as if he were going to vomit. The back of his tongue goes down and you can see easily for a second or two only. Look carefully the first time, because he may not let you try a second time. Look for and remember these three things:

The colour of his palate, pharynx, and tonsils. Are they abnormally red?

The size of his tonsils—are they normal or enlarged?

Is there any pus or membrane (18.12) on his pharynx or tonsils?

Put the spatula into a dish where it can be sterilized.

EXAMINE THE THROAT OF EVERY SICK CHILD

Sore mouth

18.3 'Agboola has a sore mouth'—caries, measles, fever, thrush, herpes stomatitis, Vincent's stomatitis, cancrum oris, vitamin B deficiency

Caries. Caries are holes in a child's teeth. In some districts many children have carious teeth and dirty infected gums. They do not usually present at a clinic until they are older and can say they have toothache (tooth pain). Regular cleaning with a brush helps to prevent caries.

18.4 The sore mouth of fever

When a child has had a severe fever for several days his mouth becomes dry and sore. The fever might be malaria, measles, or typhoid, or something else. A child's lips crack and are covered with crusts. His tongue and the roof of his mouth are covered with dirty mucus. Some diseases, such as chickenpox or measles, cause lesions in his mouth like the lesions on his skin.

THE SORE MOUTH OF FEVER

EXPLANATION. **Tell his mother to give him plenty of fluid to drink. Ask her to put half a teaspoonful of salt into a cupful of water. Ask her to wash out his mouth several times a day with this. If he is old enough, he may be able to do it himself. If he is younger his mother can do it with a piece of cotton wool and her fingers. Show her how to clean the crusts from his lips with a clean wet cloth. If they are dry and cracked, put plain ointment on them. If they are swollen and infected treat them with gentian violet.**

FEELING THE TONSILLAR LYMPH NODES

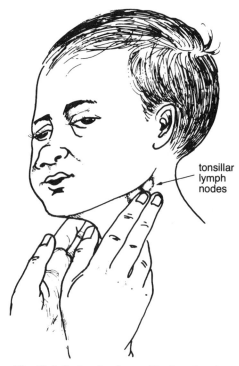

Fig. 18–3 Feeling for the tonsillar lymph nodes.

18.5 Thrush (candidiasis, moniliasis)

Thrush is caused by a fungus. The fungus grows on the mucosa of the mouth and causes white lesions. If it is severe it forms a white membrane, which looks like white cloth stuck to the mucosa. Sometimes, it makes the whole of a child's tongue white. Thrush is seldom serious, but it may stop a child sucking from the breast, or eating. Thrush can also cause mild diarrhoea. Thrush is common in newborn babies (26.55), and in children who are malnourished, or sick with some other disease, such as measles. It is also common in children who have been given antibiotics (3.13).

THRUSH

MANAGEMENT. **If a baby has stopped sucking, go to Section 26.20. Observe his growth curve carefully.**

TREATMENT. **Put gentian violet on the lesions. Show his mother how to do this. Use cotton wool and a stick. Give his mother some cotton wool, and a small bottle of gentian violet to take home. Ask her to put gentian violet on his lesions three times a day. Don't give him antibiotics, because this will make his thrush worse.**

EXPLANATION. **Tell his mother that she must go on breast-feeding him. If he is older, he must have soft foods that he can eat easily.**

Thrush

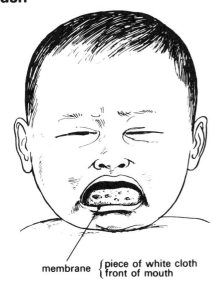

membrane { piece of white cloth / front of mouth

Fig. 18–4 A child with thrush.

18.6 Herpes stomatitis

The herpes simplex virus can cause cold sores (11.15) in a mother. Sometimes it infects her baby. It causes small

Herpes stomatitis

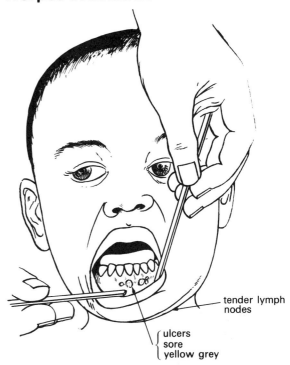

tender lymph nodes

{ ulcers
sore
yellow grey

Fig. 18–5 Herpes stomatitis is a virus disease.

painful vesicles (blisters) that burst to leave round yellow–grey ulcers on the mucosa of his mouth. We usually see the ulcers. We seldom see the vesicles because they burst so quickly. The child's lips may swell. The infection spreads to the lymph nodes under his jaw and makes them swollen and tender (lymphadenitis). He may have fever, become irritable, and stop sucking or eating. These symptoms usually come two or three days before the ulcers. There is no drug to kill the herpes virus, but the lesions heal themselves in a few days. Sometimes, they become secondarily infected by bacteria, and need treatment with an antibiotic. When a child's stomatitis has healed the virus may stay in his lips for the rest of his life. It may cause cold sores whenever he has a fever (11.15).

HERPES STOMATITIS

MANAGEMENT. **If he has stopped sucking look at Section 26.20. He may lose weight, so watch his growth curve carefully.**

TREATMENT. **Put gentian violet on the lesions. If he has a very sore dirty mouth or fever, or much swelling of his lips, give him sulphadimidine (3.14), or penicillin (3.15).**

EXPLANATION. **Show his mother how to put gentian violet onto the lesions with cotton wool on a stick. Give her some** gentian violet in a small bottle to take home. Tell her to make sure he drinks plenty of fluids, and eats plenty of soft food.

18.7 Vincent's stomatitis (Vincent's angina)

This is an acute infection of the mouth and gums which is caused by snakelike bacteria called spirochaetes (2–1). These spirochaetes are part of the normal mouth flora (2.2). A healthy child is usually immune to them, so that they do not cause disease. But, a malnourished child has less immunity, so they can multiply and harm him more easily. The child has a fever and is 'ill'. His gums are swollen and tender and bleed easily. There is pus between his gums and his teeth. If his disease is mild, there are lesions on the edges of his gums only. If his disease is severe there are yellow–grey ulcers on his gums, mouth, and tonsils. These ulcers are covered with dead tissue (sloughs) which bleed when you touch them. His mouth smells so bad that you can often diagnose Vincent's stomatitis by smelling him.

VINCENT'S STOMATITIS

TREATMENT. **Wash out his mouth every three hours with hydrogen peroxide (18.8). If you have not got this, use saline.**

Give him penicillin (3.15). Penicillin helps Vincent's stomatitis, but it does not help thrush.

EXPLANATION. **Show his mother how to wash out his mouth, and let her try to do it herself in the clinic. Explain how she can improve his nutrition.**

DIAGNOSE VINCENT'S STOMATITIS FROM THE SMELL

18.8 Cancrum (ulcer) oris (mouth)

This is a rare but very serious lesion of the mouths of malnourished children. Sometimes it is a complication of a severe infection, such as measles or typhoid. Like Vincent's stomatitis, it is caused by organisms of the normal mouth flora, especially spirochaetes.

First, the child has a sore mouth and does not want to eat. He has grey, bad-smelling, ulcers on his gums near his back teeth. These ulcers spread down to the bones of his jaws, and out to his face through the muscle of his cheeks. A black lesion forms on the skin of his face and gets bigger. Then a piece of dead tissue falls out of his cheek leaving a hole through to his mouth. Cancrum oris causes a gross deformity which can only be treated with long and expensive operations. It is one of the worst diseases any child can have. Fortunately, it is not common. To prevent it, make sure that all children are well-nourished. Diagnose and treat sore mouths early.

CANCRUM ORIS

MANAGEMENT. **Early cancrum oris can be treated in a health centre. But if the ulcer has started to spread, try to send the child to hospital.**

Eating and drinking are difficult for him, but are very important.

FLUID. **Make sure he has plenty to drink. If necessary, rehydrate him (9.20).**

FOOD. **If he cannot eat solid food, give him food through a tube, or give him an intragastric milk drip (9.24). Sometimes, he can feed himself through the hole which the lesion has made in his face.**

ANTIMICROBIAL DRUGS. **Give him penicillin (3.15) while his wound heals.**

OTHER TREATMENT. **Give him vitamin tablets (3.36). If he is anaemic, give him children's iron mixture (3.33). If he comes from a malarious district, suppress his malaria (10.7).**

LOCAL TREATMENT. **Wash out his mouth with hydrogen peroxide (about 15 ml in 100 ml of water), or saline. If necessary, use a syringe. Pineapples or papaya help to clean his mouth, if he will eat them.**

Put wet hypochlorite (3.48) dressings on his ulcers, or round the edge of the hole in his face. Cut away any pieces of dead tissue with scissors. The nerves in them will also be dead, so he will not feel any pain.

TREAT SORE MOUTHS EARLY AND PREVENT CANCRUM ORIS

Cancrum oris

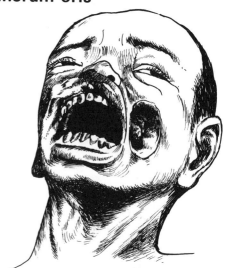

this is a marasmic child, he looks like an old man

Fig. 18–6 Cancrum oris is a complication of malnutrition.

204

18.9 Caring for a child with a sore mouth

You can usually make the diagnosis from the examination alone.

HISTORY. **Has he been given antibiotics? (These often cause a stomatitis.)**

EXAMINATION. **Examine his tongue, teeth, and gums, and the inside of his cheeks (18.2).**
  Does his mouth smell bad (*Vincent's stomatitis, cancrum oris*)?
  What do the lesions look like?
  —a white membrane or spots (thrush)?
  —round grey ulcers (herpes)?
  —swollen, tender bleeding gums (mild Vincent's stomatitis)?
  —grey, ulcerated gums (severe Vincent's stomatitis)?
  —deep ulcers on the gums, or inside the cheeks (cancrum oris)?
  Are the lesions white and easily wiped away (milk curds)?
  Have many of his teeth got holes in them (caries)?
  Or are new teeth coming into his mouth (teething)?
  If there is one ulcer, is there a sharp tooth opposite it?
  Are the lymph nodes under his jaw large and tender (lymphadenitis from any mouth infection)?
  Fever (any severe fever can cause stomatitis)?
  Is he malnourished? (Vincent's stomatitis is common in malnourished children, and cancrum oris is only seen in severely malnourished ones.)

DIAGNOSIS. **Caries (18.3)? Thrush (18.5)? The sore mouth of fever (10.3)? Herpes stomatitis (18.6)? Vincent's stomatitis (18.7)? The sore mouth of antibiotics (3.13)? Cancrum oris (18.8)?**

18.10 'Rosario's lips are sore'—fever, stomatitis, vitamin B deficiency

Any kind of fever which lasts more than a few days makes a child's lips sore. Most diseases which cause stomatitis also cause sore lips, especially the herpes virus which causes cold sores (11.15). Lack of one of the B vitamins also causes sore lips. This is worse at the corners of the mouth (angular stomatitis). If you cannot find a cause for a child's sore lips, give him vitamin B tablets.

18.11 'Amat has a sore throat and fever'—URI, tonsillitis, diphtheria

Viruses or bacteria can infect a child's throat and cause an upper respiratory infection (URI). The child has a sore throat, a nasal discharge, and usually fever. Sometimes he has mild diarrhoea also. His pharynx is abnormally red, but this is a difficult sign because a normal pharynx is red. Sometimes his tonsils are large and red and have pus on them. Often, the lymph nodes at the angles of his jaw are enlarged and tender —lymphadenitis. When a child has large red tonsils

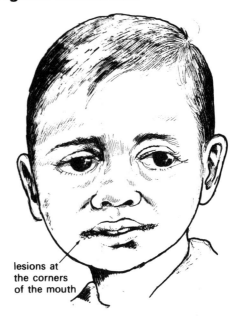

lesions at
the corners
of the mouth

Fig. 18–7 Angular stomatitis is caused by lack of B vitamins.

(especially with pus on them) we say he has tonsillitis. All other children we diagnose as URI.

Throat infections can also present as fever (10.10), febrile convulsions (15.5), swellings in the neck (19.2) or 'not eating' (18.14).

Virus infections of the throat are more common than bacterial infections. Virus infections cure themselves and antibiotics do not help. Infections with bacteria called streptococci are more serious. Streptococci can cause nephritis (23.7), or heart or joint disease. Penicillin kills them. Unfortunately we cannot easily diagnose whether a child's throat infection is caused by viruses or streptococci. You cannot give penicillin to every child with a sore throat, so follow the rules below.

18.10

18.8

TONSILLITIS, OR 'URI'

TREATMENT. **If a child has pus on his tonsils, or acute tonsillar lymphadenitis, bacteria are probably infecting him. Give him sulphadimidine, or penicillin (3.15). If possible, he needs procaine penicillin for ten days, or one injection of 'depot' penicillin.**

18.11

  If he only has a red throat, a nasal discharge, and fever without other signs, he probably has a virus infection. Antibiotics will not help. Don't give them to every child with a sore throat if it is only part of a cold. Aspirin (3.41) or paracetamol (3.42) are usually enough.
  If necessary, treat his fever (10.3).

EXPLANATION. **Tell his mother to give him soft foods and plenty to drink.**

Tonsillitis

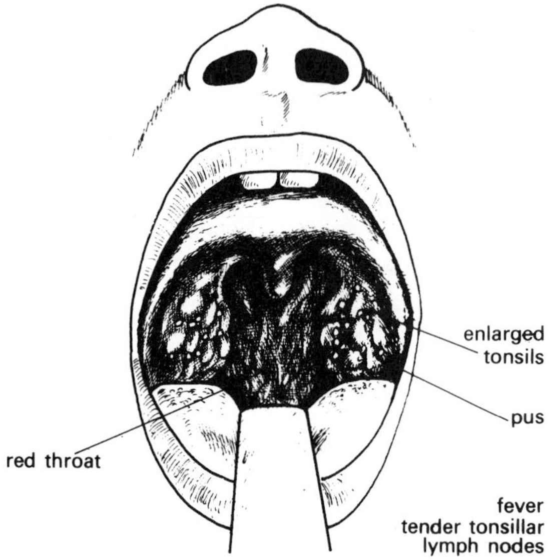

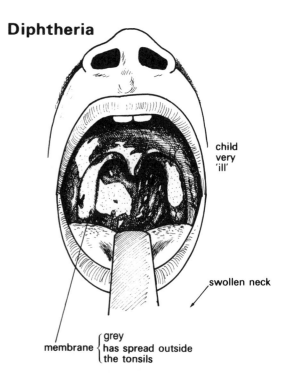

red throat

enlarged tonsils

pus

fever
tender tonsillar
lymph nodes

Fig. 18–8 Tonsillitis is an acute septic infection.

18.12 Diphtheria

This dangerous disease is caused by bacteria which grow in the pharynx and tonsils. It is spread by droplet infection. Diphtheria starts slowly and makes a child ill for a few days with fever and a cough. His fever is usually mild, but he is more ill than you would expect from a mild fever. His throat is sore and he has difficulty swallowing. Sometimes, the infection makes his neck swell like the neck of a bull—'bull neck'. His mouth smells bad, and grey lesions called diphtheritic membrane cover his tonsils. This membrane looks like pieces of dirty grey cloth stuck to the mucosa. Often, the membrane spreads outside his tonsils onto the mucosa of his pharynx. Occasionally, it causes obstructive laryngitis (8.11), so the child has difficulty breathing and speaking. Sometimes, diphtheria causes ulcers on the skin (11.7). Rarely, it presents as a bloody discharge from the nose (25.11).

The organisms which cause ordinary tonsillitis sometimes cause a purulent membrane to form in the throat. This may be difficult to diagnose from diphtheria. But other organisms seldom cause membrane spreading beyond the tonsils. Thrush can also cause a membrane, but it is white, and at the front of the mouth. Thrush does not make a child so ill.

A child with diphtheria can die from the local lesion in his throat. He can also die because the bacteria in his throat have made a toxin (poison) which harms his heart. If his heart stops working, he dies suddenly. Sometimes the toxin paralyses his palate so that fluid comes out of his nose when he tries to swallow.

A SICK CHILD WITH A MEMBRANE BEYOND HIS TONSILS PROBABLY HAS DIPHTHERIA

DIPHTHERIA

MANAGEMENT. **A child with diphtheria is very ill. You cannot treat him in a health centre, so try to send him to hospital. He needs careful nursing in bed, diphtheria antitoxin (4.2), and, perhaps, a tracheotomy (8.11). If you have to treat him yourself, give him penicillin (3.15) and treat him for obstructive laryngitis (8.11). Diphtheria spreads round a family, so his brothers and sisters need antitoxin also.**

EXPLANATION. **Explain to his mother why he is ill. If he cannot go to hospital, tell her what she can do for him. Ask her to keep him in bed for four weeks after he feels well. If he runs about too soon, he may die suddenly.**

18.13 Caring for a child with a sore throat

Whenever you see a sick child with a membrane in his throat, ask yourself—'Could this be diphtheria?' Sometimes a child has diphtheria, but there is no membrane, so diagnosis is difficult.

Diphtheria

child very 'ill'

swollen neck

grey
membrane { has spread outside
the tonsils

Fig. 18–9 Diphtheria causes a membrane in the throat.

206

HISTORY. **What other symptoms has he got? Children with a sore throat often have a cough. But if a child has difficulty breathing or stridor, go to Section 8.21.**

Did his illness come on rapidly or slowly? (Tonsillitis and pharyngitis come on rapidly; diphtheria comes on more slowly during several days.)

Has he been immunized with DPT vaccine? (This should prevent diphtheria.)

EXAMINATION. **Has he got a discharge from his nose (probably 'URI')?**

Is his neck swollen? (Diphtheria causes much more swelling than tonsillitis.)

Feel for enlarged tender lymph nodes under the angles of his jaw (18–3). (If he is not tender when you press under the angles of his jaw, he does not have tonsillitis.)

Examine his mouth and throat (18.2). Abnormally red pharynx? (Any upper respiratory infection.) (Koplik's spots? (Measles.) Tonsils large, or with pus on them? (Tonsillitis, perhaps diphtheria.) Membrane outside his tonsils, on the mucosa of his mouth or pharynx? (Probably diphtheria.) Is there bleeding when the membrane is removed with a spatula? (Probably diphtheria.)

Take his temperature. (Diphtheria causes less fever than tonsillitis.)

If he is 'ill' count his pulse. (If he has diphtheria, it may be very fast—over 120.)

DIAGNOSIS. **'URI' (18.11)? Tonsillitis (18.11)? Measles (10.6)? Diphtheria (18.12)?**

MANAGEMENT WHEN DIAGNOSIS IS DIFFICULT. **If he is 'ill' and might have diphtheria try to send him to hospital. If this is not possible treat him for it.**

The child who has stopped eating

18.14 'Yetunde has stopped eating'—any infection, painful lesions in or around the mouth, malnutrition, TB, an unhappy child, bad eating habits, or a worried mother

Very many diseases can stop a child eating, so it is a common presenting symptom. If a baby stops sucking (26.20), it is a very serious sign.

Infections. Healthy children eat well, and 'not eating' (5.15), is often the first sign of an infection. It often comes before fever. So, if a child has been eating well, and suddenly stops eating, look for signs of an infection such as measles, or otitis media.

Painful lesions in or around the mouth. A child may stop eating because he has a sore mouth (18.9), or a sore throat (18.11), mumps, or a painful lesion of his face. Occasionally, he is unable to open his mouth because he has tetanus (18.16).

Malnutrition. Children with marasmus (7.9) are very hungry, but children with kwashiorkor (7.10) are not.

'Not eating' is sometimes a presenting symptom in kwashiorkor.

Unhappiness. Sometimes, a child stops eating because he is unhappy. His mother may have given birth to a younger child, and he may be jealous, or he may have been sent away from home. Ask about his family, and look at his growth curve. Explain to his mother why he is not eating, and tell her that she must look after him with special care. Observe his growth curve carefully (5.21).

Bad eating habits. Some children eat many small pieces of food between meals and do not want to eat a normal meal. Explain to their mothers that children eat better if they are given four good meals at regular times. Food less than two hours before a meal may stop a child eating the meal.

A worried mother. Some children need less food than others, and they may not want to eat much. This may worry a child's mother, especially if she wants her children to be fat. She will usually say that he has eaten little food all his life. He may have been born small. Observe his growth curve. If he is growing, he is healthy, even if he is below the road to health (7.1). Tell her to give him good body-building food, and not to try to make him eat.

18.15 Caring for a child who is not eating

Acute infections are the most common cause for a child not eating. These infections are usually easy to diagnose. Some children have chronic diarrhoea, eat little and are malnourished.

If a mother says her child sucks milk, but will not eat any food, go to Section 25.3

If his mouth is sore go to Section 18.9.

If his throat is sore go to Section 18.13.

Symptoms of infection? Cough (8.20)? Diarrhoea (9.13)? Fever (10.10)? Worms (21.3)? If he has these symptoms, go to the sections for them.

HISTORY. **When did he stop eating? (If it is a new symptom it may be serious.)**

Look at his growth curve. (Growing normally—probably well. Growth curve flat—malnourished. Growth curve falling—malnourished, perhaps TB or chronic diarrhoea.)

Has he got any of the other common symptoms of TB (13:1) Losing weight? 'Ill'? Cough? Fever?

Is he unhappy? Has his mother given birth to another child?

Is his mother worrying about him more than necessary?

EXAMINATION. **'Ill' or 'well'? (If he is 'ill' he probably has an infection or malnutrition.)**

Is he severely malnourished? Oedema? (Kwashiorkor, 7.10.)

Examine his mouth and throat (18.2). Can he open his mouth (18.16)?

SPECIAL TEST. **Are there worms in his stool?**

DIAGNOSIS. **Any acute infection? Sore mouth or throat (18.13)? Malnutrition (7.13)? Ascaris (21.3)? Chronic diarrhoea (9.12)? TB (13.7)? Bad eating habits (18.14)? Unhappy child (25.2)? Worried mother (25.1)? Teething (25.2c)?**

MANAGEMENT IF DIAGNOSIS IS DIFFICULT. **If you find an infection, treat it.**

If you cannot find a cause, explain to his mother how she can feed him better. Observe his growth curve, and weigh him again in a month. If he is growing, explain to his mother that she need not worry. If he is not growing, and you cannot find a cause, send him for help.

The child who cannot open his mouth

18.16 'Babatunde cannot open his mouth'—infections of the mouth (18.3) or jaw, mumps, tetanus

Mumps (19.4) and infections of the mouth are in other sections. Here we will describe tetanus.

Tetanus is caused by bacteria which make a child's muscles contract. His jaw muscles contract so strongly that he cannot open his mouth and eat. Tetanus bacteria live in the gut of animals which eat grass. The bacteria are passed with the animal's faeces onto the ground. Tetanus bacteria can live for many years in earth and dust. If a child cuts himself, tetanus bacteria may go into

Tetanus of the newborn

- will not suck
- cannot open his mouth
- muscle spasms
- head bent back

tetanus bacteria have infected his umbilical cord

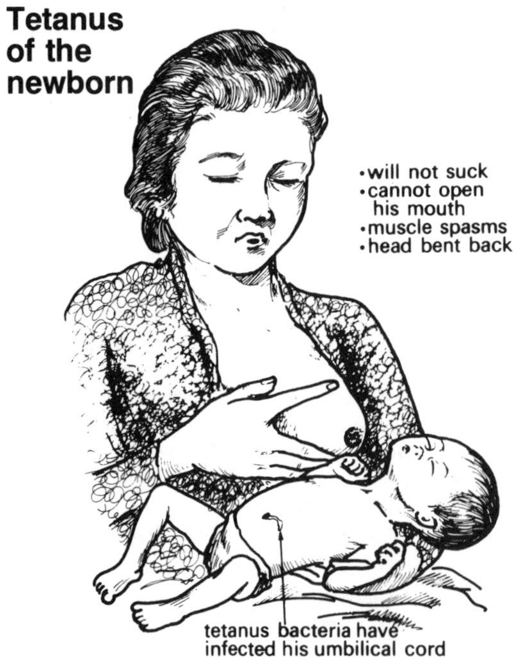

Fig. 18–10 We can prevent tetanus of the newborn.

the wound and grow. Sometimes a child has tetanus but we cannot see a cut. Tetanus bacteria can also infect the umbilical cord (26.42), carious teeth, or a discharging ear (17.10). Tetanus bacteria grow slowly. In older children the disease may not start for 20 days after bacteria have infected a cut.

Tetanus bacteria stay and grow in the local lesion. They cause disease by making a toxin (poison) which goes into a child's body. The toxin makes his muscles contract too much. At first his muscles are only stiff and painful. Later, he has strong painful contractions (spasms). Tetanus usually starts in the jaw, and a child cannot eat or suck, because he cannot open his mouth. This is his presenting symptom. As the stiffness becomes worse, his mouth stays shut. A healthy child can open his mouth wide. We can easily put three fingers in. If you cannot put three fingers in, he may have tetanus.

The stiffness soon spreads to other muscles. His back and neck bend backwards. The muscles of his face contract, so that the outer ends of his mouth and eyebrows move upwards. Later, all the stiff muscles contract in spasms. This makes him so exhausted (tired) that he dies.

Fits (15.1) also cause muscle contractions, but fits make a child unconscious. A child with tetanus stays conscious and cries with pain. Tetanus and meningitis both make a child bend backwards, but in meningitis there are no spasms.

Tetanus bacteria can infect a small cut, but they infect a large, deep, or dirty cut more easily. Earth in a cut is especially dangerous. Tetanus antitoxin can cause serious side effects (3.2), and sometimes death. So don't give it for clean cuts. Keep it for the deep dirty cuts.

PREVENTING TETANUS

EVERY CHILD. **Children who have had three injections of DPT vaccine don't get tetanus (4.9).**

MOTHERS. **Give a mother three injections of tetanus toxoid during her first pregnancy. She will make antibodies that go to her baby through his umbilical cord and give him a natural passive immunity to tetanus. Give her first dose as soon as she comes to the antenatal clinic. Give her second dose one month later. Give her third dose during the last month of pregnancy, at least two weeks before delivery. To get the strongest immunity there should be one month or more between each injection. Next time she is pregnant, give her one dose only.**

THE CHILD WITH A DIRTY CUT
Look carefully at the immunizations recorded on his weight chart.

If he has had three DPT injections. **Give him a booster injection of tetanus toxoid (or DPT or DT vaccine). If he has had any tetanus toxoid during the last year, this booster injection is not necessary.**

If he has not had three DPT injections. **Give him 3000 units** of tetanus antitoxin (3.2) and tetanus toxoid (or DPT or DT vaccine). Test for allergy (3.2). Give the toxoid and the antitoxin in different syringes on different sides of his body. Also give him one injection of depot penicillin (or procaine penicillin for 5 days). A month later give him another injection of tetanus toxoid.

THE CHILD WITH A CLEAN CUT
Treat him in the same way as with a dirty cut. But do not give tetanus antitoxin.

Tetanus is difficult to treat. Tetanus antitoxin is expensive and many children die, even though they have been given it. The most important part of the treatment is giving him enough fluids, and enough drugs to stop the spasms. In the next section we use promethazine. But diazepam (0·1 mg/kg/dose) by mouth or by injection is better. It is also more expensive.

TETANUS

MANAGEMENT
A child with tetanus needs careful nursing. If his mother will take him to hospital, and the care there is good, send him. If not, treat him at home. You may be able to save his life.

FOOD AND FLUIDS. **Pass an intragastric tube. If he is breast-fed show his mother how to express her breast-milk and give him this down the tube. If he is not breast-fed, or if his mother has not got enough breast-milk, teach her how to make an artificial feed. Explain carefully how much he needs (26.15b). Give her a syringe and show her how to inject the feed down the tube.**

TREATMENT
DRUGS TO STOP SPASMS. **On his first visit, give him an injection of paraldehyde (3.44).**

Give him promethazine syrup (1 mg/kg/dose) down his tube. Give it four times a day to stop his spasms. Don't give it more often than this. Show his mother how to measure it with a 2 ml syringe. Explain how many syringe-fuls he needs, and how many times a day she must give them.

ANTITOXIN. **Give a newborn child 3000 units intramuscularly. Test an older child to make sure he is not sensitive to antitoxin (3.2). If he is not sensitive, give him 5000 units of antitoxin intravenously and 5000 units intramuscularly.**

Newborn baby—Infected umbilicus. **Clean it, and put gentian violet on it. Leave it open as much as possible. Immunize his mother so that her next baby will not get tetanus.**

Older children—wounds. **Clean the wound. Try to get out as much dead tissue as possible, and leave it open.**

Tetanus in older children

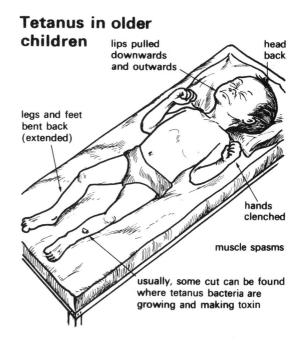

lips pulled downwards and outwards

head back

legs and feet bent back (extended)

hands clenched

muscle spasms

18.16

usually, some cut can be found where tetanus bacteria are growing and making toxin

Fig. 18–11 DPT vaccine prevents tetanus.

Ears. **Look for discharge. If necessary show his mother how to clean them.**

TREAT THE INFECTION. **If possible give him depot penicillin (3.15). If not give him procaine penicillin daily for five days.**

EXPLANATION
Explain to his mother that he must have the right amount of fluid through his tube. Ask her to bring him each day, or at least every three days.

18.17. Caring for a child who cannot open his mouth **18.17**

Diagnosis is usually easy.

HISTORY. **Has he had DPT vaccine or tetanus toxoid (4.9)?**

EXAMINATION. **How many fingers can you put into his mouth? If you cannot put three fingers in, something is abnormal.**
Swollen parotid glands (mumps)?
Examine his throat and tonsillar lymph nodes (tonsillitis).
Has he any skin lesion which might be infected by tetanus bacteria? Even a small one is enough. Discharging ear (tetanus)?

DIAGNOSIS. **A septic lesion in or around the mouth (18.3)? Mumps (19.4)? Tetanus (18.16)?**

19 Swellings

19.1 Swellings

A swelling is a part of the body which is larger than normal. Many diseases cause swellings, so they are a common presenting symptom. Swellings come in many different places. Swellings can be big or small, hard, soft, or fluctuant (full of fluid). Some swellings are tender, and other swellings are painless. You can feel some swellings, especially enlarged lymph nodes as 'lumps'. Lumps have edges you can easily feel. You cannot feel the edges of other swellings, especially cellulitis. They slowly change into the normal tissues round them. You can move the skin over some dwellings, but the skin is fixed to others. You can move some swellings over the deeper tissues under them. Other swellings are fixed to the deeper tissues.

Injuries, or acute or chronic septic infections can cause swellings anywhere in the body. Fluid in the tissues (oedema) sometimes causes swellings. Tumours occasionally cause them.

Some kinds of swellings are found in special places only. Hernias, for example, are found in the groin and abdomen. Mastoid swellings are only found behind the ear. Some of the most common swellings are in the head and neck. These swellings are in this chapter. Abdominal swellings are in the next chapter. Other swellings are in the other sections.

Swollen lymph nodes

19.2 Septic lymphadenitis

There are special lymph nodes in special places for each part of the body. The lymph nodes for most of the scalp are at the back of the neck where the hair ends. Close behind the ear there is a node for the ear and the scalp near it (17.12). The nodes for the face are in front of the ears. The nodes for the tonsils are under the angles of the jaw. The nodes for the mouth are under the front of the jaw. There are more nodes down each side of the neck. The nodes for the arm and upper part of the body are in the axilla. The nodes for the leg are in the groin (20.5).

You cannot see healthy lymph nodes, and they are difficult to feel. If you can see or feel them easily, they are swollen and diseased. Acute septic infection, chronic septic infection, and TB make them swell. Bacteria cause all these diseases.

Acute septic lymphadenitis. One or more lymph nodes become swollen and *tender*. You can usually move

THE LYMPH NODES

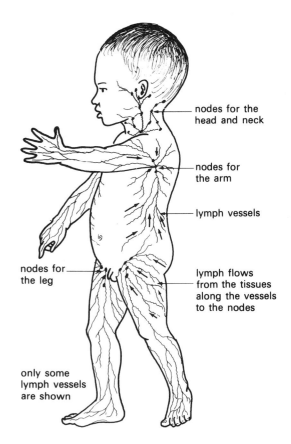

nodes for the head and neck

nodes for the arm

lymph vessels

nodes for the leg

lymph flows from the tissues along the vessels to the nodes

only some lymph vessels are shown

Fig. 19–1 The lymph nodes.

the skin over the infected node. You can usually move the node over the deeper tissues. But, if the infection has spread outside the node, you cannot do this. Occasionally, an abscess forms in a node. The abscess opens and discharges pus through the skin.

Usually, bacteria come from a septic local lesion. The septic local lesion is in the part of the body which sends lymph to the diseased node. For example, lymph from the foot goes to the nodes in the groin. So infected lesions in the foot cause lymphadenitis in the groin. Treat the child's local lesion, and treat him for a spreading septic infection (11.3).

Lymph nodes

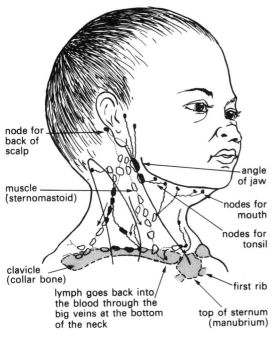

Fig. 19–1b The lymph nodes in a child's neck.

Chronic septic lymphadenitis. Many normal children have a few small (less than 1 cm), firm, painless lymph nodes. You can feel these enlarged nodes, but they are rarely big enough to see. Children have these nodes under their jaws, or in their necks or groins. The skin moves easily over them, and they move over the deeper tissues. Chronic septic lymphadenitis is caused by mild chronic infected local lesions. These lesions are in the part of the body which sends lymph to the diseased node. The lesions might be in a child's teeth, or his tonsils, or on his skin.

Chronic septic lymphadenitis is the commonest cause of enlarged nodes in the neck. It causes no symptoms, and needs no treatment, except treatment for the local lesion.

19.3 'There are large painless swellings at the side of Sudin's neck'—TB lymphadenitis

19.3

TB usually infects the lymph nodes of the lungs. Sometimes it infects the lymph nodes of the neck. Sometimes a child with TB nodes in his neck has TB in his lungs also.

TB lymphadenitis comes slowly during several months. It causes several firm painless swellings down one or both sides of a child's neck. At first these swellings feel like rubber and are separate from one another. Later they become larger, and join together. As they become larger they stick to the skin and to the deeper parts of the neck. If you don't treat them, they may open and discharge pus through the skin. TB bacilli then start growing in the skin and cause a chronic ulcer. A child with TB lymph nodes is moderately ill with fever, 'not eating', and anaemia. Sometimes, he has TB in other parts of his body, so examine him for TB (13.7).

TB lymph nodes are larger than the nodes of chronic septic lymphadenitis. If you cannot diagnose between septic lymphadenitis or TB, give him penicillin for two weeks. Observe him to see if his nodes become smaller. If he does not recover, treat him for TB (13.6). Most children with enlarged nodes in their necks do not have TB.

19.1

TB nodes of neck

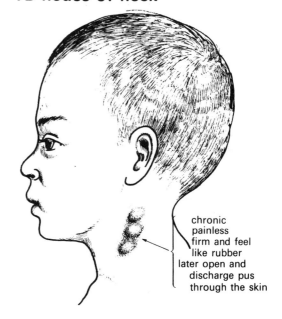

Fig. 19–2 A child with TB lymph nodes.

19.2

Some swellings of the face and neck

19.4 Mumps

19.4

This is a virus infection of the parotid glands. These glands make saliva. The parotid glands are on each side of the face, behind the jaw, below and in front of the ears. Saliva from the parotid glands goes into the mouth along small tubes.

Mumps starts with fever, and pain on eating. A child has difficulty opening his mouth. Two days later smooth soft tender swellings form in front of and below his ears. These swellings cover the angles of his jaws so that you cannot feel the angles of his jaw. You cannot easily feel the edge of the swellings. The skin moves over them, and they are fixed to the deeper tissues. Sometimes the swellings come first on one side, then on the other side. Sometimes they come on both sides at the same time.

After about a week the swellings become smaller, and after two weeks they go. Mumps leaves a strong natural active immunity (4.2), so a child seldom gets a second attack.

MUMPS

EXPLANATION. **Explain to the child's mother that mumps is not dangerous. Tell her the swellings will go by themselves in two weeks. Ask her to give him plenty to drink, and soft food that he can eat easily.**

MUMPS

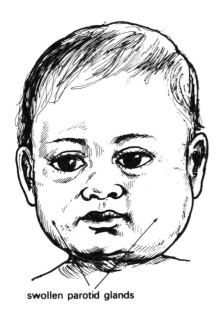

swollen parotid glands

Fig. 19–3 Mumps.

19.5 'Josefina has a swollen face'—tooth abscess

If caries (holes in the teeth) has destroyed a tooth, bacteria can spread through the tooth. They can cause an acute septic infection in the jaw. Bacteria can spread from the jaw to the cheek and cause cellulitis. Cellulitis presents as a painful tender swelling of one side of the face, like the girl in Figure 19–4. The swelling is fixed to the bone, and you cannot feel its edge. If you look into her mouth, you will find that many of her teeth have caries. One tooth will be tender if you touch it. This tooth has the abscess under it.

TOOTH ABSCESS

TREATMENT. **Give the child sulphadimidine (3.14), or penicillin (3.15), for the infection. Give him paracetamol (3.42), or aspirin (3.41), for the pain. Wait for a few days for the swelling to become less. Then someone can pull out the tooth.**

EXPLANATION. **Tell the child's mother that you can cure the swelling after the tooth is pulled out.**

Tooth abscess

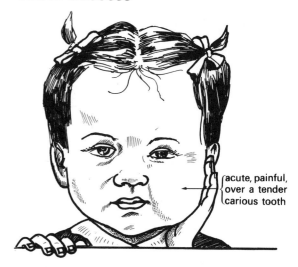

acute, painful, over a tender carious tooth

Fig. 19–4 A child with a tooth abscess.

19.6 Goitre

The thyroid gland is at the bottom of the neck, below the larynx and in front of the trachea. A healthy thyroid is small. You cannot feel it. But you can easily see and feel a swollen thyroid. We call it a **goitre**. It is a smooth painless swelling at the bottom of the front of the neck, or a little to one side of it. When a child swallows, his goitre moves up and down.

There are several kinds of goitre. Small goitres are common in girls at puberty (the time girls become women). They don't need treatment. Lack of iodine in the water causes another kind of goitre (endemic goitre). Lack of iodine is common in mountain districts. About half the school-children in some districts have a mild goitre. The mother of the child in Figure 9–23 has a

212

goitre. Goitres can be prevented by adding a little iodine to cooking salt. Or we can give every child an injection of iodized oil once every three years (4.11). An injection of 1 ml of iodized oil will usually cure an endemic goitre in a few months (3.34).

Goitre is not so important as iodine embryopathy (24.14b) which is also caused by lack of iodine.

We call a goitre Grade I if we can see and feel it with a patient's head in its normal position. It is also Grade I if it has nodules in it (small firm swellings). If more than 5 per cent of children (or 33 per cent of adults) have Grade I goitres, the community needs iodine.

Angioneurotic oedema. This is a severe kind of urticaria (11.24). Allergy (3.2) to food, drugs, or insect stings can cause it. The swellings are large (several centimetres), they come suddenly, and they usually itch. There may be swellings in any part of the body. They are usually on the face and arms. They go by themselves in a day or two. There is no protein in the urine.

Give the child promethazine. Ask his mother what drugs or unusual foods he has had. If you think a special food or drug caused the swellings, explain that he must not have it again.

Goitre

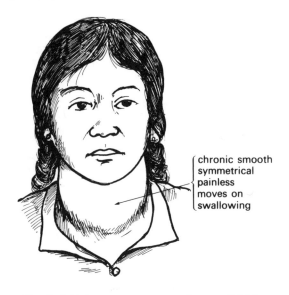

chronic smooth
symmetrical
painless
moves on
swallowing

Fig. 19–5 Goitres are very common in some districts.

Nephrotic syndrome

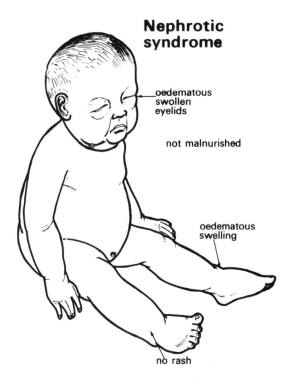

oedematous
swollen
eyelids

not malnurished

oedematous
swelling

no rash

Fig. 19–6 The nephrotic syndrome.

Swelling of the face, feet, and eyelids

19.7 'Sonji's face, both his eyelids, and his feet are swollen'—kwashiorkor, severe anaemia, acute nephritis, the nephrotic syndrome, whooping cough, angioneurotic oedema

In these diseases fluid (oedema, 7.10) forms in a child's tissues. Sometimes both his feet swell. Sometimes his face and eyelids swell also. If his disease is less severe, only his feet or only his face swell. Kwashiorkor (7.10), hookworm anaemia (22.5), whooping cough (8.17), and acute nephritis (23.7), are in other sections.

The nephrotic syndrome. A syndrome is a group of signs and symptoms. The nephrotic syndrome is a serious kidney disease. Protein from the blood goes into the urine. A child's ankles, eyelids, and face swell with fluid. Malaria usually causes the nephrotic syndrome. Hospital treatment seldom helps.

19.8 Caring for a child with swelling of his face, eyelids or feet (or his feet only)

If his conjunctivae are red or discharging he has conjunctivitis, so go to Section 16.8.

If the swelling of his face is painful, or on one side only, go to Section 19.5.

HISTORY. How old is the child? (Kwashiorkor is more common in children under three. The nephrotic syndrome is more common in children over three.)

Has he eaten special foods? Has he had any drugs? Has he been bitten by any insects? Does the swelling itch (angioneurotic oedema)?

Coughing (Whooping cough)?

EXAMINATION. Has he got a 'flaking paint rash'? Muscles

19.7

19.6

19.8

19.5

213

wasted? Underweight? Apathy? (These are all signs of kwashiorkor.)

Is he anaemic? (If he is severely anaemic, this is probably the cause of his swelling.)

Swollen fingers? Large spleen? Bossing? Mild jaundice? (Perhaps sickle cell anaemia, 22.8.)

SPECIAL TESTS. Is there much protein in his urine (L 8.3) (the nephrotic syndrome)?

Are there red cells in his urine (L 8.13) (acute nephritis (23.7), and some kinds of nephrotic syndrome)?

Measure his blood pressure. (If it is more than 140 mm/Hg he probably has acute nephritis.)

Measure his haemoglobin (L 7–1) (severe anaemia).

Are there hookworm ova in his stools (L 10.2a)? (If he has more than 40 ova in a standard stool smear, he has a heavy hookworm load, and they are probably causing his anaemia.)

Look for sickle cells (L 7.25).

DIAGNOSIS. Kwashiorkor (7.10)? Severe anaemia, especially hookworm anaemia (22.9) or sickle cell anaemia (22.8)? The nephrotic syndrome (19.7)? Angioneurotic oedema (19.7)? Whooping cough?

19.9 Caring for a child with a swelling anywhere in his body

Often, the place of the swelling will tell you the diagnosis, or the diseases which might be causing it.

HISTORY

How long has the child had his swelling? Is it becoming bigger? Slowly, or quickly? (If it is becoming bigger quickly, it is probably acute inflammation. If it is becoming bigger slowly, it is probably chronic inflammation, or perhaps a tumour.)

Are there any general symptoms? Fever? Not eating (infections)? Weight loss (chronic infections of any kind)?

Has he been injured, or bitten by insects?

EXAMINATION

Where exactly is the swelling?

Look at the swelling. Feel it. Watch his face while you do this. Is it tender? If it is, try not to hurt him. Don't touch him too much.

Are there any signs of acute inflammation? Tender? Red? Warm? If it is an acute inflammatory swelling, are the nearest lymph nodes enlarged and tender (lymphadenitis)? Take his temperature.

How big is the swelling? (Large swellings are usually more serious than small ones.)

What does the swelling feel like? Hard? Soft? Fluctuant?

Can you easily feel the edge of the swelling? Can you feel a lump?

Is the swelling in the skin? Or fixed to the skin? Can you move the skin over the swelling?

Can you move the swelling over the tissues underneath it?

If the swelling is in his face or neck, examine his mouth (18.2). If it is near his ears, examine his ears (17.3).

DIAGNOSIS

Swellings anywhere. Injury (14.5)? Acute infection, especially cellulitis (11.3)? Insect bites? Many skin diseases (11.28) can cause small swellings anywhere in the skin.

Special places. Is the swelling in one or more lymph nodes? (Acute, or chronic lymphadenitis, 19.2, or TB 19.3.) If the swelling might be TB examine him for it (13.7).

Over the 'corners' of the skull (bossing, sickle cell anaemia, 22.8)?

Over a bone (osteomyelitis, 24.5)?

In a muscle (pyomyositis, 24.5b)?

In front of and under one or both ears (mumps 19.4, tonsillitis)?

Does the swelling cover the angles of the jaw so that you cannot feel them (mumps)?

Behind the ear (lymphadenitis, mastoiditis, 17.11)?

In the eyelids? Go to Section 19.8.

In the lips (stomatitis, 18.9)?

Over the teeth (tooth abscess, 19.5)?

Over the neck of an 'ill' child (tonsillitis, diphtheria, 18.13)?

At the bottom of the front of the neck of a well child (goitre, 19.6)?

In his fingers and or toes ('hand foot syndrome' of sickle cell anaemia 22.8)?

Over the whole of the abdomen? Go to Section 20.8.

At the umbilicus (umbilical hernia, 20.7)?

Over the spine (TB 24.6)?

In the groin (hernia, lymphadenitis, 20.5)?

In the scrotum (hernia, hydrocoele, 26.59)?

In both feet, or lower arms? Go to Section 19.8.

MANAGEMENT IF DIAGNOSIS IS DIFFICULT

If the swelling might be an acute septic infection (acute, tender, fever, 'ill'), treat him for it (11.3).

If it might be TB (chronic, painless) treat him for this (13.6). If his swelling grows more while he is having TB treatment, he probably has a tumour. Hospital treatment may help.

20 Abdominal swelling, abdominal pain, vomiting

THE ABDOMEN

20.1 How the abdomen is made

The abdomen is the part of the body between the thorax (chest) and the legs. Inside it there is a space called the **abdominal cavity**. This contains the stomach and intestines, the liver and the spleen. The front and side walls of the abdominal cavity are made of muscles. The bones of the spine, the kidneys, and some more muscles make its back wall. A thin muscle called the diaphragm makes its roof. The bones and muscles of the pelvis make its floor. On this floor lie the rectum, the uterus, and the bladder.

The walls of the abdomen are covered on the outside by skin. On the inside they are covered by a sheet of thin tissue called **peritoneum**. More peritoneum covers the organs inside the abdomen. The gut is loosely joined to the back of the peritoneal cavity by a fold of peritoneum (the mesentery). The peritoneum is like the pleura. The pleura covers the inside of the ribs and the outside of the heart and lungs.

The space between the abdominal organs and the abdominal wall is called the **peritoneal cavity**. There are only a few drops of fluid in this cavity. The peritoneal cavity is like the pleural cavity. This also contains only a few drops of fluid.

20.2 'Acute abdomen'

Several serious diseases of the abdomen cause pain and vomiting, and sometimes swelling also. One of these diseases is **peritonitis**. This is an acute septic infection with pus in the peritoneal cavity. **Obstruction of the gut** is another serious abdominal disease. Organisms sometimes get out of an obstructed gut and cause peritonitis, so some children have both these diseases. Often we cannot be sure what kind of serious abdominal disease a child has. We only know that he has a serious acute abdominal disease—an **acute abdomen**. An acute abdomen must be treated by a surgical operation in hospital. If a child is not treated, he usually dies quickly. So send him to hospital soon.

ACUTE ABDOMENS ARE VERY SERIOUS

20.3 Examining the abdomen

When a healthy child lies down, his muscles relax, and his abdomen feels soft. If his spleen and liver are enlarged, you can feel them through his abdominal wall. But if he cries or moves, his muscles contract. His

THE PERITONEAL CAVITY

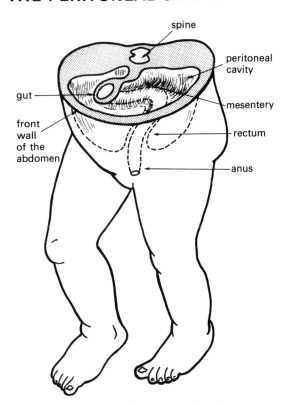

This is a drawing of the peritoneal cavity. In a living child it is filled by gut which touches everywhere, as shown in Figure 20·5

Fig. 20–1 The peritoneal cavity.

215

abdominal wall becomes hard and you can feel nothing inside his abdomen. So examine his abdomen while he is relaxed.

EXAMINING THE ABDOMEN

At some time you must undress the child. But you can start feeling his abdomen while he has his clothes on.

His abdomen must be soft and relaxed, so try to examine him lying flat. The best place to do this is on his mother's knees. If this frightens him examine him while he is in her arms, while he is sucking, or while he is standing up. If you examine him standing, put yourself behind him and let him look at her. If he cries you may be able to examine his abdomen while he relaxes between cries.

EXAMINING THE ABDOMEN

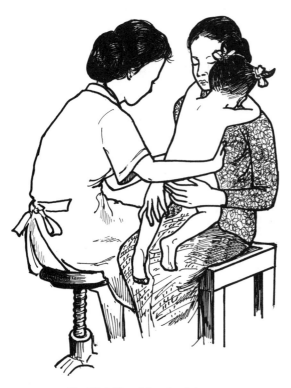

Fig. 20–2 Examining the abdomen.

Signs of an acute abdomen. When a child has peritonitis, the muscles of his abdominal wall will not relax—his abdomen wall feels hard (rigid). **Rigidity** of the abdominal wall is a sign of peritonitis. If a child's abdominal infection is less severe, there is no rigidity. But his muscles contract as you touch the infected part of his abdomen. This is called **guarding**. It is caused by his muscles contracting, so as to guard or prevent you from touching the infected place. Infection also makes his

abdomen tender when you touch it. **Tenderness** is an important sign of peritoneal infection, but it is a difficult sign to be sure about. If a child has a peritoneal infection—(1) His abdomen should be tender in the same place each time you touch it, and (2) His abdomen should always be tender when you touch it, not only sometimes. Examine another part of him and then examine his abdomen again. Try feeling his abdomen every half hour for an hour or two. Feel if the tenderness is still there, or has gone. A child with severe diarrhoea sometimes has a tender abdomen, but there is no rigidity or guarding.

Sometimes there is a third sign. If you quickly take your hand away from the tender place the child may feel an extra tenderness. This is called **rebound** ('jumping back') **tenderness**. It shows that there is inflammation of the peritoneum, and that he has an acute abdomen.

RIGIDITY, GUARDING, AND TENDERNESS ARE SIGNS OF AN ACUTE ABDOMEN

EXAMINING FOR AN ACUTE ABDOMEN

Examine him from the right. Put your right hand flat on the child's abdomen with your fingers together. Feel gently, first on one side and then on the other. Keeping your hand flat and your fingers together, slowly feel the whole of his abdomen. Feel the right lower part of his abdomen with special care, because this is a place that is often diseased.

Is there a place where the muscles will not relax, and where his abdomen feels rigid? Don't mistake the rigidity of a child who will not relax for the rigidity caused by peritoneal infection.

Is any part of his abdomen tender? Is the tenderness always in the same place? Do his muscles contract when you touch some part of his abdomen (guarding)? Does he jump (move) and feel pain as you take your hand away quickly (rebound tenderness)?

Does he lie quiet without moving? Is his pain worse if you ask him to sit up and turn over? (Both these are signs of an acute abdomen.)

A large liver or spleen. The liver and the spleen are under the ribs and the diaphragm. The liver is on the right, and the spleen is on the left. A healthy spleen is always too small to feel, but you may be able to feel the edge of a young child's liver. If he is more than two years old, a liver which is large enough to feel is abnormal.

When the liver and spleen are diseased they sometimes grow large. Malaria, typhoid, and sickle cell anaemia are the commonest causes of a large spleen. Sometimes, a child's spleen becomes so large that even his mother may be able to feel it. Large livers are less common than large spleens.

FEELING FOR THE SPLEEN

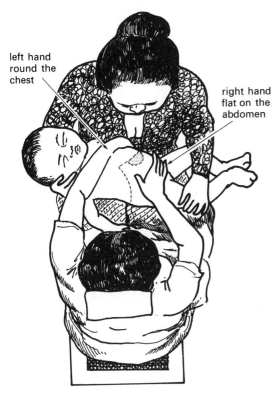

left hand round the chest

right hand flat on the abdomen

Fig. 20–3 Feeling for the spleen.

A distended bladder. A healthy bladder is too soft to feel through the abdominal wall. But if a child's urethra is obstructed, his bladder becomes tender, distended with urine, and easy to feel.

EXAMINING FOR A LARGE SPLEEN, LIVER OR BLADDER

SPLEEN. Examine the child from the right. Put your left hand under his lower left chest. Put your right hand flat on the right of his lower abdomen as shown in Figure 20–3. Keep your fingers together and the edge of your hand facing his spleen. Start with your right hand in his lower abdomen, or you may miss the edge of a very large spleen. Ask an older child to take a deep breath, then press gently into his abdomen with the flat of your hand. You may be able to feel the edge of his spleen move under your hand as he breathes. If you cannot feel anything, move your right hand a little higher on his abdomen and a little closer to your left hand. Feel again. Go on doing this until your right hand is close up under the edge of his left lower ribs. If you cannot feel anything here when he breathes, he has not got a large spleen. Use Figure 20–4 to record how big it is.

LIVER. Feel for the liver in the same way as the spleen, except that the liver is under the ribs on the right. The liver does not become so large as the spleen, so begin by putting your right hand closer under his ribs.

BLADDER. Put your hand flat on his abdomen. Using the edge of your hand, try to feel a soft round tender swelling in the middle of his lower abdomen (20–4).

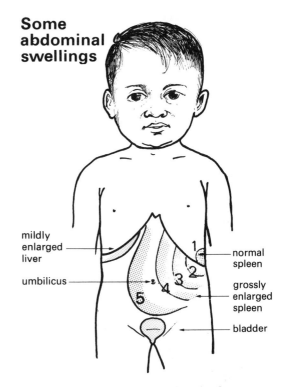

Some abdominal swellings

mildly enlarged liver

umbilicus

normal spleen

grossly enlarged spleen

bladder

Fig. 20–4 How big is the spleen?

SWELLINGS OF THE GROIN AND UMBILICUS

20.4 Hernias

20.4

A hernia is a special kind of swelling. A hernia is formed by a part of the body coming out through a hole. For example, some gut may come through a hole in the muscles of the abdomen wall. The gut makes a swelling under the skin. There are three common holes in the muscles of the abdominal wall. One hole is at the umbilicus, and the other two are in the right and left inguinal regions (groins). Hernias form in these places. A hernia does these special things.

A hernia comes and goes quickly.

A hernia gets bigger when a child coughs, cries, or runs about.

A hernia gets smaller and may go away completely when he lies down and is quiet.

You can usually *reduce* a hernia (make it go back inside the abdomen). Lie the child down and try to push the swelling back into his peritoneal cavity. A hernia soon comes back when he stands up or runs about.

20.5 'Olu has a swelling in his groin'—lymphadenitis, inguinal hernia

Inguinal lymphadenitis. Many children have a few chronic septic lesions on their legs, lower abdomen, and buttocks. Infection spreads from these to cause mild *chronic* septic lymphadenitis (19.2), in their inguinal lymph nodes. This makes the nodes swell mildly. But they do not become painful or tender, and they do not need treatment.

Infection sometimes causes *acute* septic lymphadenitis in the inguinal nodes. The nodes become swollen, painful, and tender. Occasionally, an abscess forms. Treat acute septic inguinal lymphadenitis with penicillin (11.3).

HOW AN UMBILICAL HERNIA FORMS

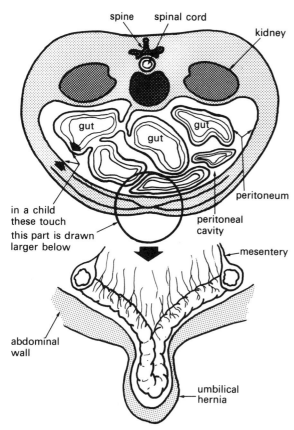

The peritoneal cavity has been drawn larger than normal to show it more clearly. In a child the peritoneum over the gut touches the peritoneum on the inside of the abdomen

Fig. 20–5 How an umbilical hernia forms.

Inguinal hernia. When a child is growing in the uterus his testes are formed high up near his kidneys. About the time of birth they move out of his abdominal cavity. They go down through special holes in his inguinal regions, and out under the skin into his scrotum. In a normal child, the holes close after the testes have come through. The gut in his abdomen cannot go down into his scrotum. Occasionally, the holes do not close. So, gut can go down towards his scrotum, or into it, and cause an inguinal hernia.

Usually, you can easily reduce an inguinal hernia. Occasionally, the gut sticks inside a hernia and you cannot reduce it. The hernia becomes tender and painful —it is **strangulated**. A strangulated hernia is serious because the gut inside it can become obstructed, or it can cause peritonitis. Obstruction and strangulation are dangerous complications of hernias.

INGUINAL HERNIA

MANAGEMENT. A child with a strangulated hernia needs an operation quickly, so send him to hospital immediately. If his hernia is not strangulated, he needs an operation during the next few months. Explain this to his mother.

Inguinal hernia

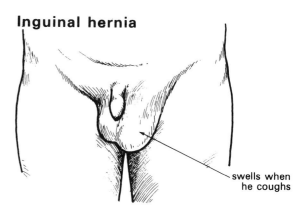

Fig. 20–6 An inguinal hernia.

20.6 Caring for a child with a swelling in his groin

Inguinal swellings are usually easy to diagnose.

HISTORY. How long has the child had the swelling? (Hernias usually come soon after birth. Acute swollen lymph nodes probably came during the last few days.)

Does the swelling come and go, or does it stay the same? (Hernias come and go and are reducible. Lymph nodes stay the same. If the swelling used to come and go, but is now firm and tender, and will not go away, it is a strangulated hernia.)

Is he 'well' (uncomplicated hernia or mild chronic lymphadenitis)? Fever (septic lymphadenitis)? Pain or vomiting (strangulated hernia)?

EXAMINATION. Look at the swelling. Can you see it? (In

chronic lymphadenitis nodes are seldom big enough to see.)

Does it go towards the scrotum (inguinal hernia)?

Feel the swelling. Is it soft (hernia)? Is it hard (chronic lymphadenitis)? Is it tender (acute lymphadenitis, strangulated hernia)?

Examine him lying down. Can you push the swelling back into his abdomen? (If it goes away completely, it is an ordinary inguinal hernia which is not strangulated. If it does not go away, and you cannot push it back, it is either a lymph node or a strangulated hernia.) Does the swelling get bigger or firmer when he coughs or cries (ordinary unstrangulated hernia)?

Is there any septic lesion on his legs, buttock, or lower abdomen, which might be causing lymphadenitis?

Fever (septic lymphadenitis)?

DIAGNOSIS. **Lymphadenitis (19.2)? Hernia? Reducible or strangulated (20.5)?**

20.7 'Budi has a swelling at his umbilicus'—umbilical hernia

Hernias sometimes form at the umbilicus where there is a weak place in the muscles of the abdominal wall. They usually go by themselves as a child grows older, and his muscles become stronger. Even a big umbilical hernia never bursts and seldom strangulates, so it is not serious. Mothers sometimes put a binder (a piece of tight cloth) round the abdomen to keep a hernia flat. This will not make it go away any quicker. Explain that the child only needs an operation if he still has the hernia when he is five years old.

SWELLING OF THE WHOLE ABDOMEN

20.8 'Sri's abdomen is swollen' malnutrition, *Ascaris* infection, a large liver or spleen, gut obstruction, fluid

A child's abdomen is normally more swollen than the abdomen of an adult. As a child grows older his abdomen becomes flatter. If his abdomen becomes abnormally swollen suddenly (acutely) during a few hours or days, his disease is probably serious. If the swelling comes on slowly (chronically) during several weeks or months, it is probably not serious.

Acute swelling. Diarrhoea sometimes causes mild swelling and pain (9.29b). Gut obstruction is the most serious cause of acute abdominal swelling. When this happens stools and gas (air) cannot get out of a child's abdomen, so it swells. He has pain, vomits, and is 'ill'.

Chronic swelling. Malnutrition (7.8) is the commonest cause of chronic abdominal swelling. It makes a child's abdominal muscles thin and weak, so that his gut falls forward. Malnutrition also harms the mucosa of his gut, so that food is not digested and absorbed normally.

AN UMBILICAL HERNIA

20.5

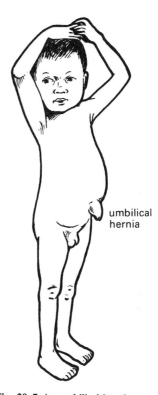

umbilical
hernia

20.7

Fig. 20–7 An umbilical hernia.

Bacteria grow and make gas in this unabsorbed food, so that his gut swells with gas.

A heavy load of *Ascaris* worms can cause abdominal swelling, so can a large liver or spleen (20.3). Many children are malnourished, like the child in Figure 20–8. They also have heavy *Ascaris* loads and large spleens caused by chronic malaria. So there are several reasons why their abdomens swell.

Occasionally, a swollen abdomen is full of fluid. This can be caused by the nephrotic syndrome (19.7), or by TB (13.1), or by a tumour.

20.8

20.6

20.9 Caring for a child with a swollen abdomen

20.9

Swollen abdomens are common, but they are seldom a presenting symptom.

HISTORY AND EXAMINATION. **Is the swelling acute (during a few hours or days)? Or chronic (during a few weeks or months)?**

Acute swelling. **Diarrhoea? (His swelling is probably not serious.) Abdominal pain or vomiting? (Both these are serious. He may have an acute abdomen, so go to Section 20.13)**

Chronic swelling. **Is he malnourished (7.13)?** *Ascaris* **ova in his stools (L 10.2)? Large spleen or liver (20.3)? Has he a** swollen face, swollen feet, or protein in his urine (the nephrotic syndrome, 19.7)?

MANAGING A CHRONIC SWELLING WHEN DIAGNOSIS IS DIFFICULT. **If he has a large spleen or liver, and you are in a malarious area, suppress his malaria (3.25).**

Measure his abdomen with a tape measure at the umbilicus. Weigh him and ask him to come back in two weeks to be measured again. If he is gaining weight, and his abdomen is not larger, there is no need to worry. If his abdomen is larger, and he is not gaining weight, try to send him for help.

If you have found nothing, tell his mother that his swelling will probably go as he grows older.

A CHILD WITH CHRONIC ABDOMINAL SWELLING

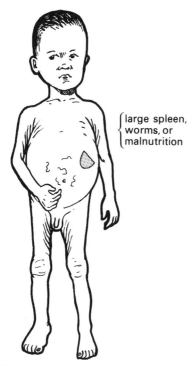

{ large spleen, worms, or malnutrition

Fig. 20–8 Chronic abdominal swelling.

ABDOMINAL PAIN

20.11 'Bakri has had abdominal pain since yesterday (acute abdominal pain)'—gut infections, other infections, acute abdomen

Abdominal pains are difficult to diagnose. Older children can say they have pain. Babies sometimes pull up their knees when they have pain, and a mother may be sure that her baby is in pain. Often she is right.

A pain which has only lasted one or two days is *acute.* Infections are the most common cause of acute abdom-

inal pain, especially gut infections causing diarrhoea (9.13), malaria (10.7), hepatitis (22.11), pneumonia (8.15), tonsillitis (18.11).

Sickle cell anaemia sometimes causes acute abdominal pain (22.8). There may also be tenderness, rigidity, and guarding.

Acute abdomen is a rare but serious cause of abdominal pain. A child with an acute abdomen usually vomits. His vomit may be green or brown. This is a serious sign. He may pass no stools, normal stools, or one or two liquid stools. But he seldom has much diarrhoea. So, if a child has abdominal pain with moderate or severe diarrhoea, his diarrhoea is probably causing his pain. He may be in danger from dehydration, but he has probably not got an acute abdomen.

20.12 'Bancombe has had abdominal pains for weeks (chronic abdominal pain)'—worms, urinary infections

These are *chronic* pains that a child has had for weeks or months. Sometimes, a child has pains all the time. More often the pains come and go in attacks. There is usually no diarrhoea or vomiting and diagnosis may be difficult. The only common and easily diagnosed cause is worm infection, especially with *Ascaris.* So examine his stools. Look for a urinary infection, especially in girls (23.4).

20.13 Caring for a child with abdominal pain

The important question to decide is—has the child got an acute abdomen? A child with an acute abdomen will probably die if you do not diagnose and treat him soon.

If he has moderate or severe diarrhoea go to Section 9.31

HISTORY. **How long has he had pain? (Acute and chronic abdominal pains have different causes.) Has he had it before? (If a child has already recovered from several attacks, this attack is probably not serious.)**

Has he any symptoms of infection? Fever? Cough? Sore throat? Jaundice? Frequency or dysuria?

Is the pain in one of his (or her) loins (urinary infection)?

Has he been vomiting (acute abdomen or an infection)? If he has been vomiting, what has his vomiting been like? (He may have an acute abdomen if he vomits much fluid suddenly and strongly, especially if his vomit is green, or brown.)

Is he constipated? Can he not pass air (gut obstruction)?

EXAMINATION. **Examine his abdomen (20.3). Look for swelling, rigidity, guarding, and tenderness. (These are serious signs of an acute abdomen, especially if he has several of them.)**

Is his spleen enlarged? Anaemia (malaria, sickle cell anaemia)?

Jaundice? Large tender liver (hepatitis)?

Examine his throat (tonsillitis).

Take his temperature (infections). Is he breathing fast (pneumonia)?

SPECIAL TESTS. **If necessary, examine his stools for ova (L 10.2), his urine for pus (L 8.11), and bilirubin (bile, L 8.8), and his blood for malaria parasites (L 7.31), or sickle cells (L 7.25).**

DIAGNOSIS. **Tonsillitis (18.11)? Malaria (10.7)? Hepatitis (22.11)? Pneumonia (8.15)?** *Ascaris* **or some other worm infection (21.3)? Urine infection (23.4)? Sickle cell anaemia (22.8)? Acute abdomen (20.14)?**

vomiting attacks every few months. A child vomits a few times, especially at night, he is mildly ill, and he sometimes has mild abdominal pain and fever. He then recovers without any treatment. Most mothers understand these attacks, and are not worried. But a young mother may bring her child to you. Often, by the time you see him, his vomiting has stopped. These children need symptomatic treatment to make sure they do not become dehydrated.

MANAGEMENT OF ABDOMINAL PAIN IF DIAGNOSIS IS DIFFICULT

'Acute abdomen'	*Less serious diseases*	
He may need an operation in hospital if he—	*He can usually be treated in a health centre or at home if he—*	**20.12**
— has severe vomiting especially if it is green or brown.	— has moderate or severe diarrhoea.	
— has abdominal swelling, tenderness, guarding, or rigidity.	— has signs of an infection.	
— has had severe pain for a short time.	— has had pains like this before.	**20.13**
— is severely 'ill' (5.15).	— is well or only moderately 'ill'.	

If a child has chronic abdominal pain, and you cannot find a cause, give him piperazine. He may have worms that you have not been able to find. If he is not better when you give him piperazine, weigh him and ask his mother to bring him to see you every month. If he gains weight and looks well, don't worry. If he does not seem well and does not grow, send him for help.

VOMITING

20.14 'Ahmad has been vomiting'—gut infections, other infections, 'vomiting attacks', acute abdomen

Usually, vomiting is not serious. Occasionally, when it is caused by an acute abdomen, it is very serious.

Gut infection (gastroenteritis). Gut infections often cause vomiting *and diarrhoea* and are usually caused by infected food (9.13). Most children recover quickly, but some become seriously dehydrated. Treat them for diarrhoea.

Infections outside the gut. Infections in other parts of the body also cause vomiting. A child may vomit when he has malaria, tonsillitis, meningitis, or a urinary infection. This kind of vomiting is easy to diagnose, if you remember to look for the signs of these diseases.

Vomiting attacks. Children and adults sometimes have short attacks of vomiting without diarrhoea for which we cannot find a cause. Some children have

VOMITING—SYMPTOMATIC TREATMENT

20.14

MANAGEMENT. There is no need to worry about a child unless his vomiting goes on for more than 24 hours, or he becomes dehydrated, or there are other signs.

EXPLANATION. Explain to his mother that his vomiting is not serious. Ask her to give him salt and sugar water (9.21) or glucose–salt solution. Tell her to give him a little fluid often.

Acute abdomen. Any kind of acute abdomen can cause vomiting. Gut obstruction always causes vomiting. The vomiting of gut obstruction is different from the vomiting of other diseases. A child with gut obstruction vomits large amounts. He may vomit so suddenly and strongly that his vomit is thrown several feet away. There may be bile in his vomit, or it may be brown like stools.

20.11

When a child's gut becomes obstructed, stools and gas cannot get out. So, he vomits, his abdomen swells and he has pain. He passes fewer stools than normal, or none (constipation). The obstruction can be caused by a strangulated hernia (20.4), by a ball of *Ascaris* worms (21.3), or because his gut has become twisted.

20.15 Caring for a child who is vomiting

If a child vomits, and has no other symptoms or signs, his illness is probably not serious. He has a mild gut infection, or has eaten too much food.

IF A CHILD HAS VOMITING AND ABDOMINAL PAIN, HE MAY HAVE AN ACUTE ABDOMEN

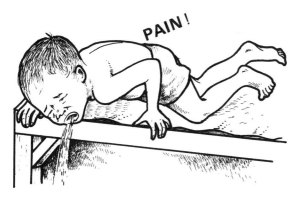

Fig. 20–9 If a child has vomiting and abdominal pain, he may have an acute abdomen.

If he is less than two months old, go to Section 26.27.
If he has moderate or severe diarrhoea go to Section 9.31.

HISTORY. **What food has he been eating? (Infected food which has stood in a warm place for some hours after cooking often causes vomiting and diarrhoea.) Has he eaten too much (overeating)?**
Does his mother sterilize his feeding bottle?
Has he had 'vomiting' attacks like this before? (If he has, he will probably recover from this attack also.)
What kind of vomiting is it? (He may have an acute abdomen if he has vomited large amounts, if he has been vomiting suddenly and strongly, or if his vomit is green or brown, and smells like stools.)
Abdominal pain (acute abdomen)?

EXAMINATION. **Is he dehydrated? (If he is dehydrated, he will need rehydration, 9.20.)**
Examine his abdomen (20.3). Swelling? Rigidity? Guarding? Rebound tenderness? (Acute abdomen.)
Tonsils inflamed? (Tonsillitis.) Inflamed ear drums? (Otitis media.) Meningeal signs? (Meningitis, 15.6.)
Jaundice? Pale stools? Dark urine? (Hepatitis may cause vomiting, 22.11.)
Temperature? (Many infections which cause fever also cause vomiting, especially malaria.)
Meningeal signs? (Meningitis sometimes presents as vomiting.)

SPECIAL TESTS. **Protein (L 8.3) or pus cells (L 8.11) in his urine (urinary infections)? If he has fever, are there any malaria parasites in his blood slide (L 7.31)?**

DIAGNOSIS. **Gut infection (9.16)? Overeating? Dirty bottle-feeding (26.15)? Tonsillitis (18.11)? A 'vomiting attack' (20.14)? Meningitis (15.6)? Cerebral malaria (10.7)? Urinary infection (23.4)? Some other infection (10.10)? Acute abdomen (20.14)?**

MANAGEMENT IF DIAGNOSIS IS DIFFICULT. **There are two important questions to decide—Has he got an acute abdomen? Has he got meningitis? If he has either of these diseases he must go to hospital. If he has neither of these diseases, he probably has some infection you can treat. If you cannot find an infection, he probably has a vomiting attack.**
A child with a vomiting attack recovers in about 24 hours. If he is not much recovered in 24 hours, he should have a lumbar puncture (15.3). If he MIGHT have cerebral malaria, he MUST have an injection of chloroquine or quinine.
Sometimes you cannot be sure that the child has NOT got an acute abdomen. If you are in doubt examine him again in two hours.
Be sure to give him symptomatic treatment with oral rehydration fluids.

21 Worms

21.1 Worm loads and cycles

Worms are so common in some districts that many children are infected. Most worms live in the gut and lay ova (eggs) which you can see in the faeces with a microscope. Worms can cause loss of weight (7.13), abdominal pain (20.13), and occasionally dysentery (9.5). Hookworms cause anaemia (22.5). *Strongyloides* causes a skin lesion called creeping eruption (11.21). Threadworms make a child's anus itch (21.5). Some schistosomes live in the bladder and cause haematuria (23.8). Worms seldom cause fever. Antibiotics don't kill them.

The number of worms living in a child is called his **worm load**. A heavy load of many worms usually causes symptoms. But a light load of a few worms seldom causes symptoms. We cannot always remove all a child's worms. But we can always remove most of his worms and cure his symptoms.

Worms are different from viruses and bacteria. One virus, or one bacteria can go into a child and multiply into millions inside his body. Worms cannot do this. Most worms multiply by going outside a child's body onto the ground (or into another animal). The worm then goes back into a child. This is called the worm's **life cycle** (life circle). For example, hookworms live in the gut and stay there by biting into its wall. Each hookworm lays many thousands of ova which are passed in the child's faeces. When ova get onto the ground they hatch and become larvae (young worms). These larvae then change into a second kind of larvae. The second larvae must go back into a child through his skin. If the larvae cannot go into a child, they die in a few days. They wait until a child walks on them with no shoes on, or sits on them with bare buttocks. Then the larvae bite through his skin, and go round his body until they find his gut. In his gut the larvae grow into adult worms, lay more ova,

THE LIFE CYCLE OF THE HOOKWORM

This does not happen if people use latrines in the right way

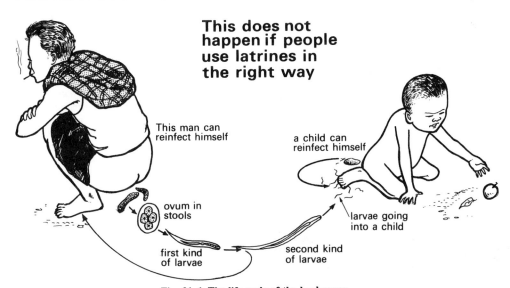

This man can reinfect himself

a child can reinfect himself

ovum in stools

larvae going into a child

first kind of larvae

second kind of larvae

Fig. 21–1 The life cycle of the hookworm.

and go round their cycle again. They spread by 'faeces to skin' infection (Path B, 2–6).

Larvae from the faeces of adults, or the faeces of other children can infect a child. He can also reinfect himself. For example, his faeces may infect the ground round his house. The hookworm larvae from the faeces can get back into him through his feet. They increase his worm load.

One larva grows into one adult worm. So the size of a child's worm load depends on how many larvae get into him.

THE SIZE OF A CHILD'S WORM LOAD DEPENDS ON HOW MANY WORMS GET INTO HIM

We can break the life cycle of worms by putting all faeces into latrines. Teaching people to use latrines is difficult, but we must try. We must teach mothers not to let their children play in a place where faeces are passed. If the ground near a child's house is already infected, he should play on a clean mat. If he is older, he must wear shoes.

SHOES PREVENT HOOKWORM INFECTION

Each kind of worm has a different cycle. *Strongyloides*, for example, also spreads from faeces to skin. But its larvae live on the ground much longer than the larvae of hookworms. The ova of *Ascaris* and *Trichuris* spread from faeces to mouth (2.7). A child becomes infected with these worms by eating infected earth. Worms can also infect him if he puts food or toys which have fallen onto infected earth, into his mouth.

HOOKWORM LARVAE GOING INTO A CHILD'S FOOT

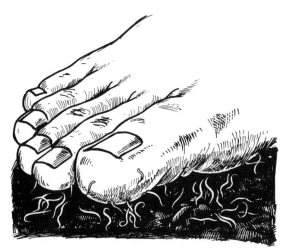

Fig. 21–2 How hookworms get in through the skin.

Worms are easy to diagnose. Use a microscope to look for their ova or larvae in faeces. To measure a child's worm load, count all the ova in a standard faecal smear (L 10.2). Put about 2 mg of faeces on a microscope slide and count all the ova in it. Less than 20 ova in a standard faecal smear is a light worm load. Between 20 and 40 ova is a moderate load. More than 40 ova is a heavy load.

There are many drugs for treating worms—see Table 3:1b and Section 3.26b.

COUNT THE OVA IN THE STOOL

21.2 'Agostinho passed a worm'—*Ascaris* (roundworm) *Taenia* or *H.nana* (tapeworm), *Enterobius* (threadworm)

If a child's mother says he passed a worm, it is usually *Ascaris*. Ask her what it looked like. Sometimes she will bring the worm for you to see. If you are not sure what kind of worm it is, look for its ova in his faeces.

21.3 Ascaris (roundworm)

These are round smooth worms about 20 cm long with pointed ends. They are very common.

Food moves down the gut from the mouth to the anus. If worms want to stay in the gut, they must swim up through the food, or hold onto the gut wall. Hookworms and tapeworms hold onto the gut wall. *Ascaris* swims. If there are only a few *Ascaris*, they usually swim quietly, and cause no symptoms. Sometimes they swim weakly and are passed in a child's faeces. Occasionally, they swim so strongly that they come out of his mouth or nose. They often do this when he has diarrhoea or vomiting from some other illness. *Ascaris* worms sometimes go into a child's larynx, or block his bile duct and cause jaundice. Occasionally, they go to his liver and help bacteria to cause sepsis there.

IF A CHILD VOMITS *ASCARIS* TREAT HIS VOMITING FIRST

Sometimes, a child has so many *Ascaris* that they make a ball of worms which obstructs his gut. You can sometimes feel this ball through his abdominal wall. A heavy load of *Ascaris* may eat so much of his food that they make him malnourished. *Ascaris* and malnutrition both make the abdomen swell. Children with a heavy *Ascaris* load often look like the child in Figure 20–8. They are moderately malnourished with a swollen abdomen. *Ascaris* can also cause chronic abdominal pain (20.12), and stop a child eating (18.15).

There are three common drugs for treating children with *Ascaris*—piperazine, bephenium, and pyrantel pamoate. These drugs stop *Ascaris* swimming, so they are passed in the faeces. Bephenium and pyrantel pamoate also kill hookworms, which is useful, because many children have both *Ascaris* and hookworms.

There is another cheap useful drug, TCE (tetrachlorethylene), which only kills hookworms. Unfortunately, TCE makes *Ascaris* swim so strongly that it swims into dangerous places, such as the liver. So we must always give a child piperazine when we give him TCE.

ASCARIS

TREATMENT. *Either,* give him pyrantel pamoate (3.30b), or bephenium (3.27). These will remove his *Ascaris,* and any hookworms he has.

Or, give him piperazine. This will remove his *Ascaris* only.

EXPLANATION. Ask the child's mother to watch his faeces, and see how many worms he passes. She may not see any worms, even though they have all gone. Explain how dangerous infected faeces are. Explain that his brothers and sisters may need treatment.

Most mothers have seen *Ascaris,* so explain how they can harm a child. Explain how they spread and how we can prevent them.

SOME CHILDREN HAVE THIS MANY ASCARIS

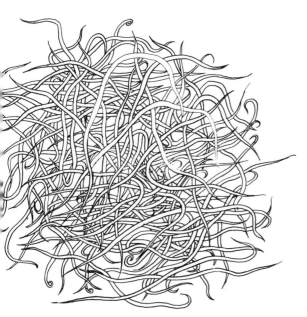

Fig. 21–3 Some children have this many *Ascaris*.

SOME WORMS

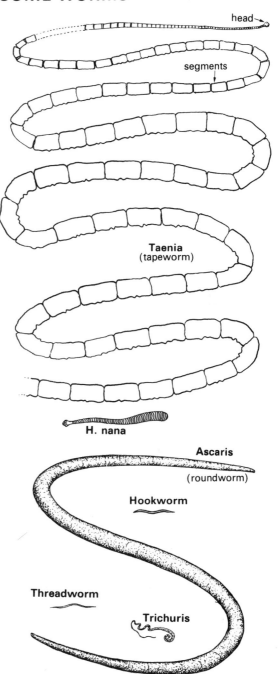

Fig. 21–4 Some worms.

21.2

21.3

21.4

21.4 Tapeworms

Several kinds of tapeworm can live in a child's gut. There are two big tapeworms several metres long—the beef (cow) tapeworm (*Taenia saginata*) and the pork (pig) tapeworm (*Taenia solium*). There is also a dwarf (small) tapeworm about 2 cm long called *H.nana*. Tapeworms are flat, not round like the roundworms (*Ascaris*). They are made of many short segments (pieces) joined

225

together. Each tapeworm has a narrow head which holds onto the wall of the gut. The segments grow out from a narrow neck behind the head. As the segments grow towards the end of a worm, they become bags full of ova which break off and are passed in the faeces. Sometimes, a mother finds a whole *H.nana* in her child's faeces. Or she may find a few segments of one of the larger tapeworms. *Taenia* segments are flat and white, and move slowly. Sometimes they come out of a child's anus while he sleeps. *H.nana* looks like a piece of thin white tape.

Taenia ova are passed in faeces onto the ground. Some of the ova are eaten by cows or pigs. The ova hatch into larvae which go to the animal's muscles (meat). They wait until the animal is killed and the meat is eaten. If the meat is well-cooked, the larvae are killed and cause no harm. But if the larvae are not killed by cooking, they infect the child who eats them. Most families can buy very little meat, and most children have a very small share of it. So these tapeworms are rare in most districts.

H.nana is different. It lives in rats. It can go from one rat to another, or from a rat to a child. But *H.nana* does not need to go through a rat. It can go from one child to another child by faeces-to-mouth infection (2.7). A child can also reinfect himself if his faeces go into his mouth. This is why heavy loads of *H.nana* are common in some districts.

Usually, a child has only one or two *Taenia*, and they cause no symptoms. Sometimes they cause abdominal pain and loss of weight. But a child may have many *H.nana*. Heavy loads of *H.nana* cause abdominal pain and bloody diarrhoea.

Treat all kinds of tapeworm with niclosamide (3.30).

21.5 'Miguel keeps scratching his anus'— *Enterobius* (threadworms)

These worms live in the gut. They look like pieces of thin white thread. Threadworms live only in people. They do not need to go into animals or onto the ground. At night the female worm comes out of the anus and lays her sticky ova on the skin around it. Sometimes, she goes into a girls' vulva and lays her ova there also (23.10). The ova make children itch, so that they keep scratching. A child may suck his fingers, eat the ova, and reinfect himself. Threadworm ova may also go into dust or spread on clothes. Often, a whole family is infected, and you may have to treat everyone in it. Threadworms are difficult to cure, and reinfection is common. But they usually become less as children grow older.

You will seldom seen threadworm ova in the faeces. But you can find the worms in a child. Bend him over his mother's knees and quickly spread his buttocks apart. You may see a threadworm before it has had time to pull itself back into his anus.

You can find the ova with a piece of clear tape ('Sellotape' or 'Scotch tape'). Put the sticky side against the child's anus, and then stick it onto a microscope slide (L

10.4). The ova from the skin round his anus stick to the tape, and you can see them with a microscope.

THREADWORMS

TREATMENT. **Treat threadworms with piperazine (3.28) once a day for a week. Or, give him pyrantel pamoate. If the itching is very bad at night, give him promethazine (3.45) before he goes to sleep.**

EXPLANATION. **Tell his mother to cut his nails very short, to wash his hands and anus after he passes a stool, and to keep his trousers clean.**

THREADWORMS MAKE CHILDREN SCRATCH

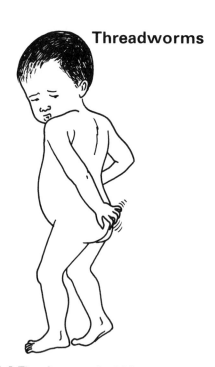

Threadworms

Fig. 21–5 Threadworms make children scratch.

21.6 *Strongyloides*

Strongyloides lays ova in the small gut. The ova hatch quickly, so you will see larvae, not ova, in a child's faeces. Heavy loads of *Strongyloides* cause bloody diarrhoea (9.5) and abdominal pain (20.12). Occasionally, larvae crawl through the skin and cause creeping eruption (11.21). If a child has even a light load of *Strongyloides*, give him tiabendazole (3.29).

226

21.7 *Trichuris* (whipworm)

Trichuris lives in the large intestine and spreads in the same way as *Ascaris*. The mouth end of a *Trichuris* worm is thinner than the tail end. This makes it look like a whip.

A light load of *Trichuris* causes no symptoms. But a heavy load can cause bloody diarrhoea (9.5), abdominal pain (20.12), loss of weight (7.13), anaemia (22.1), or prolapse of the rectum (25.7). If a child has a heavy load, give him tiabendazole (3.29).

22 The child who is pale or yellow

ANAEMIA

22.1 'Esteban is pale'—anaemia

Blood is red because it contains red cells. These are red because they contain a red substance called haemoglobin. Haemoglobin takes oxygen from the air in the lungs, and carries it to other parts of the body (8.2).

Haemoglobin in the capillaries makes a child's lips, tongue, and conjunctiva look red. If there is too little haemoglobin in his blood these parts of his body become pale (less red than normal). He is anaemic. Anaemia, like malnutrition, makes a child less able to fight diseases, such as diarrhoea and pneumonia. Infections also make anaemia worse.

Anaemia which comes slowly causes few symptoms or signs until it is severe. If anaemia comes quickly it causes symptoms when it is much milder. Anaemia makes a child's skin paler. This sign is easier to see in a white-skinned child. You can sometimes see it in a brown or black child. Occasionally, a mother says her child's lips are pale. Usually, you only diagnose anaemia when a child comes with some other symptom. So remember to examine every sick child for anaemia. A *severely* anaemic child is pale with a fast pulse, swollen feet (19.8), and fast or difficult breathing (8.21).

EXAMINING A CHILD FOR ANAEMIA

Pull down his lower lip, or one of his lower eyelids. If he is older, ask him to put out his tongue. Look at the palms of his hands. Are these parts of his body paler than normal? If you examine many children you will learn what a normal tongue, or conjunctiva, or palms look like. You can diagnose moderate or severe anaemia like this. But you can only diagnose mild anaemia by measuring the haemoglobin.

EXAMINE EVERY SICK CHILD FOR ANAEMIA

22.2 Measuring anaemia

Paleness of the lips, tongue, conjunctiva, and hands are useful signs of anaemia, but they are not enough by themselves. We must measure the haemoglobin. There are several ways of doing this (L 7.1).

We measure the number of grams of haemoglobin in a decilitre (100 ml) of blood. We write this as 'g/dl'. Healthy men have between 14 and 18 g/dl of haemoglobin in their blood. Healthy women have between 12 and 16 g/dl. A child is born with about 18 g/dl, but his haemoglobin soon falls, and it is only about 11 g/dl by the time he is two months old. After that it rises slowly until he is an adult.

A child is anaemic if his haemoglobin is less than 10 g/dl. If it is between 8 and 10 g/dl, he is mildly anaemic. If it is between 5 and 8 g/dl, he is moderately anaemic. If it is less than 5 g/dl, he is severely anaemic.

Record a child's haemoglobin on his weight chart. Put dots for his growth curve (7.1) as usual. Put a small 'H' for his haemoglobin. If his haemoglobin is 5·5 g/dl, put an 'H' on the 5·5 kg line. Draw a red line across his chart at 10 g/dl (10 kg on the chart). Healthy children are above this line and anaemic children are below it. When you treat anaemia, measure a child's haemoglobin every month. Join up the 'H's to make a haemoglobin curve. A healthy child's haemoglobin curve is nearly flat, and is always above the 10 g/dl line. An anaemic child's haemoglobin curve starts below the 10 g line, and should climb above it as you treat him. Figure 22–3 shows the haemoglobin curve of a child with sickle cell anaemia.

22.3 The causes of anaemia

Children can become anaemic in these ways:

A child's body does not make enough haemoglobin. The body makes haemoglobin from protein, iron, and a vitamin called folic acid. If a child lacks these in his food, he cannot make enough haemoglobin, so he becomes anaemic. We can treat this kind of anaemia. We can give a child iron or folic acid. Malnourished children become anaemic because they lack protein, and often iron and folic acid also. The best treatment for them is more food.

Chronic infection of any kind can also cause mild or

moderate anaemia. It stops the body making enough red cells.

Bleeding outside the body. A child can become anaemic because he is bleeding and losing too many red

EXAMINING A CHILD FOR ANAEMIA

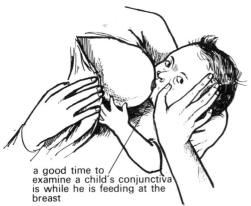

a good time to examine a child's conjunctiva is while he is feeding at the breast

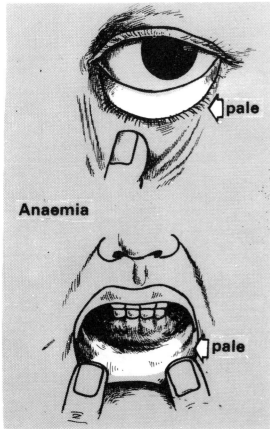

Fig. 22–1 Examining a child for anaemia.

cells *outside* his body. This happens when a newborn baby bleeds from his cord (26.38), or when hookworms bite a child's gut. The blood from hookworm bites is passed in a child's stools, so it is lost outside his body. A child with schistosomiasis loses in his urine (23.8). When a child loses blood like this, he also loses the iron in it. *So children who become anaemic because of bleeding need iron.*

HOW SEVERE IS HIS ANAEMIA?

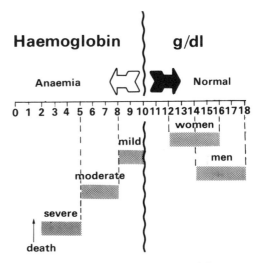

Fig. 22–2 How severe is his anaemia?

22.1

Destruction of red cells inside the body— haemolytic anaemia. Malaria and sickle cell anaemia destroy red cells *inside* the blood vessels. This causes a haemolytic (blood-destroying) anaemia. When red cells are destroyed inside the body, the iron in them is not lost. The body keeps the iron and uses it again to make more haemoglobin. *So, iron medicines are not helpful in this kind of anaemia.* They can be harmful, because sometimes there is too much iron in a child's body from all the destroyed red cells. But the body cannot use the folic acid in the destroyed red cells again. So folic acid is helpful in haemolytic anaemia.

22.3

ANAEMIA IS A SIGN, NOT A DISEASE

22.4 Iron deficiency anaemia

22.4

A child can get iron deficiency anaemia in three ways. (1) He may absorb too little iron in his food. (2) He may be born with too small a store of iron in his body. (3) He may bleed from his gut (22.5), his cord (26.38), or his bladder (23.8). Sometimes, he has several of these causes at the same time.

22.2

229

THE GROWTH CURVE AND THE HAEMOGLOBIN CURVE OF A CHILD WITH SICKLE CELL ANAEMIA

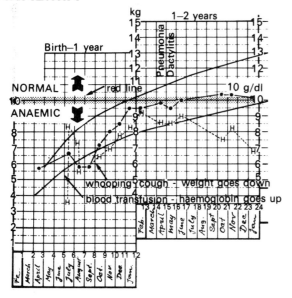

Fig. 22–3 Haemoglobin curves.

Too little iron absorbed. There is iron in fish, meat, and eggs. There is also iron in vegetable foods, such as legumes (peas, beans, and groundnuts). The iron in fish, meat, and eggs is well-absorbed, but the iron in vegetable foods is not well-absorbed. So a child who eats vegetable foods only, may not absorb enough iron. He may get iron deficiency.

Too small an iron store. A healthy mother gives her baby a good store of iron before he is born. He needs this iron store because there is little iron in breast-milk. He does not get much more iron until he starts to eat food. Unfortunately, many mothers are anaemic. They do not have enough iron themselves. So they cannot give their babies a good store or iron. Also, many babies start to eat food too late. So, a baby's first year is a dangerous time for iron-deficiency anaemia. Prevent it. Teach mothers to give their babies foods which contain iron when they are four months old.

If a baby is born too early (preterm), his mother does not have time to give him a good iron store. He soon becomes anaemic. So give preterm babies iron (26.22).

Treating children with iron. You can treat iron deficiency anaemia with ferrous sulphate (iron) tablets, or with 'children's iron mixture' or with an injection of iron dextran (3.33). Give the mixture or the injection to children of any age. But do not give a child tablets until he is more than about 20 kg. Iron dextran gives the body a store of iron, so a child usually needs only one injection. The body absorbs the iron in a mixture or tablets slowly. So give them for at least three months. A child may need it for longer. At first his haemoglobin should rise by about one gram each week. His other tissues also lack iron. So give him iron for two more months after his haemoglobin is normal.

Fortunately, iron is cheap. Iron mixture is a useful treatment for a young child, if you cannot find any abnormal signs except mild anaemia. Too much iron is dangerous, so give the right dose. Iron makes a child's stools black. This may worry his mother, but it is not important.

ALWAYS GIVE IRON FOR AT LEAST THREE MONTHS

SOME CAUSES OF ANAEMIA

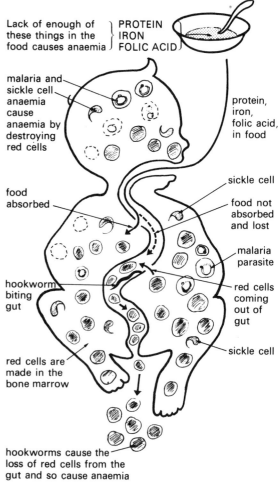

Fig. 22–4 Some cause of anaemia.

IRON DEFICIENCY ANAEMIA

TREATMENT. **Ask mothers to bring a bottle to the clinic (4–1). Put some children's iron mixture (3.33) into it. Give a child under 10 kg one teaspoon once a day. If he is over 10 kg give him two teaspoons. A child under 10 kg will need about 150 ml a month and a child over 10 kg about 300 ml. So give enough.**

EXPLANATION. **Show the child's mother how to give him iron medicine, in the right dose (3.33). Explain that he should have it for at least three months. Tell her that a larger dose will not help and may be dangerous. Explain that she must keep iron medicine or tablets in a safe place where he cannot get them (14–9).**

22.5 Hookworm anaemia

This is a common cause of iron deficiency anaemia in children who are old enough to walk. They become infected by hookworm larvae on the ground (21–2). Hookworms live in the small gut and bite its wall with their mouths (22–4). From the bite of each worm a child loses about one drop of blood each day. A few hookworms cause little bleeding, and no anaemia. His body can easily make a little more blood. But a child with a large load of hundreds of worms may lose more iron than he eats. So he gets iron-deficiency anaemia. Well-nourished children eat plenty of iron in their food. So hookworms cause anaemia more easily in malnourished children. We can easily find out how many hookworms a child has. We can count the ova in his faeces. Ask the laboratory to count the ova in a 'standard faecal smear' (21.1, L 10.2a).

There are three common drugs for hookworms—TCE (tetrachlorethylene), bephenium, and pyrantel pamoate. TCE is very much cheaper than the other two drugs. Unfortunately, it makes *Ascaris* swim into dangerous places (21.3). Also, it is not so safe as the other two drugs, especially if a child is severely anaemic. If you have no bephenium, or pyrantel pamoate, you will have to give severely anaemic children TCE. But try to raise their haemoglobin with iron first.

HOOKWORM ANAEMIA

MANAGEMENT AND TREATMENT
Severe anaemia. **His haemoglobin is less than 5 g/dl, or**

he has difficulty breathing, *or* he has swollen ankles. Try to send him to hospital. He may need a blood transfusion.
If you have to treat him yourself—
EITHER, give him bephenium (or pyrantel pamoate), and iron. Give him children's iron mixture, or iron dextran. If he is over 20 kg he can have iron tablets (3.33).
OR, give him iron only and wait until his haemoglobin is over 5 g/dl. Then treat his hookworms with TCE. Give him piperazine at the same time. He probably has *Ascaris* also (21.3).

Moderate or mild anaemia. If his haemoglobin is above 5 g/dl, treat his anaemia and his hookworms at the same time. Use any hookworm drug.

EXPLANATION. **Tell his mother why he is pale. Explain how hookworms are infecting him, and how she can prevent this. She must put his stools into a latrine. If he is old enough to walk he should wear shoes. If he is young, and if the ground around his house might be infected by hookworm larvae, he must play on a clean mat. Food containing iron will also help him, especially liver, legumes, and green vegetables.**

22.5

ALWAYS GIVE PIPERAZINE WHEN YOU GIVE TCE

22.6 Folic acid deficiency anaemia

22.6

There is folic acid in green vegetables, liver, meat, and milk. Green vegetables are cheap, but many children do not eat enough of them. So they become anaemic. Folic acid also helps the anaemia caused by malnutrition, chronic infection, and sickle cells.

A child with a haemolytic anaemia (22.3) has to make new red cells faster than normal. He needs much folic acid to make these cells. He needs more folic acid than a healthy child. If he does not get enough folic acid, he becomes more anaemic. Folic acid tablets help him.

THERE IS FOLIC ACID IN ALL KINDS OF GREEN LEAVES

22.7 Haemolytic (blood-destroying) anaemia

22.7

A child's spleen takes old or destroyed red cells out of his blood. If he has a haemolytic anaemia there are more of these destroyed cells than normal. So his spleen has

Hookworm ova in the stools

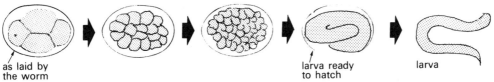

as laid by the worm

larva ready to hatch

larva

Fig. 22–5 Look for hookworm ova in his stool.

more work to do. Because his spleen has more work to do, it grows larger. So a large spleen is usually a sign of haemolytic anaemia.

When the red cells are destroyed, a yellow substance called bilirubin is made. A healthy child does not have enough bilirubin to make him jaundiced (yellow). But if he has a haemolytic anaemia, his body makes more bilirubin and he becomes *mildly* jaundiced. So, if an anaemic child has a large spleen, or jaundice, or both, he probably has a haemolytic anaemia. *The two common causes of haemolytic anaemia are malaria and sickle cell anaemia.*

Malaria. Malaria parasites destroy red cells (10.7). In some districts malaria is the commonest cause of anaemia in children between the ages of three months and five years. In these districts most children have a few parasites in their blood. Often, we cannot be sure if the parasites are causing a child's anaemia or not. So we must suppress his malaria and observe him. If malaria was causing his anaemia, his haemoglobin will rise.

ANAEMIA CAUSED BY MALARIA

ACUTE ANAEMIA. **If a child has an acute attack of malaria (10.7), and his haemoglobin is less than 5 g/dl, send him for help. He needs a blood transfusion.**

CHRONIC ANAEMIA. **This is less serious and you can treat children in a health centre. Give him chloroquine (3.25) by mouth, as for an acute attack. Then suppress his malaria for three months. Give him folic acid for at least two weeks (3.37). Many of these children have an iron-deficiency anaemia also. So iron helps them (3.33).**

EXPLANATION. **Tell his mother about malaria and how he must take his drugs.**

22.8 Sickle cell anaemia

Normal adult haemoglobin is called haemoglobin A. Some children are born with an abnormal kind of haemoglobin in their red cells called haemoglobin S. They get this from their parents. If a child gets haemoglobin S from one parent only, about half his haemoglobin is haemoglobin S. The haemoglobin in his red cells is a mixture of A and S, we say he is AS. He has a mild disease called **the sickle cell trait**. If a child gets haemoglobin S from both his parents, all of his haemoglobin is abnormal. The haemoglobin in his red cells is SS. He gets a more severe disease called **sickle cell anaemia**.

There is an easy special test for haemoglobin S. If you keep red cells containing haemoglobin S without air, they change their shape and look like cells in Figure 22–6. Some of these cells look like a sickle (a knife for cutting grass). A health centre laboratory can easily find sickle cells. The laboratory may also be able to test if a

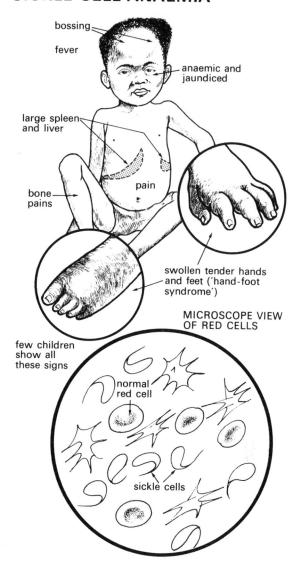

SICKLE CELL ANAEMIA

Fig. 22–6 Sickle cell anaemia.

child is AS (the trait) or SS (sickle cell anaemia) (L 7.26).

Haemoglobin S is important because sickle cells are easily destroyed. So the child becomes anaemic. Sickle cells also block blood vessels. This causes other symptoms. Haemoglobin S is very common in some communities. You will not see it in white children. If haemoglobin S is common in your district, sickle cell anaemia will be an important disease to diagnose.

Children with the sickle cell *trait* usually have no symptoms all their lives. The only abnormality they have is a positive test for haemoglobin S.

Sickle cell anaemia (SS). An SS baby is usually well until he is six months old. He then has attacks of fever, mild jaundice, and anaemia. His liver and spleen become large. When he is older his spleen may become small again. Sometimes a young child has warm, swollen, painful, hands or feet, fingers, or toes (**dactylitis**). He may have dactylitis in his hands and feet at the same time. We call this the **hand-foot syndrome**. It is most common in the first year of life. His lesions last one or two weeks and then heal themselves. When a child is about two years old bony swellings start to form at the 'corners' of his skull (occipital and temporal regions). This is called **bossing**. Dactylitis and bossing are helpful for diagnosis. Osteomyelitis (24.5) is more common in children with sickle cell anaemia.

Sometimes a child's disease gets much worse and he has a **crisis**. There are several kinds of crisis. (1) He has pain in his arms and legs, because the blood vessels in his bones are blocked. (2) His liver and spleen swell and he has abdominal pain. His pain may be so severe that you think he has an acute abdomen (20.2). There may also be tenderness, ridigity, and guarding (20.3). (3) He may suddenly become severely anaemic, because many red cells are destroyed, or because his bone marrow stops making new red cells.

SS children easily get infections. These infections often cause crises. So the best way to prevent crises is to prevent infections. If we do not care for SS children well, most of them die from infections and crises during the first few years of life.

If a child does not die, his disease becomes less severe as he grows older. When an older child is not having a crisis he is usually moderately well, and is only moderately anaemic. Sometimes however he has jaundice and pains in the long bones of his arms and legs, or in his joints. But going to school is difficult for him because of anaemia, bone pains, and jaundice.

Often there is a local word for sickle cell anaemia, such as 'nwiiwii' of the Fanti tribe in Ghana. In Ghana mothers often diagnose sickle cell anaemia themselves. Sickle cell anaemia may present as fever, anaemia, jaundice, pain in the arms or legs, as abdominal pain, as the child who is not growing normally, or as dactylitis. There is no cure for sickle cell anaemia. The best way to help these children is to keep them on the road to health and prevent infections.

SICKLE CELL ANAEMIA

BETWEEN CRISES

Immunization. **Make sure these children have all their immunizations.**

Antimalarials. **Suppress malaria with pyrimethamine, or chloroquine (3.25).**

Folic acid. **This helps the marrow to make more red cells. He may need it for several years. DON'T give iron. It may be harmful.**

Paracetamol or aspirin. **Give these if a child has pain (3.41, 3.42)**

IN CRISES

If possible send the child for help. He may need a blood transfusion if his anaemia is severe.

EXPLANATION. **If he has the sickle cell trait, *don't* tell his mother. It will worry her, and she does not need to know. If he has sickle cell anaemia, explain it to his mother. Tell her that you cannot cure it, but that you can help him. Tell her that he may get pains in his abdomen or legs, or have swellings of his fingers and toes. Tell her his symptoms will become milder as he grows older. Tell her that the best way to help him is to keep him on the road to health. If he has any symptoms, she must bring him to the clinic quickly, so that you can treat his infections early. Tell her to bring him back every month for more tablets. Put him in the special care register. Write SS on his weight chart.**

22.9 Caring for an anaemic child

Most children with anaemia present with other symptoms. You diagnose it when you examine their lips or eyelids. The causes of anaemia are not the same everywhere. Iron and folic acid deficiency and hookworm anaemia are common in most districts. But there is malaria and sickle cell anaemia in some communities only. So you may need to care for anaemic children differently from the way we describe here. Often, we cannot diagnose the cause of a child's anaemia.

HISTORY

How old is he? (Hookworm anaemia is rare under one year. The anaemia of malaria is most common between the age of three months and five years. Sickle cell anaemia is not common in children less than six months old.)

Where has he been recently? (Perhaps he has caught malaria.)

Has he been walking or playing on ground that might be infected with hookworms?

What foods does he eat? (If he is over four months, he should eat green vegetables, which contain iron and folic acid; and also legumes.)

Abdominal pain, or pain in the arms or legs of an older child (sickle cell anaemia)?

EXAMINATION. **How severe is his anaemia? Look at his lips, tongue, and conjunctivae.**

Swelling of the ankles? Difficulty breathing (signs of severe anaemia)?

Is he well or badly nourished (7.13) (mild or moderate anaemia is common in malnutrition)?

Jaundice? Look at his sclera (malaria or sickle cell anaemia). Fever? Large spleen (20.3) (malaria, sickle cell anaemia)?

Swelling of the hands or feet (dactylitis) in a young

child? Skull bossing in an older child (sickle cell anaemia)?

SPECIAL TESTS. **Measure his haemoglobin (L 7.1). Malaria parasites in his blood (L 7.31)? Sickle cells (L 7.25)?**

How many hookworm ova has he in a standard stool smear (L10.2a)?

Can the laboratory help you any more? A health centre laboratory has more tests for diagnosing anaemia (L 7.28).

DIAGNOSIS. **Is his anaemia mild, moderate, or severe? Is it caused by iron deficiency (22.4)? Hookworms (22.5)? Malaria (22.7)? Sickle cell anaemia (22.8)? Infection?**

MANAGEMENT IF DIAGNOSIS IS DIFFICULT. **If he is severely anaemic, try to send him for help.**

If he is less than one year old, iron will probably help him.

If his spleen is large, give him chloroquine, and folic acid. Then suppress his malaria for two or three months (3.25).

If his spleen is normal, give him iron for three months.

Measure his haemoglobin each month. If you give a severely anaemic child the right treatment, his haemoglobin should rise about 2 g/dl in two weeks.

RECORDING AND REPORTING. **Record his haemoglobin curve on his weight chart.**

Jaundice

22.10 'Parto's eyes are yellow'—hepatitis, haemolytic anaemia, drugs

Each red cell lives in the blood for about 120 days. Then it is destroyed and a new red cell is made. Part of the old haemoglobin is made into a yellow substance called **bilirubin**. The liver excretes this bilirubin into the gut. Bacteria in the gut make the yellow bilirubin into the brown colour of normal stools. In a healthy child bilirubin is quickly excreted. There is never enough bilirubin in his body to make him yellow. If a child looks yellow, he is jaundiced. A jaundiced child has too much bilirubin in his blood. You can see jaundice most easily in a pale-skinned child. Look for jaundice in a child's eyes. Mothers usually notice yellow eyes.

A child becomes jaundiced for three reasons. (1) Because too much blood is being destroyed and too much bilirubin made (haemolytic anaemia). (2) Because his liver is diseased (hepatitis), so that he cannot excrete bilirubin normally. (3) Newborn babies may get jaundice because their livers are too young to excrete enough bilirubin (26.23).

22.11 Hepatitis

Hepatitis means inflammation of the liver. Two viruses, hepatitis virus A and hepatitis virus B, can cause it. Hepatitis virus A causes **infectious hepatitis**. Hepatitis virus B causes **syringe jaundice**. Virus A is excreted in the bile, and goes into the faeces. It spreads from faeces to mouth in the same way as the organisms causing diarrhoea (2.7). Virus B usually spreads on dirty needles or instruments. Even a little blood from an infected child on a needle or syringe can infect another child. This is why we *must* sterilize needles and syringes every time we use them.

Infectious hepatitis (hepatitis A). A child with infectious hepatitis stops eating. This is a common symptom in many diseases (18.15). But in hepatitis not eating is sometimes so severe that it is useful for diagnosis. Even the sight or smell of food may make a child want to vomit. He usually has fever, feels tired, and has mild abdominal pain. He may present with fever before the other symptoms. After four or five days his eyes and his skin (in a pale-skinned child) become yellow. When his jaundice comes his fever usually goes. Bilirubin goes into his urine, and makes it dark like tea. Bilirubin does not go into his stools in the normal way. So his stools become pale. His liver may be large and tender.

Children do not always have these symptoms, because jaundice is milder in children than in adults. Many children with infectious hepatitis have no symptoms, or only mild symptoms, and never become jaundiced. But they are infected with the hepatitis virus, and they can infect other children. Sometimes, several people in the family get hepatitis at the same time. Most children recover without treatment. Occasionally, hepatitis kills them.

Syringe jaundice (hepatitis B). This is less common than infectious hepatitis (virus A). Syringe jaundice has the same signs and symptoms, but they are usually more serious. Symptoms start between six weeks and six months after an injection with a dirty needle. If we do not sterilize our syringes and needles, we can easily cause an epidemic of jaundice.

DIRTY NEEDLES CAUSE JAUNDICE

HEPATITIS (A OR B)

MANAGEMENT. **Most children recover without treatment. Try to send a child for help if he has any of these DANGER SIGNS: severe jaundice, much restlessness, severe vomiting, loss of consciousness (14.8), or bleeding. These signs show that his liver is seriously diseased.**

If he has been taking any drugs, stop them.

TREATMENT. **Give him vitamin tablets (3.36).**

EXPLANATION. **Tell his mother about hepatitis. Tell her to give him plenty of fluids, and any food he will eat. Tell her that he will probably recover in a few days. If he has any of the danger signs, ask her to bring him back quickly.**

22.12 Drug jaundice

Drugs sometimes cause jaundice (3.2). They may be

drugs he has been given in the clinic, such as thia-cetazone. Or his mother may have bought drugs for him in the market. So if a child has jaundice, ask his mother if she has been giving him any drugs. If the drug is stopped, he will probably recover.

22.13 Caring for a jaundiced child

If he is *mildly* jaundiced and anaemic, he probably has a haemolytic anaemia. If he is jaundiced, but not anaemic, he probably has hepatitis.

If he is less than a month old go to Section 26.23.

HISTORY. **Fever (malaria, hepatitis)?**
Several attacks of jaundice (probably sickle cell anaemia, especially if he has anaemia and a large spleen)?
Any injections between two and five months ago (hepatitis virus B)?
Drugs (drug jaundice)?
Has anyone else in the family had jaundice (hepatitis virus A)?

EXAMINATION. **Anaemic (malaria or sickle cell anaemia)?**
How severe is his jaundice (severe jaundice is probably hepatitis)?
Spleen large (malaria or sickle cell anaemia)?
Liver large and tender (hepatitis)?
Are his stools pale or his urine dark (hepatitis)?

SPECIAL TESTS. **Measure his haemoglobin (L 7.1). If he is anaemic, look for malaria parasites in his blood (L 7.31). Shake his urine. If the froth is yellow, there is bile (bilirubin) in it. If there is bile he has hepatitis, not a haemolytic anaemia (L 8.8).**

DIAGNOSIS.
Jaundice only. **Hepatitis (22.11)? Drug jaundice (22.12)?**

Jaundice and anaemia. **Malaria (22.7)? Sickle cell anaemia (22.8)?**

DIRTY SYRINGES MAY CAUSE JAUNDICE

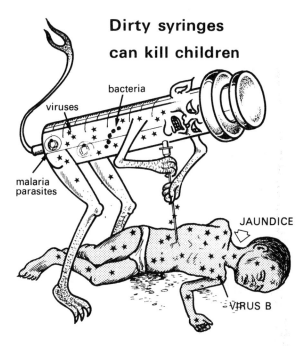

Fig. 22–7 Dirty syringes may cause jaundice.

MANAGEMENT IF DIAGNOSIS IS DIFFICULT. **If he has any of the danger signs of hepatitis (22.11), send him for help.**
If he is anaemic and jaundiced, and there is malaria in the district, give him chloroquine (3.25).

22.13

22.10

22.11

22.12

23 Urinary and genital symptoms

The Urinary System

23.1 Urinary symptoms

The three most common urinary symptoms are **dysuria** (pain passing urine), **frequency** (passing urine often), and **urgency** (wanting to pass urine quickly). Sometimes children have all three symptoms. Bacterial infection of the urinary system usually causes them. **Incontinence** is another urinary symptom. A child who is incontinent of urine cannot hold his urine, so he wets himself.

Mothers sometimes worry about the colour of their child's urine. Pale urine is always normal. A child passes pale urine when the weather is cold and he drinks much water. He passes dark urine when he is hot and sweats, when he drinks little water, and when he is dehydrated. So dark urine is usually normal also. But if a child is dehydrated (9.17), dark urine is a sign that he is not drinking enough fluid. Jaundice often makes a child's urine dark with bile (22.13). Blood (haematuria) makes it red. If there is only a little blood in the urine, we need a microscope to see it (L 8.13).

23.2 Examining the urine

Healthy urine contains no protein, blood, bacteria, or pus cells. Pus cells or bacteria in a child's urine show that he has a urinary infection. Examine the urine for pus cells and bacteria. This is useful for diagnosis. But you must take the specimen in the right way.

TAKING A CLEAN SPECIMEN OF URINE

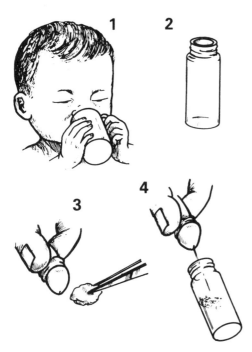

Fig. 23–1 Taking a clean specimen of urine.

TAKING A CLEAN SPECIMEN OF URINE

(1) Give the child a drink, and wait about 20 minutes.

AN OLDER BOY. **(2) Fetch a clean bottle with a wide mouth. If the urine is for culture (growing micro-organisms) the bottle must be sterile.**

(3) Pull back his foreskin and clean the opening of his urethra with a sterile swab.

(4) Ask him to pass his urine. Catch some of the urine in the bottle.

AN OLDER GIRL. **Sit her down on a latrine with her legs wide apart. Fold back the lips (labia) at the side of her urethra. Clean the opening of the urethra with a sterile swab. Catch some of the middle part of her urine in a wide clean bottle.**

BABIES. **This is more difficult. A baby often passes urine while he is being fed. His mother may be able to catch some of his urine in a wide clean bottle. Clean him first, and then explain to her what she should do. You can also take urine into a test tube or a plastic bag. Fix the tube over a baby's penis with a piece of adhesive tape. Fix a plastic bag over a girl's urethra with tape.**

Count the pus cells in the urine. This is the easiest special test for a urinary infection (L 8.11). Healthy urine contains very few pus cells. If there are more than 10 pus cells in a microlitre, the child probably has a urinary infection. Sometimes, a laboratory report tells you the number of pus cells in a high power microscope field (HPF). More than 3 pus cells in a HPF (uncentrifuged) is a sign of a urinary infection. You can see bacteria in urine when you stain a drop of it with Gram's stain (L 11.5).

Urine quickly spoils. Pus cells are destroyed and bacteria grow quickly. So, if you see bacteria in an old specimen, they may have grown after it was passed. Only bacteria in a fresh specimen must have come from inside the body. Try to examine a specimen of urine within an hour after it was passed. After three hours it will be partly spoilt. Next day it will be useless.

EXAMINE URINE SOON

USING A PLASTIC BAG TO COLLECT URINE

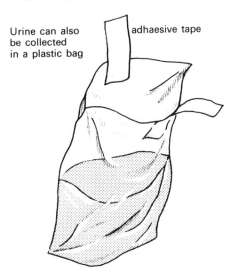

Urine can also be collected in a plastic bag

adhaesive tape

Fig. 23–2 A plastic bag for urine.

23.3 'Anna has a pain (dysuria) when she passes urine'—urinary infection, 'sores', nappy rash, threadworms.

Urinary infection is the most important cause of dysuria. Dysuria can also be caused by anything that makes a child's urethra sore, such as a vaginal infection, or a nappy rash (26.43). If a child's urine becomes too 'strong' (concentrated) in hot weather, passing urine may hurt him.

23.4 Urinary infections

Urinary infections are caused by the ordinary bacteria on the skin around the urethra. A girl has a much shorter urethra than a boy. Bacteria can get into her bladder more easily. So urinary infections are much more common in girls.

Sometimes a baby with a painfully full bladder cries *before* he passes urine. This is normal. Pain while passing urine is abnormal. Sometimes a child screams with pain when he passes urine. A girl rubs her vulva, and a boy pulls his penis. Urinary infections often cause frequency and urgency. Some children have no frequency or dysuria. Instead they start wetting their clothes, although they have already learnt to use a latrine. They wet themselves at night or in the day. They want to pass urine so urgently that they cannot get to a latrine. They are incontinent of urine.

A CHILD WHO 'WETS HIMSELF' MAY HAVE A URINARY INFECTION

Any acute urinary infection may cause frequency and urgency. These may be the only symptoms, or there may be fever, and vomiting also. Some children have pain in their loins or abdomen. Sometimes there is fever, vomiting, and abdominal pain, *but no frequency or urgency*. So remember that any child with fever and vomiting might have a urinary infection. There is only one way to diagnose a child like this—examine his urine. Look for pus in a child's urine, if you cannot find a cause for vomiting (20.15) or abdominal pain (20.13), or you cannot diagnose a fever which lasted several days (10.10).

IF YOU CANNOT FIND THE CAUSE FOR A CHILD'S FEVER LOOK FOR PUS IN HIS URINE

Urinary infections are usually caused by bacteria which are not sensitive to penicillin, so penicillin is *not* helpful. Sulphonamides are better. If an acute urinary infection is not cured quickly it becomes chronic. If a child has a chronic urinary infection, bacteria grow in his kidneys. The bacteria slowly destroy his kidneys. So he does not grow and gain weight normally. After several years he dies. So diagnose urinary infections, and treat them carefully.

Urinary infections often come back after they have been treated. This happens most often in girls, or if there is a congenital malformation (26.4) in the urinary system. Observe a child who has had a urinary infection, because he may have another infection. If boys get two or more urinary infections, or girls three or more, send them to hospital. Their urinary systems should be examined.

URINARY INFECTION

MANAGEMENT AND TREATMENT. **Give the child sulphadimidine for two weeks (3.14).**

Tell him to drink plenty of water. This washes bacteria out of his urinary system. It also stops the sulphadimidine blocking the small tubes in his kidneys.

Ask him to come to the clinic again in two weeks, so that you can examine his urine for pus cells. If there are no pus cells, stop treatment. If there are pus cells, stop the sulphadimidine and give him chloramphenicol or tetracycline for two more weeks.

Ask his mother to bring him again in one month after his symptoms have gone. Examine his urine again. If he still has pus cells in his urine, he needs more treatment, so try to send him to hospital.

23.6 'Eri has passed red urine (haematuria)'—schistosomiasis (bilharzia), acute nephritis, urinary infection, sulphonamides.

Most symptoms, such as a cough, diarrhoea, or fever, are common in all districts. But haematuria is different—it is common in some districts and rare in others. Where haematuria is common, it is usually caused by schistosomiasis (23.8). Acute nephritis occasionally causes haematuria, so does a urinary infection (23.4), or sulphonamides (3.14).

23.7 Acute nephritis

In this kidney disease a child passes red blood cells, protein, and casts (L 8.9) in his urine. His eyelids swell and his blood pressure is higher than normal, but he does

HOW SCHISTOSOMES SPREAD

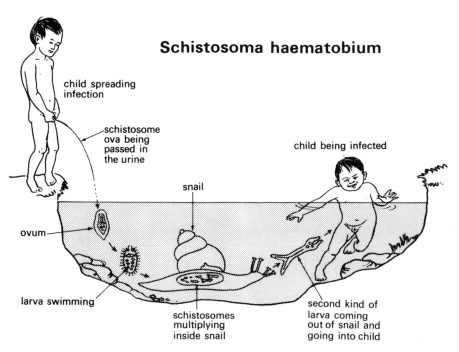

Schistosoma haematobium

child spreading infection

schistosome ova being passed in the urine

child being infected

snail

ovum

larva swimming

schistosomes multiplying inside snail

second kind of larva coming out of snail and going into child

Fig. 23–4 How *Schistosoma haematobium* spreads.

Observe him carefully. If he does not gain weight and is being well-fed, send him for help. He may have a chronic urinary infection.

EXPLANATION. **Tell his mother why he is ill, and why he must come to the clinic often. Explain that he must finish his treatment, even if he seems to be recovered.**

Put him on the 'special care register' (6.3) and try to visit him at home. Write URINARY INFECTION on his weight chart.

not have frequency or dysuria. Most children recover in a few days or weeks without treatment. Occasionally, a child dies. Sometimes, nephritis becomes chronic.

Acute nephritis usually begins about two weeks after a child has had a throat or skin infection with streptococci (a kind of bacteria). He may still have streptococci in him, so penicillin is helpful for killing them. Streptococci sometimes cause secondary infection when a child has scabies. So secondarily infected scabies can cause acute nephritis.

ACUTE NEPHRITIS

TREATMENT. **Give him procaine penicillin daily for ten days, or one injection of depot penicillin (3.15). Send him for help if he has these danger signs—passing very little urine, difficult breathing, or fits.**

EXPLANATION. **Tell his mother why he is ill, and why he may need to go to hospital.**

23.8 Schistosomiasis

In some parts of the world is a worm called *Schistosoma haematobium* lays ova in the veins of the bladder. These ova have a sharp point for making a hole in the wall of a vein. The ova come out of the veins of the bladder into the urine. The injured veins bleed into the bladder, so that a child passes blood and ova in his urine. Sometimes he has frequency and dysuria also. If he has many worms, he may lose so much blood that he becomes anaemic (22.3). Schistosomiasis is so common in some districts that school-children think it is normal to pass blood in their urine.

Schistosome ova hatch into larvae when they get into the water of a pond or a river. If the right kind of snail is living in the water, the larvae go into the snail, and multiply. Some days later many young schistosomes come out of the snail into the water. When a child washes or swims in the water, the schistosomes go through his skin into him. They go round his body until they find the veins in his bladder. Then they grow into adult worms, lay more ova, and so start their life cycle (circle, 21.1) again.

We can prevent schistosomiasis by breaking the worm's life cycle. We can kill snails and treat patients. We can stop the ova in infected urine getting into water. Everyone, especially children, *must* pass their urine into a latrine, and *not* into water.

Diagnose schistosomiasis. Look for ova in a child's urine with a microscope. Mildly infected children need no treatment. But if a child has haematuria, give him niridazole (3.31) or metrifonate. Severe infections can harm his kidneys and kill him.

23.9 Caring for a child with urinary symptoms—dysuria, frequency, urgency, incontinence, haematuria.

HISTORY. **If a child comes with any one of these symptoms, ask about all the others. Don't use the words dysuria, incontinence, frequency, or urgency. Ask instead if he has pain, wets himself, passes urine often, or has to pass it in a hurry.**

Dysuria? Frequency? Urgency? Incontinence (urine infection)?

Haematuria (schistosomiasis, nephritis)?

Fever or vomiting with these other symptoms (urine infection)?

EXAMINATION. **Look at his clothes. Do they smell of urine? Is there blood on them (haematuria)?**

Is there any infected lesion near the opening of his urethra? (Even a small lesion near the opening of his urethra may cause dysuria, but none of the other urinary symptoms.) 23.6

If he passes urine during the examination, notice what it looks like and if it is painful.

SPECIAL TESTS. **Examine his urine for pus cells (L 8.4) and bacteria. Count the pus cells (L 8.11). Stain a drop of (uncentrifuged) urine with Gram's stain and look for bacteria. If there is schistosomiasis in the district look for the ova of Schistosoma haematobium (L 8.15).** 23.8

23.7

DIAGNOSIS. **Urinary infection (23.4)? Acute nephritis (23.7)? Sores on the vulva or urethra (23.10)? Schistosomiasis (23.8)?**

The Genital System

23.10 'Her vulva is sore'—nappy rash, dirt, threadworms, foreign body, 'ordinary vulvovaginitis', or gonococcal vulvovaginitis. 23.10

Small girls sometimes have a sore vulva. A girl's mother may notice a vaginal discharge (pus coming from her vagina) or red skin near the vagina. She may notice the girl rubbing herself, or the girl may cry when she passes urine. A sore vulva may cause dysuria, but it does not usually cause frequency or make a girl wet herself.

A girl's vulva may become sore if she is dirty, and not washed enough. Threadworms (21.5) or a nappy rash (26.43) can also cause a sore vulva. Occasionally, a girl puts a foreign body into her vagina. This causes a discharge, sometimes with blood. Put your little finger into her *rectum*. Feel for the foreign body in her vagina through the front wall of her rectum.

Sometimes the skin of a girl's vulva and vagina become infected—**vulvovaginitis**. Pus comes from her vagina. Her vulva is red, sore, and sticky. She may have pain in her anus, and dysuria also. Vulvovaginitis is usually caused by ordinary bacteria. Sometimes it is caused by gonococci. Adult women with gonorrhoea (26.40) usually have few symptoms. But if gonococci infect small girls, they cause acute vulvovaginitis. Sometimes a man infects her. Usually, she is infected from her mother by dirty towels, or because they sleep in the same bed. A laboratory may be able to find gonococci in a swab of pus. Treat these children with procaine penicillin. If necessary treat their parents also (26.40). 23.9

If a girl has vulvovaginitis caused by ordinary bacteria, sit her in a bath of permanganate (11.6) several times a day. Dry her well after the bath. No other treatment is necessary. If her vulvovaginitis might be gonococcal, give both treatments.

23.11 'Parto's foreskin is too tight'—phimosis 23.11

A mother often worries about her son's foreskin. Tell her that he may not be able to pull back his foreskin until he is four years old. Tell her not to try.

Table 23:1   Some diseases of the urinary system

	Pain passing urine	Swelling of the eyes and feet	Urine red with blood	Protein in the urine	Pus cells in the urine	Schistosome ova in the urine
Urinary infection	Usually	Never	Sometimes	+	Always	Never
Schistosomiasis	Sometimes	Never	Often	+	Sometimes	Always
Acute nephritis	Never	Sometimes	Often	+ +	Never	Never
Nephrotic syndrome	Never	Severe	Never	+ + + +	Never	Never

Sometimes, a mother thinks that the hole in her child's foreskin is too small. Explain that if he passes urine with a good stream, the hole is big enough. If the hole really is too small (phimosis), urine comes out too slowly. His foreskin swells with urine, and he cries when he tries to pass it. He may need a small operation to make the hole bigger.

Sometimes a child's foreskin becomes pulled back over the end (glans) of his penis. His foreskin will not go back again (paraphimosis). He may need an operation in which a cut is made in the top of his foreskin.

Circumcision. This is an operation to remove a child's foreskin. Circumcision is rarely necessary, but many people like it. If a child is circumcised, sterilized instruments must be used. If dirty instruments are used, he may get a severe septic infection of his penis, and septicaemia. He can also get syringe jaundice (22.11) or tetanus (18.16), or severe bleeding.

23.12 'Lupo has a discharge from his penis'—gonorrhoea

Small boys sometimes get gonorrhoea from infected towels in the same way that small girls get vulvovaginitis. Treat them with penicillin (3.15). Treat their parents also (26.40).

24 The child who does not walk or talk

24.1 Has he stopped walking, or did he never start?

A child who cannot walk presents in two ways. (1) Sometimes a child has never walked and is now past the age when he should have started walking. (2) Sometimes a child started walking normally, but has now stopped walking, or has begun to limp (walk abnormally). A child who has stopped walking is easier to care for, so we describe him first.

All these diseases can stop a child walking—(a) severe general infection, (b) malnutrition, especially kwashiorkor, (c) injury, (d) polio, (e) a septic infection on the skin of his leg, (f) a septic infection in his leg muscles (pyomyositis), (g) a septic infection in a bone (osteomyelitis), or, (h) TB of a bone or joint.

24.2 Examining a child's arms, legs, and back

Before you can diagnose why a child has stopped walking, you must learn how to examine him.

EXAMINATION

Examine both sides of a child's body together. If one side is different from the other, one side is abnormal. Look for weakness, wasting, and swelling. Touch him to find out if he has a tender lesion. Move each joint as far as it will go in every direction. Is there less movement in a joint than there should be, or pain on moving it?

LEGS

A young child. Look for weakness by watching him play. Ask his mother to make him do what he can, such as crawling or kicking. Tickle (gently scratch), or pinch his legs and see if he moves them away.

Put his legs together. Bend his knees. Bend his hips up over his body. Then, keeping his hips bent, open his legs out wide. This is a good way of testing for a hip lesion. If one of his hips is abnormal, you cannot open out his leg normally on that side, because you cause pain.

Older children. If he can walk, ask him to walk. Ask him to stand on one leg and then on the other leg. Ask him to stand on his toes.

Lie him on a couch and put his legs together. Look at and feel them carefully. Wasting? Swelling? Tenderness? **24.1**

Bend each joint as far as it will go in every way. Don't forget his hips. Pain? Lack of movement?

Move his abnormal leg around. Compare it with his other leg. Is its tone (1.10) normal, increased (hypertonic), or reduced (hypotonic)?

Find out how strong he is by keeping his knee straight and asking him to bend it. Do the same with the other knee. Are they the same? Then keep his knee bent and ask him to straighten it. Do the same with his ankles and hips. Are any of these movements weaker on one side than the other? Perhaps both sides are abnormally weak? **23.12**

Examine his hips in the way described above for a young child.

ARMS **24.2**
Examine these in the same way as his legs.

BACK

Stand him up, or sit him up. Look at his back. Any swelling? Is it straight? Are both sides of his back the same? Can he stand and touch his toes? Can he bend first to his right then to his left?

Gently hit his back with your fist. Start at the top of his spine, and go down to the bottom, hitting each bone in turn. Is there any tender place (TB spine)?

THE CHILD WHO WAS WALKING BUT HAS NOW STOPPED

24.3 Injury **24.3**

Sometimes, a child hurts his leg when his mother is not looking. She may not know he has had an injury, and he may be too young to tell her. Perhaps you cannot see the injury, but it may be too painful for him to walk. So she brings him to you and tells you that he has stopped walking. If you see a child like this, examine him carefully for signs of an injury. He will soon start walking when his pain is less.

EXAMINING A CHILD'S LEGS

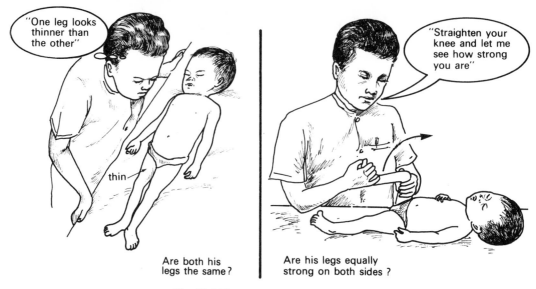

Fig. 24–1 Examining a child's legs.

ASKING A CHILD TO TOUCH HIS TOES

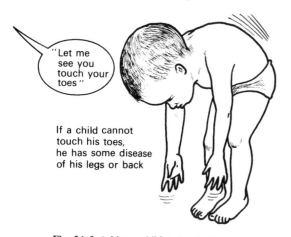

Fig. 24–2 Asking a child to touch his toes.

24.4 'Ram's leg is weak.'—Polio (poliomyelitis)

A virus causes polio. It infects the gut and spreads by 'faeces-to-mouth' infection in the same way as the organisms causing diarrhoea (2.7). Sometimes the virus spreads to a child's nerves, and injures them. The injured nerves go to muscles. These muscles become paralysed (weak), and wasted.

Most children are infected with polio virus at some time. Most children have no symptoms. Some children have a few days of fever with painful tender muscles, and then recover. Occasionally, the polio virus causes a virus meningitis (15.6). These children have a headache, vomiting, a stiff neck, and meningeal signs. These symptoms last a few days and then the child recovers. Very occasionally an unfortunate child has fever and meningeal signs, and then becomes paralysed in part of his body. Paralysis is most common in a child's legs. Part of his leg, a whole leg, or both his legs may be paralysed. Sometimes his arms are paralysed. Rarely his diaphragm and the muscles which move his ribs become paralysed. He dies because he cannot breathe.

Acute polio

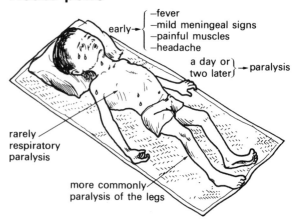

Fig. 24–3 Acute poliomyelitis.

242

The antibodies in mother's milk prevent young babies getting polio. Children most often get polio when they are between one and two years old, and are beginning to walk.

Acute polio. Polio usually presents as the child who has a weak leg and is not walking. He may have been well when the weakness began. Or he may have had a fever, neck stiffness, or mild diarrhoea for a few days. The paralysis stops getting worse when the fever stops. During the next six weeks, some of his nerve cells recover, and his leg becomes stronger. About one third of the children with paralysis recover during this time. The other children have some weakness for the rest of their lives.

Chronic polio. During the next year, other muscles near the weak ones learn to do more work. A paralysed leg becomes a little stronger. Weak muscles cannot move joints normally, so a child's leg may stay bent all day. If he is not treated, his leg becomes fixed in an abnormal position. He is deformed and he has a contracture. A contracture prevents a child using his normal muscles, and makes his disability worse. A paralysed leg does not grow normally, so he grows up with a short, thin, deformed leg. If both a child's legs are deformed by contractures, he has to walk on his hands and knees like the boy in Figure 1–9. A contracture can only be treated by a surgical operation.

Preventing polio and deformities. No child should get polio. We can prevent it by immunization (4.8b). If a child gets polio, we cannot make his injured nerves and muscles grow again. But we can prevent him becoming deformed by contractures, and we can help him to use his muscles. If his legs are very weak a splint may help him. Drugs and injections *don't* help. Injections may be harmful. An injection early in the acute stage while the child has fever may help to *cause* paralysis. So we must not give unnecessary injections.

POLIO

MANAGEMENT
If he has any difficulty breathing, his respiratory muscles may be paralysed, so send him for help quickly.

Most children with polio can be cared for at home. If both legs are weak, or if his weakness is not much better in two months, try to send him to hospital. A splint, like that in Figure 24–5, may help him to walk, and prevent deformity. If he is already deformed, he may need an operation.

TREATMENT
Acute polio. If his muscles are painful give him aspirin or paracetamol.

EXPLANATION
The first six weeks. Tell his mother to rest his leg. As soon as his fever has gone his mother must move his weak leg

through all its normal movements. She must do this for five minutes five times a day. Explain that this may hurt him. Explain that it will prevent deformity and help him to walk later. If necessary, help her to make simple splints to prevent his strong muscles pulling his leg into an abnormal position.

MUSCLES THAT ARE COMMONLY PARALYSED BY POLIO

'Old' polio

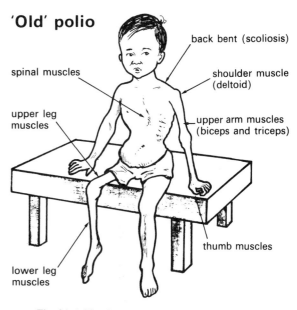

Fig. 24–4 Muscles commonly paralysed by polio.

After six weeks. He can begin to walk on his weak leg. Tell his mother to go on moving it five times a day as before. She must not let him sit all day in the same position. Teach her to help him to use his normal muscles.

His father may be able to make wooden bars for him to pull himself up with. He can hold onto these while he is learning to walk again. Tell his mother to help him to do as much as he can for himself. Most children with polio learn to walk, but they may walk abnormally, or need a splint.

Tell her not to waste money on injections, because there are no drugs for curing polio.

24.4

ANYTHING WHICH CAUSES PARALYSIS CAN ALSO CAUSE CONTRACTURES

24.5 'Suraji has fever and severe pain in his leg (or arm)'—osteomyelitis

24.5

Occasionally, bacteria go from a septic lesion on a child's skin, to his bones. Bacteria can also go from his gut to his

Splints for polio

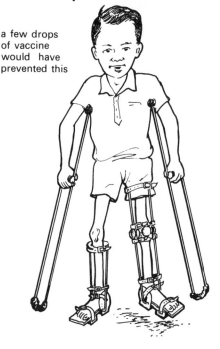

a few drops of vaccine would have prevented this

Fig. 24–5 A polio child in a splint.

bones. Bacteria cause an acute septic bone infection called osteomyelitis. Usually there is only one lesion, but there may be several. Osteomyelitis can cause septicaemia and kill a child. It is more common in children with sickle cell anaemia (22.8).

The child is 'ill' with a high fever. Sometimes he presents as a fever before there are any local symptoms. Osteomyelitis causes a painful tender local lesion in one of his long bones, usually in his leg. His leg may be so painful that he cannot walk, or move it, or let anyone else bend it. After some days an abscess forms. The lesion becomes warm, red, and swollen. If he is treated late, pus may come out from the abscess through a hole (sinus) in his skin.

Bacteria in a bone abscess are difficult to kill, because antibiotics cannot easily get to them from the blood. So we must give big doses of antibiotics for a long time. Treat osteomyelitis for six weeks. If treatment starts too late or stops too soon, a child's lesion may become chronic. Osteomyelitis may last for years. Pus discharges from the hole in the child's leg, and the bone is destroyed. He has fever and he becomes very thin. The only way to cure him may be to cut off his leg. So you must diagnose osteomyelitis *early* and give enough antibiotics for long enough. Start treatment in the first four days. If you start treatment later the child will probably need an operation later to let out the pus.

OSTEOMYELITIS

MANAGEMENT. **Try to send the child to hospital. If you have to care for him yourself, do it like this.**

SPECIAL TESTS. **If possible, measure his haemoglobin, X-ray his bone and culture the pus.**

TREATMENT
Penicillin. **Give 600 mg of benzyl penicillin intramuscularly or intravenously every three hours for two days. Then give it six hourly for four weeks.**

AND chloramphenicol
Under five years. Give 1 ml of suspension per kilo (25 mg/kg) every six hours for three days. Then give him ½ ml of suspension per kilo (12 mg/kilo) every six hours for six weeks.
Over five years. Give him chloramphenicol in the doses in Figure 3–12 for six weeks.
If he still has fever, swelling, or much tenderness after 48 hours' treatment, try again to send him to hospital. He probably has an abscess and needs an operation to let out the pus.

TREAT OSTEOMYELITIS FOR SIX WEEKS, OR THE CHILD MAY LOSE HIS LEG

24.5b 'Banjoko has a painful swelling in his thigh' —pyomyositis

This is a disease of older children and adults. Sometimes, bacteria make a very large abscess in a child's muscles—pyomyositis (pus in the muscles). This acute disease causes fever, rigors, and 'not eating'. There is a firm, tender, warm swelling in a muscle anywhere in his body. Sometimes the swelling is fluctuant. Often there is more than one swelling. If the abscess is in a child's lower leg, he cannot walk—moving his leg is too painful. Pyomyositis often presents with fever and pain before the swelling has begun. If you don't treat the abscess, pus discharges through a hole (sinus) in his skin. Sometimes you cannot be sure if the swelling started in a bone (osteomyelitis) or a muscle (pyomyositis). So diagnosing between these two diseases may be difficult.

PYOMYOSITIS
MANAGEMENT. **Usually, we must open the abscess, so send him for help.**

TREATMENT. **Give him penicillin (3.15), or tetracycline (3.17).**

24.6 'Anatoly has pain and swelling in his back'—TB of the bones and joints

TB bacilli sometimes spread from a child's lungs and cause chronic TB abscesses in his bones or joints. His spine or hips (13.2) are most commonly infected. A TB abscess of the spine usually presents as a swelling over the spine (24–7). Later the spine becomes bent. Sometimes a TB abscess presses on the spinal cord and causes paralysis.

Pain from a TB hip abscess may stop a child walking, or make him limp. Sometimes, a swelling forms over the lesion or in the muscles near it. TB is a chronic infection, so the symptoms come slowly. The child has a mild fever for some weeks. He also has any of the general symptoms of TB, such as loss of weight (13:1).

TB OF THE BONES AND JOINTS

SPECIAL TESTS. **Try to send the child to hospital for an X-ray. This is the only way to make a sure diagnosis.**

MANAGEMENT AND TREATMENT

TB spine. **If he can walk, treat him for TB. Plaster jackets (splints for the spine) usually don't help. If he cannot walk send him to hospital. He probably needs an operation to drain the abscess.**

TB of other joints. **Treat him for TB.**

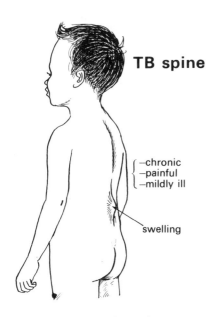

TB spine

—chronic
—painful
—mildly ill

swelling

Fig. 24–7 TB of the spine.

24.7 Caring for a child who has stopped walking or started limping, or who has a weak or painful arm.

Any severe acute or chronic infection, such as chronic diarrhoea, can stop a young child walking. You can diagnose his disease from his other symptoms. So we will not list all the diseases he might have. If you treat one of these diseases, TB for example, he will start walking when he recovers. Sickle cell anaemia can stop a child walking. It causes dactylitis (22.8) in his toes, or pains in

his legs. Occasionally, a child stops walking because he has a disease of his brain (such as meningitis), which makes him backward (24.9).

HISTORY. **Did it come suddenly (polio, osteomyelitis, pyomyositis, injury)? Or slowly (TB)?**
  What happened to him just before he stopped walking (fever, polio, osteomyelitis)? Fits (meningitis, fever)? Injury?
    Immunized against polio?
    Other symptoms (any severe general disease)?
    Has he had an injection in his weak leg recently (polio)?
    Are his other milestones normal?

EXAMINATION. **Any septic lesion on his leg?**
  'Ill' with a high fever (osteomyelitis)?
  Meningeal signs (polio, or meningitis)?
  Malnourished? Oedema (kwashiorkor)?
  Examine his legs and back (24.1).
  Any signs of injury, such as bruising?
  Weak, hypotonic, slightly, tender muscles (acute polio)?
  Weak wasted muscles (chronic polio)?
  Acute tenderness or swelling over a bone (osteomyelitis)?
  Acute tenderness and swelling of a muscle (pyomyositis)?
  Chronic swelling over a bone joint, or a muscle near it (TB or chronic osteomyelitis)?
  Anaemia? Large spleen (sickle cell anaemia)?

DIAGNOSIS. **Septic lesion on his leg? Any severe illness (10.10)? Severe malnutrition (7.13)? Injury (14.5)? Polio (24.4)? Sickle cell anaemia (22.8)? TB (24.6)? Osteomyelitis (24.5)? Pyomyositis (24.5b).**

MANAGEMENT IF THE DIAGNOSIS IS DIFFICULT. **If the child is 'well', and will not move his leg, he may have an injury or polio.**
  If his illness is acute with high fever and a tender lesion over a bone, treat him for osteomyelitis.
  If his illness is chronic with pain and low fever, examine him for TB. If necessary, treat him for it (13.6).

24.8 'Sirun's leg (or arm) is thin'—malnutrition, polio, leprosy, or chronic disease of the bone

24.8

Malnutrition makes a child thin all over. It does not cause contractures and is easy to diagnose.

24.7

CARING FOR A CHILD WITH A THIN LEG OR ARM
Was he immunized against polio?
  Did his leg become thin after an illness (polio)?
  Has he any anaesthetic skin lesions (12.3) or thickened nerves (leprosy)?
  Any lesion of a bone or joint?

24.6

DIAGNOSIS. **Malnutrition (7.13)? Polio (24.4)? Leprosy?**

THE CHILD WHO IS LATE WALKING OR TALKING

24.9 'Pablo is late walking'—the backward child

There is a right or normal age for a child to start smiling and holding things. There is a right age for him to smile, sit, stand, walk, and talk. Growing up and doing these things at the right time is called **development**. The age for doing each thing is called a **milestone**. It is like a stone beside a road which tells us how many miles (or kilometres) we have come. A child who does not pass his milestones at the normal age is backward. He is going along the road too slowly. A very backward child who is a long way behind his milestones is **mentally deficient** (lacking in mind). He may grow up disabled, so that he cannot do a normal job, or have a normal life.

Backwardness usually presents as late walking, because this is when a child's mother needs help. He is getting heavy. She may be pregnant again, and she does not want to go on carrying him. She may have noticed that he was late with his earlier milestones, but said nothing about it.

24.10 Diagnosing backwardness

Normal children do not develop at exactly the same speed. Some normal children start walking when they are ten months old. Other children do not walk until they are eighteen months. Some children never crawl, but walk straight away. Others don't say a word until they are two years old and then suddenly talk well. 97 out of every 100 children, sit by the time they are 9 months old and walk by the time they are 18 months old. A child who has not passed a milestone at the age when 97 per cent of children have passed it is late with that milestone.

If a child is late with one milestone only, but is normal for the others, he is not backward. He may be normal, or he may have a lesion in another part of his body. For example, if he is walking normally but not talking, he may be deaf, so test his hearing (17.7). If he sat up normally, and is beginning to talk but cannot walk, he may have an abnormality of his legs (24.2). But, if a child is late with several milestones, he is backward.

USE SEVERAL MILESTONES TO DECIDE ABOUT A CHILD'S DEVELOPMENT

Table 24:1   Development

The age at which most (97 per cent) children pass their milestones.

Smiling	6 weeks
Sitting without help	9 months
Walking without help	18 months
Saying single words	21 months
Talking in sentences	36 months

There is much mild backwardness in every community. Parents often hide backward children. They want to protect them and do not want other people to see them. About three children in a hundred are too backward to keep up with other children of the same age in school. Two of these three children can learn something if they go to a special school. The third child cannot learn anything in school.

A BACKWARD CHILD IS LATE WITH MORE THAN ONE MILESTONE

24.11 Helping a mother with her backward child

If a child's brain is badly made or harmed, there is no curative treatment which will make it work normally. But we can help many of these children to have a nearly normal life, and we can help their mothers. Many backward children have symptoms, such as fits, for which there is useful symptomatic treatment. If a mother teaches her backward child in the right way, he can learn to do many useful things. He can be a help at home, instead of needing to be watched all the time. If he can learn to wash, feed, and dress himself, and use a latrine, this will help his family.

THE BACKWARD CHILD

MANAGEMENT. **Most backward children must be cared for at home. Sometimes there is a special school where they can go.**

TREATMENT. **If a child has any symptoms, be sure to treat them.**

Fits. **Phenobarbitone (3.43) may help him. Try to give him only enough to stop them, without making him too sleepy.**

Not sleeping. **If he cries at night and wakes the family, promethazine may help.**

Contractures. **If he might get contractures, his mother must move his arms and legs through their full movements several times each day (24.4).**

EXPLANATION. **Don't tell his mother he is backward until you are sure. Don't tell her all at once. First tell her he *might* be backward. Later, tell her he probably is backward. Explain that his backwardness is not her fault. She must not blame herself for it, or be ashamed of it, or hide him. Try to help her in the difficult job of looking after him. Let her feel that she can always come and talk to you.**

Tell her that she must be very patient teaching him. She may have to show him many times what to do, and what not to do. She must teach him more carefully, more slowly, and more often than her other children. She must not do everything for him. Doing everything herself may be easier than teaching him, but it will not help him to learn.

Tell her that there is no drug treatment for backwardness, so she must not waste her money buying

MILESTONES AND THE WEIGHT CHART

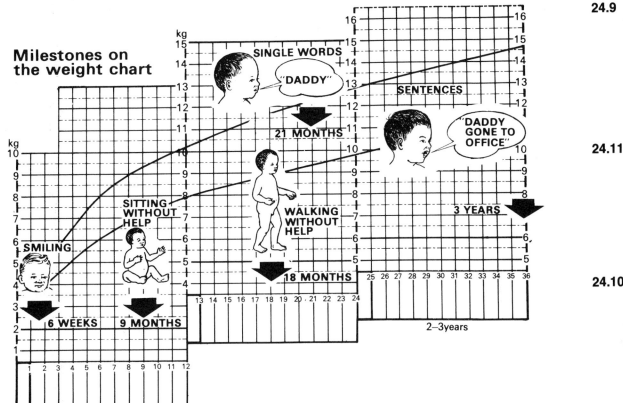

Milestones on the weight chart

Fig. 24–8 Development and the weight chart.

drugs. **Visit him at home, and make sure he is on the special care register.**

LOOK FOR HIDDEN BACKWARD CHILDREN

24.12 Some causes of backwardness

A child is backward because his brain is not working normally. His brain may have been badly made while he was in the uterus, or some disease may have harmed it afterwards. Some children are backward because they have had some illness, or because they have not been loved enough.

Diseases which harm a child's brain. If a child is born too early, his brain has not had enough time to finish growing. A child's brain can be harmed at birth, by injury, or asphyxia (26.6). Soon after birth it can be harmed by jaundice (26.23), or hypoglycaemia (26.42). Sometimes, a child is normal until fits (15.1), meningitis (15.6), or cerebral malaria (10.7) harm his brain and make him backward. These diseases may also cause paralysis. They can make the muscles in his arms and legs hypertonic (spastic). Children whose brains have been harmed like this have **cerebral palsy** (24.15). Sometimes, they have epileptic fits also (15.8).

Badly made (malformed) brains. Lack or iodine before birth (iodine embryopathy, 24.14b), or lack of thyroid (cretinism, 24.14), or Down's syndrome (24.13) all cause backwardness. Often, we know that a child is backward and that he must have a malformed brain. But we cannot diagnose what disease is causing it.

General illnesses. Malnutrition and infections, such as chronic diarrhoea or TB, may prevent a child walking at the normal time. In some districts 3 per cent of children walk late because of these diseases. When we treat a child like this he quickly learns to walk, but he may grow up less clever (N 2.2a).

Lack of love. If parents do not love a child enough and play with him enough, he may be mildly backward. The children without parents in a children's home are often backward. Sometimes they are malnourished also.

24.13 Down's syndrome (mongolism)

When we can find a cause for backwardness, it is often Down's syndrome. About one baby in 700 is born with Down's syndrome. It is much more common in children born to mothers over 40 years old.

When you have seen a few children with this syndrome, you will be able to diagnose it easily. The children all look like one another. They might all be the brothers or sisters of the child in Figure 24–9. You can diagnose Down's syndrome at birth, but diagnosis is easier when a child is a few months old. His muscles are hypotonic, and his body bends so easily that you can put his feet behind his ears. He has narrow sloping eyes with folds across the inner ends of his eyelids (epicanthic folds). The top (bridge) of his nose is flat, and his eyes are far apart. He has a small mouth and a big tongue, so that he keeps his mouth open and his tongue sticks out. The back of his head is flatter than normal. His fingers are short, so his hands look wide. Sometimes he only has one fold across the palms of his hands, instead of the normal two folds. He is not as strong as a normal child and dies more easily. Don't diagnose Down's syndrome from one or two of these signs. *He should have most of them* before you can be sure he has Down's syndrome.

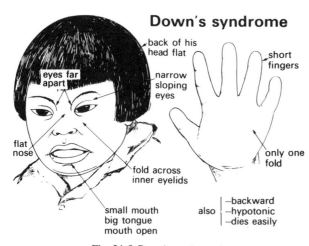

Down's syndrome

back of his head flat

eyes far apart

narrow sloping eyes

short fingers

flat nose

fold across inner eyelids

only one fold

small mouth big tongue mouth open

also | –backward | –hypotonic | –dies easily

Fig. 24–9 Down's syndrome.

24.14 Cretins

In some ways cretins look like children with Down's syndrome. The bridges of their noses are flat. They have open mouths and big tongues. But they are different, because they have swollen eyelids, and thick dry skin and hair. They do not have epicanthic folds, and they have normal palms with two folds. The backs of their heads are normal. A cretin is constipated and cold. He does not move much, and he has an abnormally low voice. A child with Down's syndrome is warm, and has

normal movements, stools, and voice. Cretins are rare, but they develop normally if you diagnose them early and give them thyroid tablets. Send them for help.

24.14b Iodine embryopathy

A baby must get enough iodine from his mother while he is in the uterus. If he does not get enough iodine, his brain does not grow normally. He gets a disease called iodine embryopathy. A child with iodine embryopathy is always backward. He may be deaf, mute (unable to talk), have a squint (eyes looking in different directions), and have a facial palsy (26.60). He may walk abnormally. He may be shorter than normal (dwarfed). He may also have some of the same signs as a cretin. Sometimes his mother has a goitre.

Iodine embryopathy is common in districts which lack iodine in their soil and water. Lack of iodine also causes endemic goitre. So you will only see iodine embryopathy in districts where endemic goitre is common. If there is plenty of iodine in a district, you will never see iodine embryopathy or endemic goitre. We can easily prevent iodine embryopathy. We can add a little iodine to the cooking salt. We can also inject women with iodized oil every three years. If 5 per cent of the children, or 10 per cent of adults have a Grade I goitre (19.6) or larger, there is severe iodine deficiency in the district. We must prevent iodine embryopathy in these districts.

If goitres are common in your district, give every backward child iodized oil (or some other kind of iodine). It may make him grow. It may also help an older backward child enough to let him work.

WE CAN PREVENT IODINE EMBRYOPATHY

24.15 'Ali is backward and his muscles are stiff'—cerebral palsy

We saw in Section 24.11 that many diseases can injure a child's brain and cause cerebral palsy. Children with cerebral palsy do not recover and do not become worse. Their brains can be harmed in two ways.

Some parts of the brain are used for moving the muscles, and other parts for thinking. Cerebral palsy can harm one part, or both parts of a child's brain. If only the part which moves muscles is harmed, a child's muscles contract, so that they become hypertonic (stiff and tight). A child like this is **spastic**. He may be late standing and walking, because he cannot make his muscles move normally. But if the thinking part of his brain is normal, he will be normal in thinking. If the thinking part of his brain is injured, he will be backward in every way.

When a spastic child is very young his muscle tone may be normal or even hypotonic. He becomes spastic (hypertonic) as he grows older. Increased tone of the muscles on the inside of his legs make them cross one another like a pair of scissors (24–10). Some spastic children have slow twisting movements of their arms and legs, so that they cannot keep still.

Try to find out how much of a spastic child's back-wardness is caused by the stiffness of his muscles. Find out how much is caused by injury to the thinking part of his brain. This may not be easy, but it is important, because we can help a clever child more easily.

CEREBRAL PALSY

A spastic child

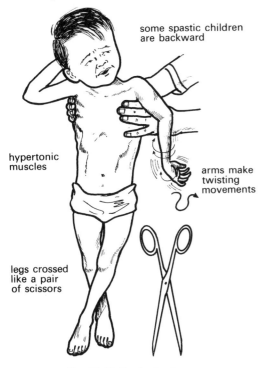

some spastic children are backward

hypertonic muscles

arms make twisting movements

legs crossed like a pair of scissors

Fig. 24–10 Cerebral palsy.

24.16 Caring for a child who is late walking or talking

Often, we cannot diagnose why a child is backward. When we can make a diagnosis, it is usually Down's syndrome, or cerebral palsy.

HISTORY

MILESTONES. **How old is he? What can he do? Ask about all his milestones.**

Is he late with one milestone only? (If he is only late talking he may be deaf. if he is only late walking he may have a disease of his arms or legs.)
Late with several milestones? (If he is, he is backward.)

FEEDING DIFFICULTIES. **Did he have difficulty feeding in the first few weeks of life? (This is an early sign of the backward child, especially the child with cerebral palsy.)**

PAST ILLNESSES. **Any illnesses in the past, which might have harmed his brain? Birth injury (26.6)? Was he abnormally 'floppy' (hypotonic) immediately after birth? (Spastic or Down's syndrome.) Meningitis (15.6)? Cerebral malaria (15.7)? (He may have been normal with his early milestones and then had a disease which harmed his brain.)** 24.13

LOVE. **Has he been well-loved and cared for? (Lack of love is a cause of mild backwardness.)**

MOTHER'S AGE. **How old was his mother when he was born? (Down's syndrome is much more common in mothers over 40.)**

EXAMINATION

MILESTONES. **Ask his mother to show you what he can do. This can be difficult. Many children will not talk in a clinic, even to their mothers.**

DOWN'S SYNDROME. **Open mouth and large tongue? Eyes narrow and far apart? Bridge of nose flat? Folds across the inner ends of the eyelids? Back of the head flat? Short fingers? Only one fold on the inside of his hands? Hypotonic? Can you put his feet behind his ears?**

CRETIN. **Open mouth and large tongue? Swollen eyelids? Thick, dry, cold skin and hair?**

CEREBRAL PALSY. **Hypertonic muscles? 'Scissors' legs (24–10, mildly spastic)? Twisting movements of the arms and legs (severely spastic)?**

IODINE EMBRYOPATHY. **Goitre common in the district? Deaf? Unable to speak? Squint? Small? Facial palsy? Walks abnormally? Signs of cretinism?**

DEAF. **If he is late talking, especially if this is his only late milestone, test his hearing (17.7). Examine his ears. Children with iodine embryopathy are often deaf. If a child is late talking, but is normal in every other way, he may be deaf.** 24.15

DISEASE OF HIS LEGS. **Examine them (24.2). He may have some disease of his legs which prevents him from walking.** 24.16

CHRONIC INFECTION AND MALNUTRITION? **Look at his weight chart.**

DIAGNOSIS

How backward? **Mildly? Moderately? Severely?**

Cause of late walking or talking. **Chronic infection? Malnutrition? Lack of love? (All these three cause *mild* backwardness only.) Deaf (not talking only)? Some disease of his legs (not walking only)? Some brain disease we cannot diagnose (a common cause of backwardness)? Cerebral palsy following birth injury, hypoglycaemia, jaundice, fits, meningitis, or cerebral malaria (24.15)? Down's syndrome (24.13)? Cretin (24.14)? Iodine embryopathy (24.14b)?** 24.14

25 Some other problems

Family problems

25.1 The worried mother

Some symptoms, such as fits (15.1), are serious. All mothers should worry about these serious symptoms. Other symptoms such as constipation are seldom serious, but often cause worry. Mothers think about the symptoms in their children in different ways. For example, one mother may think that a discharging ear is normal. Another mother may be very worried about it. Mothers who do not worry about their children are a problem to us. It is difficult to help these mothers to care for their children in the right way. Mothers who worry too much are a problem also.

Poor mothers with many children and too much work may not have time to worry. But richer mothers have more time to worry about their children, especially the first child. A richer mother may come to the clinic every week about a symptom in her first baby. She might come because he is not passing a stool every day, or because he is 'not breathing regularly'. Both these things are normal, but because they only happen to some children, mothers think they are abnormal. We have tried to tell you which things are normal, and which are not. If you know this, you can comfort a mother and tell her that her child is normal. But if a mother comes with a normal symptom, don't tell her that her visit was not necessary. She needed to visit you, and you have helped her.

25.2 The unhappy child—some behaviour diseases

These are the diseases of what a child does, or how he behaves. They are less common than malnutrition, infections, or accidents. A child behaves abnormally if he is not loved and cared for in the right way. His abnormal behaviour is his way of saying he is unhappy. He may be unhappy because his mother does not care for and play with him enough, or because he is jealous of his newborn baby sister. Because he has been sent away to live with his grandmother. Because his father is unkind to him. Or because his parents fight or get drunk.

A child can behave abnormally in all these ways—not eating (18.15), crying too much, wetting his bed when he is older (enuresis), not sleeping, not speaking normally

(stammering), stealing, not going to school, or by getting severe attacks of angry crying (tantrums). The best way to help a child like this is to explain to his parents why he is behaving abnormally. Explain that they may have caused his abnormal behaviour. Tell them that punishing a child will probably make his behaviour worse. For example, if a child wets his bed they should not beat him. Don't make him wash his bed clothes as a punishment.

25.2b The 'ill child'

Occasionally, a mother will say that her child is not well, but she does not tell you any other symptoms. He may be irritable and restless with the signs of a child in Stage C or D of Table 5:2. If he has any special symptoms, such as cough, go to the section for that symptom. If he has no special symptoms, and he has been 'ill' for a few hours or days only, go to Section 10.10 (fever). If he has been 'ill' for a few weeks, go to Section 13.7 (TB).

Some problems in the gut

25.2c 'Abdul is teething'

When a child's teeth are growing, we say he is teething. When healthy teeth grow through a child's gum they do not make him ill. Teething does not cause fever, fits, diarrhoea, colic, coughs, bronchitis, rashes, not sleeping, or ear rubbing. But teething sometimes makes a child restless, or makes him rub his gums, or suck his thumb, or stops him eating (18.15).

25.3 'He sucks milk, but won't eat any food'

A baby should start to eat porridge and other foods when he is four months old. A baby less than a year old likes eating new foods. A child more than a year old eats new foods less easily. So try to make a baby eat several good foods before he is a year old.

Sometimes, a mother does not give her baby new foods early enough. She comes to you and says that her one- or two-year-old child will not eat anything except breast-milk. This is serious, because mother's milk by itself is not enough for an older child. Tell her to give him porridge when he is hungry, *before* she feeds him from the breast. If she tries hard, he will eat. Occasionally, a mother may have to stop breast-feeding an older child to make him eat.

Breast-feeding for a long time never *causes* 'not eating'.

25.4 'Something has stuck in Maria's throat'—choking

Occasionally, a foreign body, such as a piece of food, a sweet, or a toy, obstructs a child's throat, so that he chokes (8.18). He coughs and his face becomes cyanosed (blue). Remove the foreign body quickly, or he will die.

CHOKING
Turn him upside down and hit him on the back. He will probably cough out the foreign body. If it does not come out, you may be able to get it out with your finger. If this does not work, and he is cyanosed, send him for help quickly.

Choking

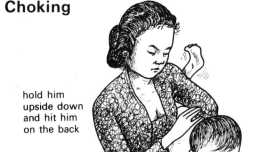

hold him upside down and hit him on the back

sweet

Fig. 25–1 Something has stuck in his throat.

25.5 'Parto has eaten a button'—swallowed foreign body

Children often swallow foreign bodies, such as buttons, toys, or beads. Small foreign bodies are usually passed in the faeces without difficulty in a few days. A long sharp foreign body, such as a needle, may make a hole in a child's gut, and cause peritonitis. Occasionally a foreign body obstructs his gut. Obstruction is serious. So observe him carefully. If he has no symptoms, do nothing. If he has pain or vomits, send him to hospital quickly. He may need an operation.

25.6 'Amin's stools are hard'—constipation 25.6

If a child does not pass faeces, or passes hard faeces, he is constipated. Constipation is the opposite of diarrhoea. Any sick child who is not eating passes less faeces than normal. So, most children with fever are constipated. Mothers often worry about this. But when a child eats again, he will pass faeces normally. He needs no treatment. If a well child is constipated, tell his mother to give him more fruit and vegetables. 25.4

Hard faeces are painful. Sometimes a child keeps them in his rectum, so they get harder and even more difficult to pass. Occasionally, passing a large lump of faeces tears a child's anus and causes an anal fissure (sore). Ask his mother if he passes blood. Look at his anus to see if you can find a sore. Tell her to give him plenty of fruit, or a few spoonfuls of liquid paraffin. This will make his stools soft. If the fissure does not heal, he may need hospital treatment. 25.1

For constipation in babies, go to Sections 26.29 to 31.

Constipation is not serious unless there is also severe abdominal pain (20.13), swelling (20.9), or vomiting (20.15).

**CONSTIPATION IS NOT SERIOUS
UNLESS THERE IS SEVERE ABDOMINAL
PAIN, SWELLING, OR VOMITING**

25.7 'A red lump has come out of his anus'—rectal prolapse, polyp, intussusception 25.7

A child's rectum sometimes prolapses (falls out) from his anus. He comes to the clinic with a soft red swelling with a hole in it. Sometimes a mother says the lump comes out when he passes a stool. She may have pushed it back, so there is nothing to see. Sometimes, he has had a swelling for some days, and the prolapsed rectum is ulcerated (sore) and bleeding. He may be frightened, and his mother worried. Prolapse is not serious. You can easily push the swelling back inside. Prolapse of the rectum is common in malnourished children, especially if they have diarrhoea. Sometimes, a prolapsed rectum is covered with *Trichuris* worms that have helped to cause it.

There are other red swellings at a child's anus. The swelling may be a polyp (tumour), or a part of the gut which has come from higher up (intussusception). A polyp comes out when he passes faeces, and goes up again afterwards. These swellings are rare. 25.2 25.5 25.3

PROLAPSED RECTUM
TREATMENT. **Make him less frightened by giving paraldehyde (3.44), or phenobarbitone (3.43). Ask his mother to cut her nails short. Ask a helper to hold him. Bend up his knees. Then show his mother how to take some toilet paper or a wet cloth and gently push back the swelling. If she is using paper, let it stay in his anus until he next**

passes a stool. This will help to stop his rectum prolapsing again. If the swelling is difficult to push back, or if it comes down again quickly, hang him over a bed with his feet up ('the gallows position'). When you have pushed it back, let him stay there for a few hours.

Prolapse

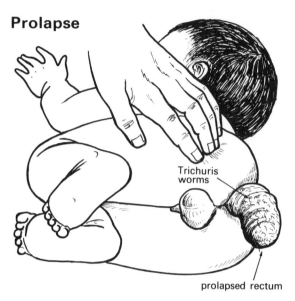

Fig. 25–2 Prolapse of the rectum.

If there are *Trichuris* worms (21.7) on the prolapsed swelling, or if he has diarrhoea (9.31), or constipation (25.6), treat him. If he does not recover in a few months, send him for help. He may need an operation.

EXPLANATION. **If he is below the road to health, explain to his mother how she can improve his nutrition.**

25.7b Blood in the stool

This is usually caused by diarrhoea. If a baby is less than a week old go to Section 26.33. Look at the child's stools carefully.

Watery diarrhoea stool mixed with a little blood —probably bacillary dysentery (usually dehydrated). Measles can also cause a bloody diarrhoea.

Soft stool with bright blood and mucus—probably amoebic dysentery (usually not dehydrated).

Blood, or blood and mucus without diarrhoea. If he has abdominal pain, abdominal swelling, or vomiting (20.2), he may have an intussusception (9.15).

Blood only. Perhaps an anal fissure (25.6).

25.8 'He always vomits when he goes in a bus' —travel sickness.

Promethazine (3.45) often helps these children. Give it to him half an hour before the journey starts.

A few more problems

25.9 'The skin round my little girl's ear-ring is red'

Parents often put gold rings into the ears of young girls. If the gold is pure, they rarely cause trouble. But cheaper rings made of less pure gold may cause inflammation. If a mother brings you her child with the signs of inflammation round an ear-ring, take it out. When the inflammation has gone, a new ring of purer gold will probably not cause any trouble.

25.10 'Sugeng's nose is bleeding'

Nose bleeds are more common in older children. Sit the child forwards over a bowl. Tell him to sit quietly and to pinch his nose tight. Ask him to bite on something soft, such as a cork or a bandage, so that he cannot swallow. If the bleeding does not stop in an hour, try to send him for help.

Nose bleeding

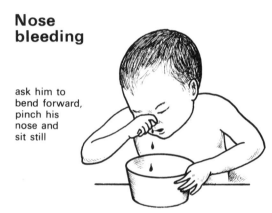

ask him to bend forward, pinch his nose and sit still

Fig. 25–3 Nose bleeding.

25.11 'There is a discharge from one side of Fifi's nose'—foreign body, diphtheria of the nose

A cold causes discharge from both sides of the nose. Foreign bodies and diphtheria (18.12) cause discharge from one side only. In diphtheria the discharge is usually bloody.

Foreign bodies in the nose are more common than foreign bodies in the ear. The foreign body may be a seed, a piece of maize, a small button, or anything.

FOREIGN BODY IN THE NOSE

Hold the normal side of his nose shut. Ask him to blow hard. If this does not remove the foreign body, hold his head still (18–1) and remove it with a wire hook. Remove it in the same way as you remove a foreign body from the ear—see Figure 17–12. If necessary, you can use forceps. Syringing the nose does not help. If there is a purulent discharge because of secondary infection, give him an

antibiotic. Removing the foreign body will probably make his nose bleed. This bleeding soon stops.

25.12 'Ade has pains in his arms or legs'

Mild pains in the arms and legs are common and not serious. Many fevers cause pain in the arms and legs. Any injury (fracture)? Fever, tenderness, and swelling over a bone (osteomyelitis)? Fever, tenderness and swelling over a muscle (pyomyositis)? Anaemia and a large spleen (sickle cell anaemia)?

25.9

25.12

25.10

25.11

25.8

26 The newborn baby

HIS FIRST HOUR

26.1 The healthy newborn baby

A healthy baby breathes and cries as soon as he is born, and he quickly becomes pink. During the first quarter of an hour he breathes irregularly. Sometimes he stops breathing for half a minute. Sometimes he 'grunts'. A grunt is any noise which a newborn baby makes when he breathes. There may also be some insuction (8.9). After the first quarter of an hour he breathes more regularly—between 30 and 50 times a minute. But he may not breathe completely regularly until he is about a year old. At birth his heart rate is about 180. After an hour it falls to between 120 and 150. He coughs or sneezes when you suck out his mouth. He has good muscle tone (1.10), and he moves his arms and legs about, especially if you touch him. During the next hour these movements become less and he goes to sleep.

Any of these things are *abnormal* in a newborn baby—

Not breathing as soon as he is born.

'Grunting' or insuction after the first quarter of an hour.

Hypotonia ('floppy' arms and legs).

Not moving his arms or legs by himself.

Not moving his arms or legs when you pinch him.

Not coughing or sneezing when you suck out his mouth.

A white or blue face and body (blue hands and feet are normal if he is cold).

A pulse which you cannot feel or hear, or a pulse which is less than 100.

26.2 Normal birth

When a baby is born, first make sure he is breathing, then tie his cord.

BIRTH

As soon as the baby is delivered, note the exact time. Hold him with his head a little lower than his legs, so that the fluid drains from his respiratory system.

If someone is helping you, show her how to hold him

while you suck him out. First suck out his mouth, then his nose with a sterile, wide, soft, rubber catheter, or rubber bulb (3:2). Give one strong, long, suck. Don't push the catheter too far down his throat, because this will not help. A normal baby will breathe and cry.

If he does not breathe and cry, hit the bottoms of his feet. Listen to his heart with a stethoscope. Feel if his umbilical cord is beating. Count his pulse.

If he is not breathing 2 minutes after he was born, and his pulse is less than 100, go to Section 26.3. He needs mouth to mouth resuscitation—QUICKLY!

When he is breathing keep him lower than the uterus for a few minutes, so that blood can flow towards him down his cord.

Feel his cord. After it has stopped beating for a few minutes, clamp it with two sterile artery clamps. Cut his cord between the clamps with sterile scissors. Then tie his

A HEALTHY NEWBORN BABY

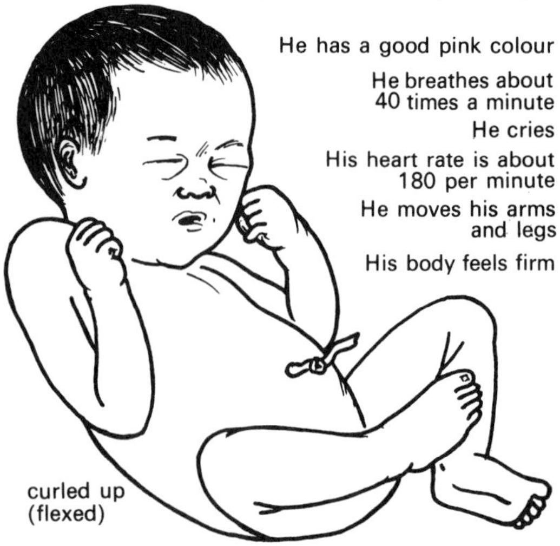

When you suck him out, he coughs

He has a good pink colour

He breathes about 40 times a minute

He cries

His heart rate is about 180 per minute

He moves his arms and legs

His body feels firm

curled up (flexed)

Fig. 26–1 A healthy newborn baby.

CLAMPING THE CORD

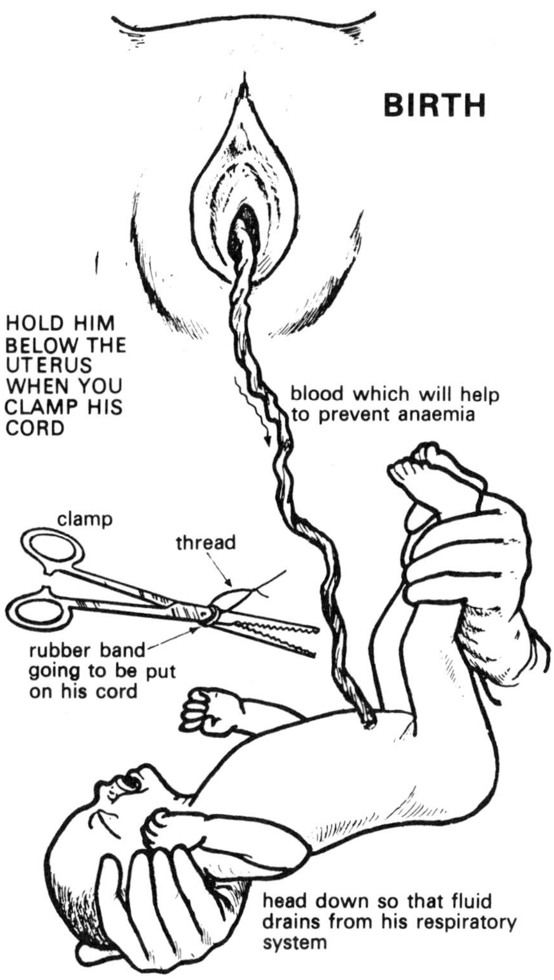

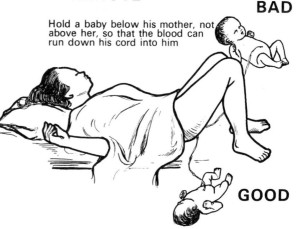

BIRTH

HOLD HIM
BELOW THE
UTERUS
WHEN YOU
CLAMP HIS
CORD

blood which will help
to prevent anaemia

clamp

thread

rubber band
going to be put
on his cord

head down so that fluid
drains from his respiratory
system

Fig. 26–2 Clamping the cord.

cord twice, 5 cm from the umbilicus. Use sterile tape, string or rubber bands (26–4). After you have tied his cord, take off the artery clamp.

Clean his eyes from the nose side outwards with a piece of sterile cotton wool. Put some chlortetracycline eye ointment (3.17) or a drop of silver nitrate (3:1) into them. This will prevent gonococcal conjunctivitis (26.40).

Quickly wipe the blood and the meconium (faeces) from his body.

Give him an injection of vitamin K.

If there are other babies, tie a label round his ankle with his mother's name on it. Then he will not get mixed up with the other babies.

Wrap him in a clean cloth and give him to his mother. If he sleeps by himself, make sure he is warm.

If his mother's membranes (coverings in the uterus)

were torn before birth, harmful organisms may have got to him and his placenta. Organisms make a smell as they grow. So, if there is a bad smell as he is born, give him penicillin and streptomycin (26.24), or ampicillin (3.16).

EXPLANATION. **Teach his mother how to look after him, and especially how to care for his cord (26.34).**

The catheter, forceps, scissors, artery clamps, and tape must be sterile. If they are not sterile, the baby may get an acute septic infection, or tetanus.

We hold a baby below his mother, because this helps to prevent anaemia. Blood goes from his placenta down into him (26–2).

Leave 5 cm of cord below the tie, because part of a baby's gut sometimes goes into his cord. You may harm his gut if you tie his cord too close to his umbilicus. Make two ties to stop bleeding, because one tie might come loose. Even a small bleed is dangerous. The cord gets smaller as it dries, so sterile rubber bands are better than string or tape, but they must be strong and elastic. You can make these bands easily (26–4). Cut a rubber ring from the right size of rubber tube (3 mm bore, 2 mm wall).

26.1

26.3 'He has not started to breathe'—asphyxia

26.3

Asphyxia means not breathing. If a newborn baby does not breathe, resuscitate him quickly (make him breathe). If he does not breathe in 4 minutes, lack of oxygen may harm his brain and cause cerebral palsy (24.15). If you are in a health centre, try to get a high sloping couch or shelf made. Then you can put the baby on it with his head low while you are resuscitating him. If

HOLD HIM LOWER THAN THE UTERUS FOR HALF A MINUTE

BAD

Hold a baby below his mother, not above her, so that the blood can run down his cord into him

26.2

GOOD

Fig. 26–3 Hold him lower than the uterus for half a minute.

255

you are in a home, use any sloping place which you can find. Put him on the bed or a table with some folded cloth under his body.

MOUTH TO MOUTH RESUSCITATION

Clamp and cut his cord quickly. But if necessary his cord can wait.

Bend his head gently back over a rolled up towel. Put your lips over his mouth AND NOSE.

Blow in gently. Blow with small breaths about 40 times a minute. DON'T BLOW FROM YOUR LUNGS. BLOW FROM YOUR CHEEKS ONLY. You need very very little air to blow up the lungs of a small baby. If you blow too hard, you will burst (break) his lungs. His chest should move as you blow, as if he was breathing himself. Most babies start breathing with your first two blows. So, stop after two blows and see if he breathes. He should start breathing, and become more pink. His heart should beat faster.

If he does start breathing, go on blowing. Go on trying to resuscitate him for 15 minutes, or for as long as his heart is beating. If his heart has stopped beating for five minutes, he is dead.

If you have oxygen, give it to him through a thin rubber tube which is put into your own mouth. When he has started breathing, leave him with this tube pushed a short way (1 cm) into his nose.

If he has several of the abnormal signs in Table 26:1, he is sick. Go to Section 26.6. Don't let him get cold!

IF A BABY DOES NOT BREATHE IN FOUR MINUTES HE MAY GET CEREBRAL PALSY

26.4 Examining a newborn baby

The babies of healthy well-nourished mothers weigh about 3·5 kg. The babies of poor mothers usually weigh about 3 kg. These babies may be smaller because their mothers are malnourished or anaemic, or have malaria of the placenta (10.7). The average birth weight of the babies in a community can tell us how healthy and well-nourished its mothers are. The average birth weight is a good index (measure) of the development of that community. If development is good and mothers are healthy, it is about 3·5 kg. If development is poor and mothers are malnourished, it is 3 kg or less.

A newborn baby breathes through his nose. He cannot breathe easily through his mouth until he is about a month old. Normal newborn babies often hiccough and yawn. Sometimes, they sneeze, even if they have not got a cold.

Several signs are normal in a newborn baby, but they may worry his mother. For example, slightly swollen eyelids are normal. A little bright red blood in the sclera of his eyes is also normal.

The part of a baby's head which comes out first during birth is swollen with fluid. This swelling is called **caput**. He may bleed into it, so that it is bruised. If his face comes first, it may be so swollen with caput that he looks deformed. Caput is not serious, and soon goes.

During labour the shape of a baby's head changes so that he can be delivered more easily. We call these changes in shape **moulding**. Moulding makes his fontanelles difficult to feel. It sometimes pushes the edge of one of his skull bones over the others. You can feel this edge as a hard line on his skull. Moulding is not serious, and all these signs go by themselves in a few days.

Sometimes, a baby is born with a round swelling (**cephalhaematoma**) on one side of his head (26–7). Bleeding under the cover of one of his skull bones causes this. A cephalhaematoma has a thickened edge, and feels softer in the middle. It usually grows larger for the first four days after birth, and then slowly goes during several months.

Table 26:1 Signs in a newborn child			
	Normal	**Mildly abnormal**	**Very abnormal (Asphyxia)**
Heart rate	More than 100	50–100	Less than 50, or you cannot feel it or hear it
Breathing	Regular, cries	Slow and irregular	Not breathing
Muscle tone and movement	Moves his arms and legs. His body feels firm	Normal muscle tone, lies with arms and legs bent. He only moves a little when you slap his feet	Hypotonic, lies in any position you put him in. Does not move when you slap his feet
When you suck out his throat with a mucus extractor	He coughs, sneezes, and cries loudly	His face moves	Nothing happens
Colour of face and body	Pink	Blue	Pale and blue
Treatment	*Nil*	*Suction. Slap his feet*	*Suction, mouth-to-mouth resuscitation*

PUTTING A RUBBER BAND ON THE CORD

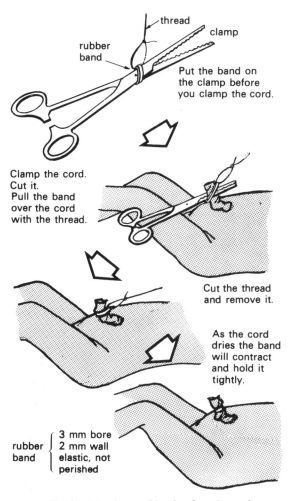

thread

clamp

rubber band

Put the band on the clamp before you clamp the cord.

Clamp the cord.
Cut it.
Pull the band over the cord with the thread.

Cut the thread and remove it.

As the cord dries the band will contract and hold it tightly.

rubber band { 3 mm bore
2 mm wall
elastic, not
perished }

Fig. 26–4 Putting a rubber band on the cord.

CEPHALHAEMATOMA

TREATMENT. **Inject 1 mg of vitamin K into the baby's thigh. A large cephalhaematoma causes an iron-deficiency anaemia (22.4). So give him intramuscular iron (3.33) or 'Children's iron mixture' (3.33) for two months.**

Never try to take the blood out of a cephalhaematoma, because bacteria may get into it and kill him.

EXPLANATION. **Tell his mother that the swelling will go slowly by itself.**

Occasionally, there are mistakes in the way a baby's body is made—**congenital malformations**. This is the time to look for them. He may have abnormal ears, or

MOUTH-TO-MOUTH RESUSCITATION

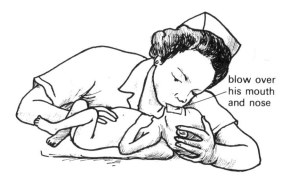

blow over his mouth and nose

Fig. 26–5 Mouth to mouth resuscitation.

extra fingers (26.54), or birth marks (24.46), or perhaps something more serious.

EXAMINING A NEWBORN BABY

Examine him in a good light, with warm washed hands. Take off his blanket, but don't let him get cold.

Rub his cheek. Does he turn towards your finger and try to suck (the rooting reflex)? Take him in your arms and quickly lower him, as if you might drop him. Do both his arms reach out and try to catch something (the Moro reflex)? A normal child more than 24 hours old does both these things. If a baby does not do them, he is sick.

26.4

USING OXYGEN

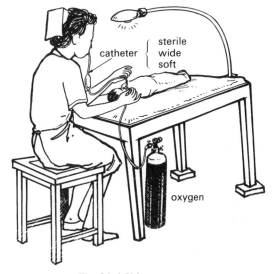

catheter { sterile
wide
soft }

oxygen

Fig. 26–6 Using oxygen.

257

Examine him from head to toe for abnormalities. Look at his head, eyes, ears and mouth. Look for a cleft in his palate (26.51). Look for injuries to his arms and shoulders (26.61). Has he any extra fingers (26.54)? Look at his sex organs and feel for his testes. Look at his back. Abnormalities of the bottom of the spine (spina bifida) are common. Is his anus normal (26.31)? Are his feet normal (26.52)? Can he move his hands and feet?

Weigh him and put him to the breast.

EXPLANATION. Tell his mother what you have found. If he is strong and healthy tell her so. Make anything abnormal as mild as possible, but do not say he is healthy if he is not. If you have found anything serious, try not to tell her until she is well again after her delivery. If she already has several children, talk to her about family planning.

26.5 Bathing and sleeping

You do not need to bath a baby for the first week or more after he is born. Give him his first bath after his cord falls off. Wipe the blood and meconium off him, and cover him with clean cloth. A newborn baby is covered with vernix (grease). Vernix is useful; it helps to protect him from infection. Don't wash it off; it will soon go by itself. Later, his mother can bath him every day. In

CEPHALHAEMATOMA

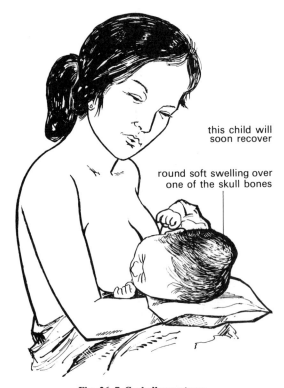

this child will soon recover

round soft swelling over one of the skull bones

Fig. 26–7 Cephalhaematoma.

LET HIM SLEEP ON HIS SIDE

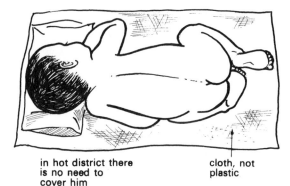

if he sleeps on his side fluid will fall out of his mouth and not go into his lungs

in hot district there is no need to cover him

cloth, not plastic

Fig. 26–8 Let him sleep on his side.

the first few days of life change his nappy often, and clean his buttocks. This is more important than bathing. When his mother baths him, he needs a towel of his own.

Put a newborn baby to sleep on his front or on his side with his knees bent. Like this, he breathes and sleeps easily, and cries less. If he vomits, fluid does not go into his lungs. Put him on a cotton cloth; don't put him on plastic. Let him sleep with his mother.

26.6 The sick newborn baby

Several abnormal signs show that a newborn baby is sick—
— a blue or white body
— not sucking strongly
— vomiting
— fits
— weakness
— muscle tone which is too high (hypertonic), or too low (hypotonic)
— a high sharp cry
— a swollen fontanelle
— fast breathing (more than 60 times a minute)
— grunting
— insuction
— absent Moro or rooting reflexes (26.4), or reflexes which are weaker on one side than the other
— a baby moving his limbs abnormally quickly if you touch him.

A sick baby may have several of these signs. Almost anything that harms a newborn baby can cause them. For example, if his brain was injured during birth, he may have abnormal reflexes, hypotonia, or hypertonia, and a high sharp cry. If he breathed meconium into his lungs, he may have a special kind of pneumonia. This causes grunting and other respiratory signs. If his mother was given drugs during labour, he may be weak and he may not want to suck.

THE SICK NEWBORN BABY

Hold him very carefully. Let him rest as much as possible. Keep him warm (26.25).

Suck out any mucus from his mouth and throat.

Give him 1 mg of vitamin K intramuscularly.

Tube-feed him with expressed breast-milk until he can suck for himself (26.18).

EXPLANATION. **Tell his mother that he is weak and needs extra care for a few days. Let her do as much as possible for him herself.**

FEEDING AND SOME OF ITS DIFFICULTIES

26.7 Breast-feeding

Breast-fed babies are more fortunate than bottle-fed babies. If mothers bottle-feed badly, their babies die from marasmus or diarrhoea (N 8.1). Even if mothers bottle-feed well, their babies are sick more often than breast-fed babies. *Their babies get more diarrhoea and respiratory infections.* So we must make sure that mothers breast-feed. We must not do anything which stops breast-feeding. If your clinic has advertisements for bottle-feeding, take them down. Other people follow what important people do. So try to persuade the wives of important people in your community to breast-feed.

**DON'T ADVERTISE BOTTLE-FEEDING.
BREAST-FEED YOUR OWN CHILDREN**

Let a baby try to suck from the breast as soon as he can. Many babies can suck immediately they are born. Early

THE VICIOUS CIRCLE OF NOT SUCKING AND NO BREAST MILK

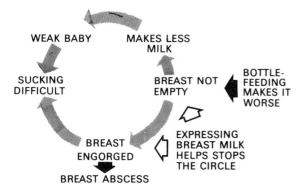

Fig. 26–9 **The vicious circle of not sucking and no breast-milk.**

breast-feeding helps to make more milk come into a mother's breasts. It also helps to prevent sore nipples and breast abscesses. It gives a newborn baby the fluid and energy food which he needs. It helps to make jaundice less. Early breast-feeding also helps a baby to gain weight sooner. The first yellow fluid that comes into the breasts is called **colostrum**. It is good for a baby, and contains antibodies (4.2), which help to prevent infection.

A breast-feeding mother has two people to feed—herself and her baby. So she *must* eat plenty of food. If she does not eat enough food, she will become malnourished. She will not have enough milk to give her baby.

Let a mother keep her baby near her, and feed him when he is hungry. At first, let him suck from each breast for five minutes. He may take only a little milk for the first day or two, but even this is good for him. Don't feed him by the clock, let him feed when he wants to. *Let her take him to bed with her and feed him at night.* Most village mothers know how to breast-feed. We don't need to teach them. If you need to teach a mother, teach her like this.

26.5
26.7

BREAST FEEDING

Only teach this if a mother has difficulty.

Sit her on a low chair with a back to lean against. Let her hold her baby in the way she finds easiest.

Hold him against her breast. When his mouth opens to search for the breast, put the whole nipple *and much of the areola* into his mouth. He cannot suck from the nipple only. He will start sucking when the nipple touches the roof of his mouth.

26.6

**BREAST-FEEDING IS MUCH BETTER
THAN BOTTLE FEEDING**

26.8 Expressing breast-milk

26.8

When breast-feeding is normal, a mother's breasts make as much milk as her baby needs. If he is hungry and empties them, they make more milk. If he does not empty them, they make less milk. If he stops sucking completely, her breasts 'think' that no more milk is wanted, and stop making milk. In this way a strong baby gets exactly as much as he needs. But, if a baby is weak, he cannot suck enough milk, and a vicious circle starts (7.5). His mother's breasts are not emptied, so that they make less milk. Because there is less milk for him he becomes weaker. This makes him go round the circle again.

**IF A BABY SUCKS MORE,
THE BREASTS MAKE MORE MILK**

There is also a second vicious circle. A breast takes several days to stop making milk, or to make less milk. If a baby stops sucking, his mother's breasts may become too full of milk. They become swollen, tender, and painful. They are **engorged**. The nipple of an engorged breast will not go into the child's mouth. He hurts his mother when he tries to suck. So he sucks less milk, and her breasts become more engorged. This is dangerous, because bacteria can easily go into an engorged breast and cause a breast abscess.

A mother can break both these vicious circles by expressing (pressing out) the milk from her breasts. Milk taken from the breasts in this way is called **expressed breast-milk,** or **EBM**. A baby can drink it in any of the ways in Section 26.18. Expressing milk empties breasts, so they go on making milk. Expressing milk also stops breasts becoming engorged. A mother can express her milk with her hands, or with a breast pump. A breast pump is a glass tube with a swelling to catch the milk, and a rubber bulb (ball) to suck it out. Breast pumps are the best way to express milk when a breast is tender, or a nipple is sore. Breast pumps are cheap and easy to use, but mothers must sterilize them each time they use them. Keep some breast pumps to sell or lend to mothers.

EXPRESSING BREAST MILK

Ask the child's mother to wash her hands.

USING HANDS AND A CUP. Find a clean bowl or cup, a table, and a chair.

Show her how to hold up her left breast with her left hand. Show her how to press it with her right hand from the edge towards the nipple. Then show her how to squeeze the part behind her nipple between her thumb and first and second fingers. After she has done this two or three times, milk will start to come out into the bowl. She must do this many times and press on each part of both breasts, especially any hard parts. The breast is made of several segments (parts) like the pieces of an orange. Empty EACH segment. Emptying all the milk from one breast takes about ten minutes.

USING A BREAST PUMP. **Wash and sterilize a cup and a breast pump. Put the open end of the pump over the nipple touching the skin all round. Press the bulb empty, and then let go. The nipple goes into the pump and milk comes out into the swelling on the bottom of the tube. Each time the swelling fills with milk, empty it into the cup.**

Harmful organisms can grow in expressed breast-milk in the same way as in cow's milk. So give the milk with a sterilized cup and spoon, or down a sterilized tube. Breast-milk soon goes sour. So if a mother wants to keep it for a few hours, she must boil it. Tell mothers to express their breast-milk about five times a day.

A FULL BREAST STOPS MAKING ANY MILK

EXPRESSING BREAST MILK

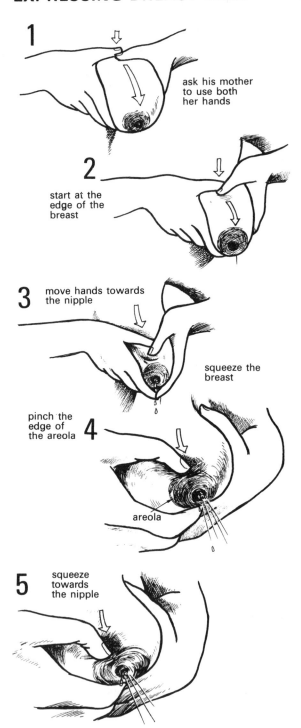

1 ask his mother to use both her hands

2 start at the edge of the breast

3 move hands towards the nipple

squeeze the breast

pinch the edge of the areola

4 areola

5 squeeze towards the nipple

Fig. 26–10 Expressing breast-milk.

A breast pump

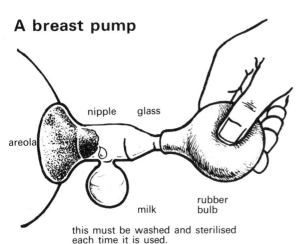

this must be washed and sterilised each time it is used.

Fig. 26–11 Using a breast pump.

SOME BREAST LESIONS

26.9 'My nipples are flat'

Some women have short flat nipples. Flat nipples are common, especially in mothers who are having their first child. Most nipples are **protractile** (you can pull them out). A few nipples are not protractile (you cannot pull them out). A baby can feed from a protractile nipple, but he needs help at first. If a nipple is not protractile, a baby has more difficulty. If he cannot suck enough milk, give his mother a nipple shield for a few days. A nipple shield is a glass tube with a rubber teat on it which fits over a nipple. As a baby sucks, he pulls his mother's nipple into

A FLAT NIPPLE

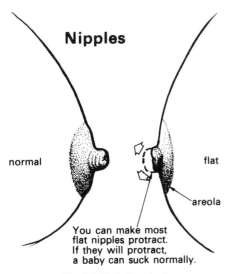

You can make most flat nipples protract. If they will protract, a baby can suck normally.

Fig. 26–12 A flat nipple.

the glass, and milk comes out of her breast. His sucking helps her nipples to become longer. In a few days he can suck from her nipples without a shield. His mother will not have difficulty with her later children.

FLAT NIPPLES

PREVENTION
Examine a mother's breasts when she first comes to the antenatal clinic. If her nipples are flat, examine them to see if they will protract. If they will protract, explain to her that her baby will be able to suck, but he may need help. Teach her to press her nipples and pull them longer between her two thumbs. Look at Figure 26–13. If she does this for five minutes twice a day during her pregnancy, her nipples will grow longer.

PREVENTING FLAT NIPPLES

26.9

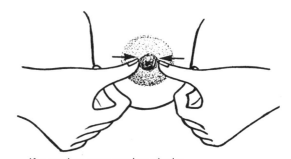

If a mother squeezes her nipples like this several times each day during pregnancy, they will get longer and her baby can suck more easily.

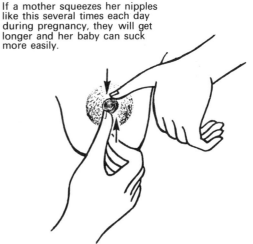

Fig. 26–13 Preventing flat nipples.

TREATMENT
Help the baby to suck. Show his mother how to press her areola together before she puts it into his mouth. If her breast is engorged, express some of the milk. Let him try to suck again when her breast is softer.

261

NIPPLE SHIELDS. If a baby cannot suck from a flat nipple, show his mother how to use a nipple shield (26–15). Make sure the teat has a hole in it. Press the nipple shield close against her breast so that air cannot get past it. Put the teat inside the baby's mouth so it touches his palate. This makes him suck. Tell her to boil her nipple shield each time she uses it. This is easier if she has several nipple shields. Or she can keep them in a bowl of hypochlorite (26.15). This will sterilize them.

Let him try to suck from her breast without a nipple shield sometimes, especially when her breasts are nearly empty. In a week or two he should be able to suck by himself. Her next baby will probably be able to suck without a nipple shield.

Keep some nipple shields to lend to the mothers who need them.

26.10 'My breasts are swollen'—engorged breasts

Sometimes a mother's breasts make more milk than her baby needs. Sometimes he is too weak to suck them empty. If a breast is not emptied normally it becomes painful, and swollen with milk. It is engorged. The skin of an engorged breast is tight. So a baby cannot get enough of the areola into his mouth to suck. Sometimes sucking is very painful for his mother; so she does not want him to try. Prevent and treat engorged breasts. Keep them empty.

USING A NIPPLE SHIELD

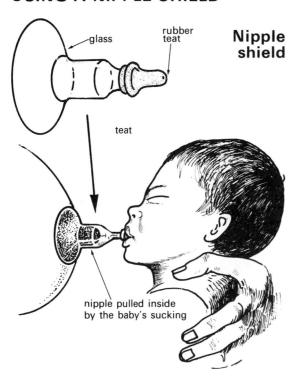

Fig. 26–15 Using a nipple shield.

'My breasts are swollen and I have fever.' Sometimes a mother with engorged breasts has a very short fever for 24 hours. She has no local signs of infection and does not need an antibiotic. Give her paracetamol and observe her carefully. She may have a breast infection later (26.12).

ENGORGED BREASTS
Teach a mother to express (26.8) her milk when her breasts feel painfully full. If there is a tender lump in her breast, show her how to press it carefully until it is soft. If breast-feeding is painful, teach her to use a nipple shield. As soon as her breasts are softer, her baby will be able to suck normally again. If necessary, feed him the expressed breast-milk by one of the ways in Section 26.18.

She only needs an antibiotic if there are signs of infection (26.12).

KEEP BREASTS EMPTY

26.11 'My nipple is sore (or cracked)'

If a baby bites a nipple with his gums it becomes sore. He usually does this because the nipple is not completely inside his mouth. Sore nipples are more common when a mother's nipples are short, or if her breasts are swollen.

SORE NIPPLES
PREVENTION. If a baby cannot suck normally don't let him suck for more than about five or ten minutes without help. Keep a mother's breasts empty—use a nipple shield or a breast pump. One wash with soap is enough each day. Let nipples dry in the air after a feed. Or, put a piece of clean cloth over them under her dress.

TREATMENT. Sucking is usually too painful, but the sore breast must be emptied. Empty it by hand, or with a pump (26.8) or let the baby suck through a nipple shield. Put gentian violet, or chlortetracycline ointment on the sore. Let him suck from the other breast. As soon as her sore nipple has healed, teach her how to put the whole of it inside her baby's mouth when he feeds. Make sure that his gums bite on the areola behind the nipple. Don't let a sore nipple cause her to end breast feeding and start artificial feeding.

EMPTY BREASTS TO PREVENT ABSCESSES

26.12 'My breast is painful and tender, and I have fever'—acute septic infection, breast abscess

Bacteria sometimes go into a mother's breast through a cracked nipple. They cause an acute septic infection. Part of a breast becomes swollen, painful, red and warm. She has fever and tender lymph nodes (acute septic lymphadenitis, 11.3) in her axilla. If you don't treat her an abscess may form.

BREAST INFECTION
Give the mother penicillin (3.15), tetracycline (3.17), or sulphadimidine (3.14). If her abscess becomes fluctuant, it must be cut open (11.5). The cuts must be radial—look at Figure 26–16. If the infection is in more than one segment, more than one incision is needed.

If possible, let her baby go on sucking from the infected breast. Do not let him suck if (1) the nipple is cracked, (2) there is pus coming out of the nipple, or (3) there is an open lesion near the nipple. If there is one of these three things, keep the breast empty, and throw the milk away. Emptying a breast helps it to heal quicker and go on making milk.

26.13 'My baby was born yesterday and my breasts are empty'

Tell this mother not to worry. A mother's breasts make little milk during the first few days after birth. They may not be full of milk for five days. A baby is born with plenty of water in his body; he does not need to drink much during the first few days. He normally loses some weight at this time (26.21). But he must suck so he gets some colostrum, and sucking helps the milk to come into the breasts. *Don't let her start bottle-feeding.* If she bottle-feeds badly he may die from diarrhoea. Also, if he has a bottle he sucks less from her breasts. So her own milk takes longer to come. He may start to like a bottle and he may not want to suck from the breasts.

EMPTY BREASTS
Let him suck from her breasts as often as he wants to. This helps them to make more milk. Try not to give him any extra feeds. If he must have a small extra feed, give it to him once or twice a day, after he has sucked. Give him boiled water or sugar water, or a half strength artificial feed (26.15). Don't give him so much feed that he does not want to suck from his mother.

TRY NOT TO GIVE NEWBORN BABIES EXTRA FEEDS

26.14 'My baby is crying because I have not got enough milk'

The mother of a two- or three-month-old baby sometimes says she has not got enough milk. If this is true, he may have to have animal milk or porridge. Before you start to give animal milk (or porridge before the fourth month), make *sure* there is not enough breast-milk. Try hard to increase it.

If a baby has sucked enough milk, he is quiet for about three hours after a feed. He has a swollen abdomen and after the first week he gains about 25 g a day. If he is getting too little milk, his abdomen is less swollen, and he gains less weight. He wakes early crying with hunger. Crying *immediately* after a feed is not usually a sign that he is hungry. Sometimes, he cries because his stomach is painfully swollen with air which he swallowed during his feed. Crying after a feed does *not* mean that he should start bottle-feeding. Let out the air in his stomach—hold

26.14

26.10
26.13

26.11

ENGORGED SEGMENTS IN THE BREAST

The breast

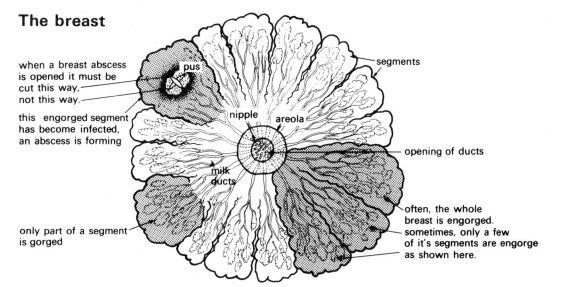

when a breast abscess is opened it must be cut this way, not this way

pus

this engorged segment has become infected, an abscess is forming

nipple

areola

segments

milk ducts

opening of ducts

only part of a segment is gorged

often, the whole breast is engorged. sometimes, only a few of it's segments are engorge as shown here.

26.12

Fig. 26–16 Engorged segments in the breast.

him upright with his abdomen against your shoulder. Hit his back gently. Let him sleep with his face down. This will help him. Swallowed air is a more common problem in bottle-fed babies.

CRYING IMMEDIATELY AFTER A FEED IS *NOT* A SIGN OF HUNGER

NOT ENOUGH MILK

Examine the baby's weight chart. If he is gaining weight (26–19b), he is getting enough milk. So don't tell his mother to start artificial feeding.

If he is not gaining enough weight, he needs more milk, or porridge, or both. Try to increase his mother's milk before you tell her to give him porridge.

Increase the milk. Let him feed more often for a week. He should feed about every two hours. If he sucks more, her breasts may make more milk. His mother should eat and drink and rest more. This is difficult for most mothers. Perhaps another woman, or his grandmother can breast-feed him? Give his mother chlorpromazine (50 mg three times a day for ten days). This often helps to increase her milk. Sometimes a mother can get more milk from her breasts with a breast pump after her baby has sucked.

If his mother has only a little breast-milk, she must continue breast-feeding her child. The little breast-milk she has is good, and she may have more later.

Porridge. If you cannot increase his mother's milk give him porridge. Most babies can eat porridge when they are a month old.

SOME BREAST-MILK IS BETTER THAN NONE

26.15 Artificial feeding.

Artificial feeding means feeding a baby with animal milk (N 8.1). It needs plenty of time, money, water, fuel, and a good kitchen. Most mothers do not have enough of these things, so they *must* breast-feed their children. Even if they have all these things, breast-feeding is better for a baby than bottle-feeding.

Bottle-feeding is dangerous because it may cause—

STARVATION. Babies who do not get enough milk do not grow normally. They often get marasmus (7.9).

INFECTION. Harmful organisms like growing in milk. They grow quickly in warm dirty feeding-bottles. If even a little milk stays in a bottle after a feed, organisms will grow in it. These organisms cause diarrhoea and vomiting. Mothers can clean and sterilize cups and spoons more easily than feeding-bottles. So cup-and-spoon feeding causes diarrhoea less often.

A breast-fed baby can feed whenever he wants to. If he and his mother are healthy, he will not suck too much or too little milk. But an artificially fed baby needs five feeds a day. His feeds must not be too strong or too dilute (weak). His mother must sterilize his cup or his bottle after EVERY feed. A feeding bottle is NOT a plastic breast that a baby can suck whenever he is hungry!

BREAST-FEEDING IS ALWAYS BEST. CUP-AND-SPOON FEEDING IS BETTER THAN BOTTLE-FEEDING

ARTIFICIAL FEEDING

STERILIZING

BOILING. Wash the bottles and teats. Use several bottles and a pan with a lid. Boil the bottles and the teats. Pour out the water and leave the bottles and teats in the pan until you want them.

HYPOCHLORITE. Use any domestic hypochlorite bleach. Put enough water to cover the bottles in a plastic bowl. Add two teaspoonfuls (10 ml) of bleach to each litre of water.

After every feed wash the bottle and teats clean with a brush.

Put the bottles and teats under the hypochlorite solution and empty all the air bubbles from them.

Leave the bottles and teats in the hypochlorite solution for at least one hour, or until the next feed.

At the next feed wash your hands. Pour the solution out of the bottle and make fresh feed. You need not rinse the hypochlorite out of the bottle.

Make new hypochlorite solution every day.

FEEDING

If the baby's mother has any breast-milk, let him suck from her, before he has his artificial feed. Even a little breast-milk is helpful.

Use boiled water and boiled cups, spoons, or bottles. Use fresh boiled cow's milk, or the cheapest full-cream dried milk powder. You can use evaporated milk. Don't use condensed milk, because it contains too much sugar. Don't use skim milk. It contains no fat.

USING ANIMAL MILK. You can make animal milk more like mother's milk like this. Mix three parts (cups etc.) of cow's or goat's milk with one part of boiled water. Mix one part of buffalo milk to one of boiled water. Add one heaped teaspoonful of sugar to each cupful of milk.

USING FULL-CREAM MILK POWDER. Add SEVEN LEVEL teaspoonfuls of milk powder to a cupful of cold boiled water. Mix well with a fork and add ONE HEAPED teaspoonful of sugar to each cupful of milk. Don't make the feeds too strong, because this can make a baby very ill. Don't make them too weak, or he won't grow.

Give him a few teaspoonfuls of fruit juice (vitamin C) every day to prevent him getting scurvy.

SOME IMPORTANT POINTS. **Start porridge at 4 months. Try to stop bottle-feeding and change to a cup and spoon as soon as possible.**

Teach mothers to buy enough milk for the whole month on the day their husbands are paid. A newborn baby needs 2 kg of milk each month. A four-month baby needs 3 kg.

If a mother cannot boil a bottle, ask her to wash it and leave it upside down to drain.

Empty, wash, and sterilize a bottle after EVERY feed.

Glass feeding-bottles are better than plastic ones.

Don't put a baby's medicines in his feeding-bottle.

Don't put milk feeds in a vacuum flask (thermos).

The hole in the teat must be big enough. Hold the bottle upside down. There should be a steady flow of milk.

DON'T MAKE HIS FEEDS TOO STRONG OR TOO WEAK

26.15b 'How much milk does my bottle-fed baby need?'

If a breast-fed baby sucks well, looks well, and sleeps well between feeds, he is getting enough milk. But if a baby is artificially fed, you must know how much milk he should have.

From the age of 7 days, a normal (3 kg) baby needs 150 ml of milk every day (24 hours) for each kilo he weighs. Most cups hold about 200 ml, so 150 ml is about ¾ of a cupful. Older babies need five feeds a day. Small young babies need six, seven, or eight feeds.

Divide the total amount he needs into five (or more) feeds, and give them to him every three or four hours. So a 3 kg baby will need $3 \times 150 = 450$ ml of feed each day. At each feed he needs 450 ml divided by 5 = 90 ml. This is about half a cupful. The exact amount is difficult to measure and is not important. In the first few days a baby cannot drink so much. He may only drink about half this amount. Let him take what he wants.

HOW MUCH MILK?

HOW OFTEN? **Feed him five times a day (small babies 6, 7, or 8 times).**

CUP AND SPOON. **Give a newborn baby half a cupful of milk at each feed. Give a five-month-old baby a cupful at each feed.**

BOTTLE. **Give him 30 ml at each feed for each kilo he weighs. For example, a 7 kg child needs $7 \times 30 = 210$ ml at each feed.**

AN ARTIFICIALLY FED BABY NEEDS 150 ml/kg/DAY

FOUR WAYS OF FEEDING A BABY

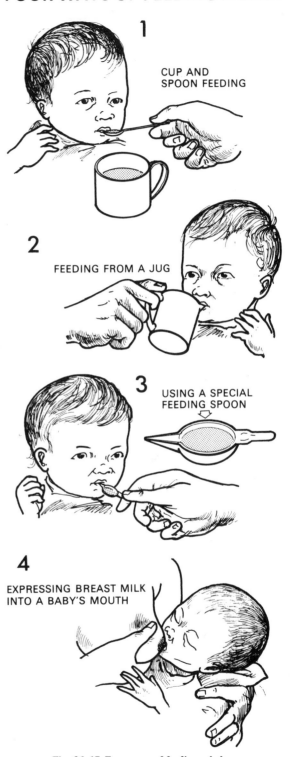

1 CUP AND SPOON FEEDING

2 FEEDING FROM A JUG

3 USING A SPECIAL FEEDING SPOON

4 EXPRESSING BREAST MILK INTO A BABY'S MOUTH

26.15

Fig. 26–17 Four ways of feeding a baby.

265

26.16 'When does a baby need extra water?'

The breast-fed baby. He needs extra water only if the weather is very hot and dry, or he has fever (10.3), vomiting (26.27), diarrhoea (26.32), or jaundice (26.23). If he drinks too much water, he may not want to suck milk. If he needs extra water, give him boiled water after feeding, or when he cries between feeds.

The artificially fed baby. Ordinary full-cream milk powder contains more salts than mother's milk. A baby excretes these in his urine. He needs to pass plenty of urine to excrete these salts, so he must drink enough water. Give him a drink of water *between his feeds.* This is specially important if the weather is very hot or if he has fever, etc. Some special baby milks contain fewer salts, but they are too expensive for most mothers.

He is in special danger if he does not drink enough water, and his feeds are too strong. He is drinking many salts and other substances in his feed. But he is not drinking enough water to excrete the salts. He may get hypernatraemic (too much salt in the blood) dehydration with fits (9.18).

ARTIFICIALLY FED BABIES NEED EXTRA WATER

26.17 'I have not got enough breast-milk, and I don't have enough money to buy milk powder'

What can this mother do? Tell her to let her baby suck all the milk that he can from her breasts. She must feed herself well and drink plenty of fluid, so that she makes more milk. Tell her to give him *soft* porridge once or twice a day. She must give him porridge more often if she has no breast-milk. Make the porridge from fine flour and add some protein food to it, such as sieved beans or egg. If necessary she can make a 'milk' from groundnuts, or coconuts pounded in water.

This is not the best way to feed babies, but it is better than bad bottle-feeding. Children should start eating porridge when they are four months old. But mothers can give porridge earlier if necessary. Good staples (rice, maize, wheat, or Irish potatoes) make better porridge than poor staples (cassava, bananas, sweet potatoes, or sago, N 4.3).

26.18 Eight ways of feeding a baby

Some ways are better for older babies and some ways are better for younger babies. Use the way which works best. Feed a newborn baby a little at a time. If his mother pours too much fluid down him too fast, he will drown.

EIGHT WAYS OF FEEDING A NEWBORN BABY WHO CANNOT SUCK

ONE—WITH A CUP AND TEASPOON. **His mother must sterilize the cup and spoon (N 8.6). If this is difficult, she**

FOUR MORE WAYS OF FEEDING A BABY

5 Feeding with a dropper

6 Feeding with a cotton wick

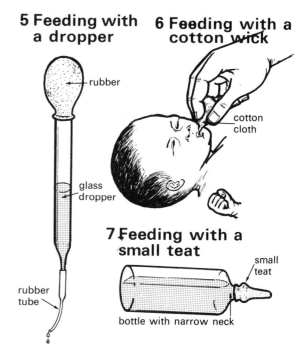

7 Feeding with a small teat

8 Tube feeding

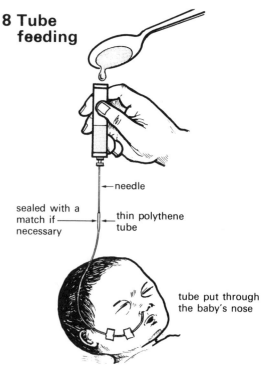

Fig. 26–18 Four more ways of feeding a baby.

must wash them clean, and *DRY* them and leave them in the sun.

TWO—FROM THE POINTED LIP OF A JUG. This is useful for younger babies. A young baby cannot suck milk from the front of his mouth. The pointed lip of a jug puts milk further into his mouth, and lets him drink more easily.

THREE—WITH A SPECIAL BABY'S FEEDING SPOON. This is like a jug, but it is better, because the point is longer.

FOUR—EXPRESSING BREAST-MILK INTO A BABY'S MOUTH. Some mothers express their milk into their baby's mouth. If he is very weak, and might get too much milk, they express it with the nipple pointing upwards.

FIVE—WITH A DROPPER. This is useful for very small babies. Make a dropper with a thin rubber tube from a bicycle valve. Give him the milk, a few drops at a time, under his tongue.

Take the rubber tube and teat from the dropper. Wash and, if possible, boil the tube and the dropper and teat before you use them again.

SIX—USING A COTTON WICK. Roll up a small piece of cotton cloth, put it in the milk, and let the baby suck it. Then wet it with more milk, and let him suck again. If necessary, feed him one drop at a time.

SEVEN—FROM A BOTTLE WITH A SPECIALLY SMALL TEAT. A very small baby, who cannot suck from an ordinary teat, may be able to suck from a smaller teat. You can use the teat from a dropper, like in Picture 5, Figure 26–18, and cut a small hole in it for the milk. A teat like this will not fit onto an ordinary baby's bottle, so use a bottle with a smaller neck. Make sure that his mother washes and boils the bottle and teat after every feed.

EIGHT—TUBE-FEEDING. You can find this in Section 9.24. Get some thin plastic tube, a syringe, and a needle which will fit both the syringe and the tube. Boil the syringe, the needle and the tube.

Cut off a piece of tube which will go from the baby's eyes to the bottom of his chest. Fit the needle into one end of it. If the tube is loose, flame it, soften it, and squeeze it round the needle (9–17). Gently push the other end of the tube through his nose and down into his stomach. Look into his mouth to make sure that the tube is not curled up in his pharynx.

Do the tests in Section 9.24 to make sure that the tube is in his stomach. If, by mistake, you put milk into his trachea, it will probably kill him.

Pour the milk into the barrel of the syringe, and let it go down the tube by itself. Don't push it down with the plunger.

If he possets after feeding (26.27), give him smaller feeds more often.

Some mothers learn to tube-feed their babies (18.16). Has his mother any questions to ask?

DON'T DROWN HIM

26.19 'He will not start to suck'

26.16
26.19

Sometimes, a newborn baby will not start to suck. Some of the reasons for this are in him, and some of the reasons are for his mother.

THE BABY WHO DOES NOT BEGIN TO SUCK

DIAGNOSIS.

In himself. **Very small (26.22)? 'Sick' after a difficult delivery (26.6)? Cleft palate (26.51)?**

In his mother. **Are her breasts engorged (26.10)? Are her nipples flat (26.9)?**

TREATMENT. **Treat any cause you can find. Teach his mother to express her milk. Help her to feed it to him by one of the ways in Section 26.18. Make sure he is warm.**

26.20 'He has stopped sucking'

26.20

Sometimes, a baby who has been sucking normally, stops sucking, or sucks weakly. He can stop sucking for

CUP AND SPOON FEEDING IS BETTER THAN BOTTLE FEEDING

26.17

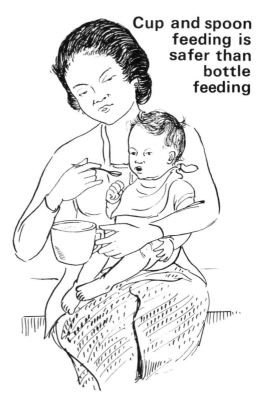

Cup and spoon feeding is safer than bottle feeding

26.18

Fig. 26–19 Cup-and-spoon feeding is better than bottle-feeding.

three reasons: (1) some mild feeding difficulty (the most common reason); (2) some disease of his nose, mouth, or throat; (3) some serious general disease such as tetanus, septicaemia, or pneumonia (the least common reason).

THE BABY WHO HAS STOPPED SUCKING

HISTORY AND EXAMINATION

Mild feeding difficulty. **The baby is 'well'.**
Engorged breasts (26.10)? Milk coming out so fast that the baby chokes? Tell his mother to express some breast-milk before feeding.
The baby will suck from a bottle but not from the breasts? Stop the bottle, and he will soon start sucking from the breast.

Nose and throat. **A cold (8.7)? Thrush (18.5)?**

Serious disease. **Signs of an acute septic infection? Septicaemea (26.24) Pneumonia (26.26)? A swollen fontanelle (meningitis 15.6)? Dehydration (26.32)? Jaundice (26.23)?**
Has tetanus caused spasms in his muscles, so that he cannot open his mouth to suck (26.37)? Tetanus usually begins between the fourth and the fourteenth days of life.
Take his temperature. Fever? Hypothermia (26.25)?

TREATMENT. **Treat any cause you can find. If his nose is blocked, clean it with a cloth, a rubber bulb (3–18), or by sucking it (2–7).**
Feed him, if necessary by tube (26.18). Express his mother's milk.
If there is any serious cause, send him for help.

MANAGEMENT IF DIAGNOSIS IS DIFFICULT. **If he is not well, treat him for septicaemia (26.24).**

NOT SUCKING IS A SERIOUS SIGN. 'IS HE SUCKING NORMALLY?' IS A VERY IMPORTANT QUESTION

26.21 'He is not gaining weight'

Many healthy babies lose weight during the first days of life. They pass urine and stools, and only drink a little milk. A baby may not get back to his birth weight for ten days. If a baby breast-feeds as often as he wants, and as long as he wants, he loses less weight. He is usually back to his birth weight by the seventh day. All this is normal. Only worry if a baby loses more than 10 per cent of his birth weight. 10 per cent of a 3 kg baby is 300 g. After the first ten days, a healthy baby gains about half a kilo (500 g) a month for six months. Baby A in Figure 26–19b did this and went straight up the road to health. Baby B only gained about a quarter of a kilo each month and soon got marasmus. So watch children's weight curves carefully. *Not growing normally is serious in young babies.* When a

HE IS NOT GAINING WEIGHT

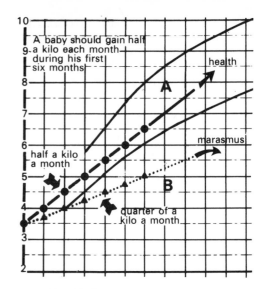

Fig. 26–19b He is not gaining weight.

child is older than nine months, it is less serious. Diagnose failure to gain weight early.

A HEALTHY BABY GAINS HALF A KILO A MONTH DURING HIS FIRST SIX MONTHS

NOT GAINING WEIGHT

If he is not sucking well, go to Section 26.20.
Goes to sleep normally after a feed, but wakes up and cries too soon afterwards? He is probably not getting enough milk, so go to Section 26.14.

DIFFICULTIES WITH ARTIFICIAL FEEDING. **Is he having the right milk in the right amount, in the right way (N 8.1, 26.15, 26.15b)?**

DIFFICULTIES WITH BREAST FEEDING? **Is he fed often enough (at least every 3 or 4 hours), and for long enough (ten minutes each side)?**

BECAUSE OF OTHER FOODS. **Is he eating other foods, such as banana, or other fluids, such as tea, which do not help him grow? They may stop him wanting to suck from the breast.**

ABNORMALITIES? **Examine him carefully (26.4). Cleft palate (26.51)? Birth injury (26.6)?**

MANAGEMENT IF DIAGNOSIS IS DIFFICULT. **Watch his growth curve carefully for a few weeks. Is he gaining half a kilo a month? Sometimes a baby's growth curve is below the lower line, but rises and follows it. He is small but healthy.**
If management is difficult, give him an extra feed of

animal milk or porridge (7.2). Give it *after* he has sucked from the breast.

Has his mother any questions to ask?

26.22 'He is so small.' The low birth weight baby

Babies over 2 kg are usually quite strong. Babies below 2 kg need special care.

A newborn baby can be small for two reasons. He may have been born too early (before 37 weeks)—the **preterm** baby. Or he may have been born at the normal time, but he may have been malnourished in the womb—the **small-for-dates** baby. Some babies are small for both these reasons.

We can usually diagnose if a small baby is preterm or small-for-dates. We look at his heels and feel his breasts and his ears. These two kinds of babies have different problems and need different treatment.

Small-for-dates babies. These babies were malnourished while they were in the womb. A small-for-dates baby may have been malnourished because his placenta was harmed by malaria, or because his mother was malnourished during pregnancy. He may be small-for-dates because he is a twin, because his mother smoked too much, or because pregnancy was complicated (pre-eclampsia, or antepartum haemorrhage). We can give pregnant mothers drugs to prevent malaria. And we can teach them to feed themselves better during pregnancy, especially during the last few months of pregnancy. Preventing small-for-dates babies is important. Soon after birth and later these babies die and become sick more often than normal babies. They also have more infections.

Often, these babies don't start breathing by themselves; they need resuscitation. But, when they have started breathing they breathe normally. They often get hypoglycaemia (too little sugar in the blood), which causes fits. Because they are malnourished they need plenty of milk. They can get this by themselves if they are sucking. But if they are tube-fed we must give them extra milk.

Small-for-dates babies are different from preterm babies. Small-for-dates babies who are full term (39 weeks) have creases (folds) in the skin over their heels. They have breast nodules (lumps) which feel more than 5 mm in diameter. We can easily feel the cartilage (hard substance) in their ears.

PREVENT SMALL-FOR-DATES BABIES

Preterm babies. These babies have no creases on the balls of their heels. Their breast nodules are less than 5 mm, and there is no cartilage in their ears.

Preterm babies have all the problems of a newborn baby, but the problems are much worse. These babies

IF HE IS VERY WEAK, TUBE FEED HIM

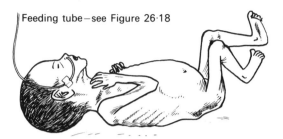

Feeding tube—see Figure 26·18

Fig. 26–20 If he is very weak, tube-feed him.

are too young to live happily outside the uterus. Bacteria which do not harm adults can easily infect them. Their skin is thin and pale and they have no fat under it to keep them warm. They need plenty of food because they are growing fast. But they suck weakly and have small stomachs, so they have difficulty sucking enough. Milk easily flows into their lungs, but they cannot cough it out. They have difficulty breathing. Preterm babies lack iron for making haemoglobin, so they become anaemic (22.1). They have weak blood vessels which bleed easily. They often get jaundice, which is more dangerous in them than in larger babies. Their muscles are hypotonic. They lie with their legs and arms stretched out, instead of bent (flexed) like a normal baby.

Hospital care can help small babies, but even in good hospitals many of them die. In bad hospitals most of them die. We can help mothers to care for small babies at home. A small baby may be safer at home than in a bad hospital. He will probably live if we feed him well, keep him warm, and prevent infection.

THE BABY WHO WEIGHS LESS THAN 2 kg

DELIVERY. **Suck out his mouth very carefully. Give him 1 mg of vitamin K by intramuscular injection.**

Look at his heels. Feel his breasts and his ears.

THE SMALL-FOR-DATES BABY. **He has creases on the balls of his heels. His breasts *feel* more than 5 mm in diameter. You can feel something firm and stiff (cartilage) in the edges of his ears.**

He may need mouth-to-mouth resuscitation. When he has started breathing, he will probably breathe normally.

THE PRETERM BABY. **He has no heel creases, and no ear cartilage. His breasts are less than 5 mm in diameter.**

He will probably start to breathe by himself, but he very easily stops breathing. *Watch him carefully.* If he stops breathing suck him out quickly. This will probably start him breathing again.

BATHING. **Don't bath a small baby. Wipe him clean. Weigh him gently and quickly. Lie him with his head on one side. Move him as little as possible.**

WARMTH. **Keep him warm. See Section 26.25.**

269

PREVENT INFECTION. **Always wash your hands before you touch a small baby, especially if you have just touched another baby.** Don't forget this, even if water is difficult to find. Health workers easily carry harmful organisms from one baby to another.

FEEDING. **Let a small baby feed as soon as he is born. Don't let a preterm baby wait, because he may get hypoglycaemia (26.42). Lift up his head a little for a quarter of an hour after a feed.** Milk will be less likely to flow out of his stomach.

Let a small baby try to suck from the breast. If he cannot suck, feed him in one of the eight ways in Section 26.18. If he is fed at home, a dropper may be useful. If he is very weak, tube-feed him. Try to change the tube after three days. It can stay in for a week.

The preterm baby. **Give him expressed breast-milk every two hours (eight times a day) like this—**

Weight	First day each feed	Increase each feed each day	Maximum each feed at 10 days
less than 1400 g	4 ml	4 ml	40 ml
1400 g to 1800 g	6 ml	6 ml	60 ml
more than 1800 g	8 ml	8 ml	80 ml

Example. On the first day a preterm baby weighing 1600 g needs 6 ml at each of his eight feeds. On the second day he needs 6 + 6 = 12 ml. On the third day he needs 12 + 6 = 18 ml. On the tenth day, he will need 60 ml.

The small-for-dates baby. **He needs more milk to start with. Give him twice as much milk (8, 12, or 16 ml) on the first day. From the second day onwards give him the same increase as above.**

Example. On the first day a 1600 g small-for-dates baby needs 12 ml at each feed. On the second day he needs 12 + 6 = 18 ml. On the tenth day he too will need 60 ml.

If you are feeding a small baby down a tube, measure the milk with a syringe. **If he vomits, give him smaller feeds more often.**

As soon as a small baby is a week old, give him half a mixed vitamin tablet each day.

When he is 2 weeks old, give him one injection of 2 ml of iron dextran, OR ONE drop of iron mixture (3.33) each day. This prevents anaemia. *Give him one more drop each day until* **he is getting five drops twice a day. Go on with this until he is eating mixed food.**

ALWAYS WASH YOUR HANDS BEFORE YOU TOUCH A NEWBORN BABY

26.23 'His skin and eyes are yellow'—Jaundice

Sometimes a baby's liver cannot excrete enough biliru-

THE SMALL-FOR--DATES BABY

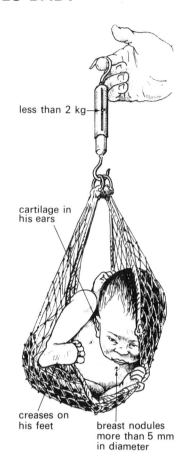

less than 2 kg

cartilage in his ears

creases on his feet

breast nodules more than 5 mm in diameter

bin into his bile (22.10). The bilirubin stays in his blood, and makes him jaundiced (yellow). Severe jaundice harms a baby's brain, so it is serious.

EXAMINATION

Look at the baby's sclera. This is where you see mild jaundice first most easily. When jaundice is worse his skin becomes yellow.

Stretch his skin between two fingers. This presses out the blood so you can see the yellow colour more clearly. **Mild jaundice makes only the skin of his head yellow. As his jaundice gets worse it goes further down his body. So look for it in his forehead, chest, abdomen, knees, and feet. If his knees are yellow his jaundice is serious. Jaundiced feet are even more serious.**

About half of all babies get *mild* jaundice between the second and fifth day of life. This is called **physiological** (normal) **jaundice**, it needs no treatment.

Jaundice is dangerous if it starts too early, if it gets too deep, or if it lasts too long (2 weeks or more). Jaundice is also dangerous if the baby shows other signs, such as sleepiness or not sucking.

Jaundice in the first 24 hours. This is always serious. His red blood cells are being destroyed too quickly, and he will become anaemic. He has haemolytic (red cell destroying) disease of the newborn, and needs hospital treatment quickly.

PREVENT INFECTION BY WASHING YOUR HANDS

Wash your hands

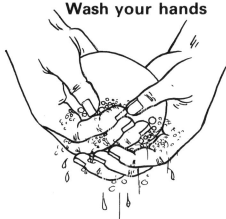

Wash your hands before touching a newborn baby

Fig. 26–21 Prevent infection by washing your hands.

Jaundice between the second and fifth day. This is usually physiological jaundice and is not serious. It may take two weeks to go completely. But it can become serious and harm the brain of a small baby. Prevent it—feed a small baby early with enough breast-milk, if necessary by tube (26.18). If his jaundice becomes severe, send him for help.

Jaundice after the fifth day. Often, physiological jaundice has not completely gone by the fifth day. This is not serious. But if jaundice which started before the fifth day is still getting worse after the seventh day, it is serious. Jaundice which *begins* after the fifth day, and especially after the seventh day, is also serious. Septicaemia may cause it. So look for signs of infection, especially umbilical sepsis.

**IF JAUNDICE STARTS AFTER
THE FIFTH DAY, LOOK FOR SIGNS
OF INFECTION**

JAUNDICE

HOW SERIOUS IS IT? **How old was he when his jaundice began? (It is serious if it started in the first 24 hours. Often you do not see a child in the first 24 hours. So you do not know when it started.)**

Look for jaundice in his forehead, chest, abdomen, knees, and feet. (The lower down his body his jaundice goes, the more severe it is.)

Is his jaundice getting better or worse? (If it is getting better, it is probably not serious.)

Drowsy? Sucking weakly? Abnormally hypotonic or hypertonic? Weak Moro or rooting reflexes (26.4)? Abnormal movements? Pale? (These are all serious signs in a jaundiced baby.)

A JAUNDICED BABY

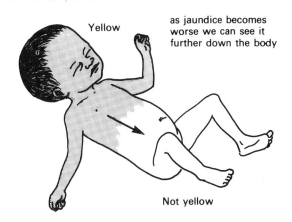

Fig. 26–22 A jaundiced baby.

IS HE INFECTED? **Septic skin lesions? Pus on his umbilicus (26.34)? Other signs of septicaemia such as vomiting, or fits (26.24)?**
Hypothermia (26.25)?

MANAGEMENT. **If he is seriously jaundiced, send him for help.**

TREATMENT. **If he might have septicaemia, treat it (26.24).**

Bilirubin is excreted in the urine, so make sure he has plenty of fluids. If he is drowsy and not sucking, tube-feed him. Give him sugar-water (26.42) from a spoon after he has fed from the breast.

Phenobarbitone 5 mg twice a day may help.

Light helps some kinds of jaundice. If possible let him sleep undressed in a bright place. But he must not become too cold or too hot, and the sun must not burn him.

JAUNDICED BABIES NEED PLENTY OF FLUID

26.23

271

Septicaemia

26.24 A difficult diagnosis

A newborn baby cannot easily fight the harmful bacteria which infect him. In an older child or an adult, bacteria usually stay in a local lesion. In a newborn baby they spread very easily and cause septicaemia. Sometimes, in a newborn baby bacteria cause septicaemia, and don't cause any local lesion first.

Pyogenic bacteria do not get into a baby while he is in the uterus. They don't get in during a normal delivery. Bacteria only get into a baby before birth if the membranes break many hours before birth (26.2). After a baby is born, bacteria need a day or two to grow in him. So septicaemia is most common after the second day, during the first month of life.

THE FIRST MONTH IS THE MOST DANGEROUS TIME FOR SEPTICAEMIA

A health worker carries bacteria on his hands, throat, and nose. These bacteria can cause septicaemia. Instruments and towels also carry bacteria from an infected baby to a healthy baby. This is especially dangerous when there are many babies together. So wash your hands, and dry them on a clean towel, or on a baby's sheet, before you touch him. If you have even a small septic lesion on your skin, you should not care for babies.

The signs of infection in a newborn baby are different from the signs in an older child. A baby may be abnormally **pale**, or **sleepy**. He may **suck badly**, or have **abdominal swelling, diarrhoea, vomiting, jaundice, fits** or **cyanotic** (blue) **attacks**. A new baby cannot easily keep his body at 37°C. He cannot always warm himself to make a fever if he is infected. So temperature is not helpful in diagnosis, because it may be low, or normal, or high.

A birth injury (26.6) can also cause some of these signs, such as sleepiness, not sucking, fits, or cyanosis. So, if a baby has these signs at birth, they are probably caused by a birth injury. But, if he is normal at birth, and they only begin afterwards, they may be caused by septicaemia.

Many healthy babies have at least one of the signs of septicaemia during the first few weeks of life. But if a baby has *several* signs, he probably has septicaemia.

A NEWBORN BABY WITH SEVERAL ABNORMAL SIGNS MAY HAVE SEPTICAEMIA

SEPTICAEMIA

MANAGEMENT
Try to send him for help.

TREATMENT

ANTIMICROBIAL DRUGS. **If you have to treat him yourself, give him ampicillin, or penicillin and streptomycin. You can use a small dose of tetracycline (8 mg/kg, or 6 drops of the mixture every six hours), but it is not a good antibiotic for small babies. Only use benethamine or benzathine penicillin, if you have nothing else. Don't use chloramphenicol until a baby is a month old. If you have to use it, give him ¼ ml (5 drops) of mixture (5 mg) for each kilo he weighs every six hours.**

Babies need small doses, so measure them carefully. Too much penicillin or streptomycin is dangerous. Many injections are not good for small babies. If a baby is less than a month old, give penicillin *twice* a day. Older babies can have penicillin four times a day in the doses in Figure 3–12.

Penicillin. **Give him 30 mg/kg of benzyl penicillin *twice* a day. Don't give more than this. If he is 3 kg, he needs 3 × 30 = 90 mg twice a day. Usually 150 mg are dissolved in 1 ml. ½ ml contains 75 mg, so a little over ½ ml is the right dose.**

OR give him procaine penicillin (150 mg, ½ ml) daily.

AND streptomycin. **Give him 20 m/kg *once* a day. If a child weighs 3 kg, he will need 3 × 20 = 60 mg at each dose. If you only have 1 g ampoules, dissolve one of them in 10 ml of sterile water. This has 100 mg in 1 ml.**

To give	Inject
50 mg	0·5 ml
100 mg	1·0 ml
150 mg	1·5 ml
200 mg	2·0 ml

OR ampicillin alone. **Give 125 mg (half a 250 mg vial) *twice* a day. If he is under two kg, give him half this.**

FEEDING. **If he sucks weakly, feed him by intragastric tube (26.18). Make sure he has enough fluid.**

WARMTH. **Keep him warm.**

WASH YOUR HANDS BEFORE YOU TOUCH A NEWBORN BABY

Hypothermia

26.25 'He is too cold'

A small or sick baby easily becomes cold, so that his temperature falls below 25°C, and he has hypothermia (10.4). He can easily become cold soon after delivery, so wrap him up quickly. A room which feels hot to us feels cold to a baby, so put him in a warm room.

A baby easily becomes cold at night, so let him sleep close to his mother. He also becomes cold if he is wet, so don't bath him too soon. Babies lose much heat through their scalps, so keep their heads warm.

A cold baby is weak, he sucks badly, and he does not gain weight (26.21). His hands and feet swell, they feel cold, and they go blue, but his face and arms may stay pink. If you take his temperature with an ordinary thermometer, the mercury may not go up into the scale. A special low-reading rectal thermometer shows that his temperature is less than 35°C. If a baby becomes very cold, the fat under his skin goes hard (sclerema) and he dies. Sometimes he bleeds into his lungs, so that blood comes out of his mouth.

HYPOTHERMIA

WARMTH. **A baby's mother should hold him close to her. This is the safest way to keep a baby warm. When this is not possible, cover him with a soft cloth and a blanket. Put a bottle of warm water each side of him—but not touching him. *Small babies easily burn,* so cover these bottles with a blanket or a towel. Every three hours, empty *half* the water out of one or other of the bottles, and fill it with boiling water.**

Take his rectal temperature daily (10.1). If it is more than 38°C, or less than 36°C, take his temperature four-hourly. If he is colder than 36°C, give him another bottle and another blanket. If he is hotter than 38°C, take one of the bottles away, or fill it up less often.

FOOD. **If he cannot suck, feed him with expressed breast-milk by tube or dropper (26.18).**

ANTIBIOTICS. **Many babies with hypothermia also have septicaemia, so treat him for it (26.24).**

EVEN IN WARM COUNTRIES BABIES DIE FROM HYPOTHERMIA

Abnormal breathing

26.26 'He is not breathing normally'

Small babies do not show the signs of lower respiratory disease as clearly as older children do. Lower respiratory

Keep babies warm

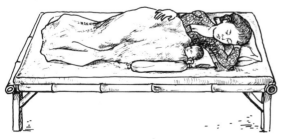

Fig. 26–23 Keep babies warm.

disease is often difficult to diagnose. But any of these signs are abnormal—cyanosis, grunting, breathing more than 50 times a minute, breathing less than 30 times a minute, breathing very irregularly, or stopping breathing for more than half a minute (apnoeic attacks). Abnormal breathing is common after a difficult labour, or a birth injury, or if a baby inhales meconium (26.29), or if he is preterm.

Sometimes a baby breathes easily at birth and his breathing becomes abnormal later. If a child breathed normally at birth but starts to breathe abnormally after the second day, he probably has pneumonia.

DIFFICULT BREATHING

OBSTRUCTED MOUTH OR NOSE. **Is there blood, milk or meconium in his nose or throat? If there is suck it out.**

Is his nose blocked with mucus? Remove it gently with a rubber bulb or small catheter, or ask his mother to suck it out with her mouth. A few drops of sterile saline may help. Put them into his nose to loosen the mucus and then suck them out again.

PNEUMONIA. **This usually starts after the first 24 hours. Give him antibiotics as for septicaemia (26.24). If he is cyanosed give him oxygen (26–6).**

PRETERM BABY. **These babies often have difficulty breathing. Send them for help.**

WORRIED MOTHER. **Babies do not breathe as regularly as older children. A baby may not breathe completely regularly until he is a year old. He may take a few quick breaths and wait a little before breathing again. This is normal. If he is sucking well, and there are no abnormal signs, such as fast breathing, 'grunting', insuction, or cyanosis, he is well. Explain this to his mother.**

Disease of the gut

26.27 'He brings up fluid'—posseting and vomiting

Babies easily bring up milk out of their stomachs. Occasionally this is serious vomiting. Usually it is posseting (regurgitation) which is normal.

Posseting. A baby often brings up some milk when he has a full stomach, or if he has swallowed air with his feed. A young mother may be worried by this, because even a spoonful of milk looks a lot. It is normal. It usually means that he has drunk more milk than he needs. Explain this to her and show her how to help him bring up his air (26.14, 26–24).

Vomiting. When a baby vomits he brings up much more fluid than when he possets. He usually has other signs at the same time.

A gut infection can cause vomiting. This usually

causes diarrhoea also. An infected umbilicus, skin sepsis, septicaemia, or meningitis can also cause vomiting.

Obstruction anywhere in the gut can cause vomiting. If the obstruction is near the baby's anus, he has a swollen abdomen. He only passes a little meconium or none (26.29). If the obstruction is near his mouth, he passes a normal amount of meconium. His abdomen is only mildly swollen. If his oesophagus is obstructed, he immediately vomits everything which he is given by mouth. He becomes cyanosed. Saliva comes out of his mouth, because he cannot swallow it. If the lower end of his stomach (pylorus) is obstructed, he starts vomiting about a month after birth. If his gut is obstructed after his bile duct has joined it, his vomit is green with bile.

VOMITING

Is the baby vomiting, or only posseting?

POSSETING. **There is usually only a little fluid. He is gaining weight and sucking well.**

VOMITING. **There is much fluid. It is serious, if he is—pale, or hypotonic, or losing weight, or dehydrated, or not sucking, or if his vomit is green or yellow, or red with blood, or if**

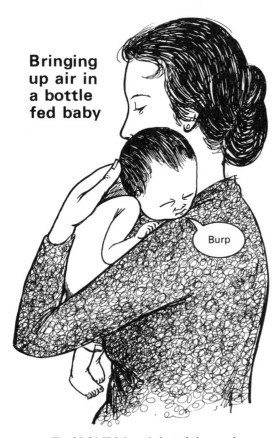

Bringing up air in a bottle fed baby

Burp

Fig. 26–24 Helping a baby to bring up air.

his abdomen is swollen, or if his vomit is thrown a long way out of his mouth, or if he has not passed meconium.

WHAT IS CAUSING HIS VOMITING?

Swallowed meconium. **This happens during the first two days only. His vomiting is mild and there are no serious signs. Give him some sugar and water to drink.**

Birth injury or prematurity. **Does he have fits, or a swollen fontanelle (15–9)? Small babies vomit easily (26.22).**

Infection. **Diarrhoea (26.32)? Thrush (26.55)? Skin sepsis (26.47)? A septic umbilicus (26.36)? Other signs of septicaemia (26.24)? Meningitis?**

Gut obstruction. **Green vomit (lower gut obstruction)? Swollen abdomen? Vomit thrown a long way out of his mouth (most kinds of gut obstruction)? Passing meconium (upper gut obstruction)? Not passing meconium (lower gut obstruction)?**

Put ointment on your little finger and put it into his anus. His anus may be blocked by meconium.

Pyloric stenosis. **If he starts vomiting when he is 3–5 weeks old, he may have pyloric stenosis (obstruction to the lower end of his stomach). These babies are hungry and active until they become dehydrated. They vomit with great force. A baby's pylorus swells. You can feel it as a swelling about the size of your little finger in the place shown in Figure 26–36. Pyloric stenosis is serious, but it can be treated by an easy surgical operation. Try to send the baby to hospital. His stomach becomes swollen with fluid. So put a tube into his stomach (9.24) and suck it empty before you send him. If he is severely dehydrated, give him intravenous fluid (9.27).**

26.28 'He has vomited blood'

Find out how much blood he vomited, and when he vomited it. This will tell you how serious his vomiting is. A baby sometimes swallows his mother's blood during birth. If he vomits blood during the first 24 hours after birth, it is probably her blood. If he vomits a little blood later on, the blood may have come from a crack in her nipple. But if he vomits much blood between the second and fifth days after birth, the blood is probably his own. He probably has haemorrhagic disease of the newborn, so go to Section 26.33.

ALL BABIES WHO VOMIT BLOOD NEED VITAMIN K

26.29 Normal faeces

A baby's first faeces are green–black. They are called meconium. During the next few days they become soft, yellow, and sour smelling. The faeces of a healthy breast-fed baby are sometimes watery. The faeces of a bottle-fed baby are usually harder. Some healthy babies pass faeces after every feed, and others only once in four days. Sometimes a healthy baby passes faeces four times on one day and then none for a few days. Bottle-fed babies, and babies on mixed food pass more faeces. Many babies cry and move about while they are passing faeces, as if they had pain. *All this is normal,* so mothers should not worry about any of these things.

26.30 'My baby's faeces are hard'

Constipation, like diarrhoea, is more common in bottle-fed babies than in breast-fed babies. A bottle-fed baby may pass such hard faeces that they scratch his rectum and make it bleed a little (25.6). Tell his mother to make his faeces softer—she can give him fruit juice or soft fruit.

If a mother has not got enough milk, her baby's faeces may become hard. He may also not gain weight. So watch his growth curve. Don't give him purgatives (bowel-opening medicines). If his mother wants treatment for him, tell her to give him boiled water with a spoonful of sugar once a day.

26.31 'He has not passed any faeces'

If a baby passes meconium during birth, he may not pass any more for two or three days. He should pass meconium during birth, or during the first 24 hours. If he has not passed meconium he may have a congenital obstruction of his gut (26.27). This will soon make his abdomen swell and make him vomit bile. His gut may be obstructed anywhere, but the anus is the most common place. Try to put a rectal thermometer (or your little finger covered with ointment) into his rectum. If you can do this, there must be a hole through his anus, and it is not obstructed. If a baby has signs of obstruction, send him for help.

NEVER GIVE A NEWBORN CHILD MEDICINE TO MAKE HIM PASS FAECES

26.32 'My baby has diarrhoea'

Gut infections are the most common cause of diarrhoea, especially if a baby is bottle-fed, or given dirty food. Infections in some other part of his body can also cause diarrhoea (9.10).

DIARRHOEA

PREVENTION. **Breast-feeding prevents diarrhoea. Make sure that everything that goes into a baby's mouth is clean. Give him clean food and boiled water.**

HISTORY. **Has he been given porridge or other foods when he is too young (less than four months old)? (This often causes diarrhoea, especially if the foods are infected.)**

EXAMINATION. **What other signs has he? Thrush (18.5)? Signs of a septic infection, such as an infected umbilicus, or skin sepsis?**

Signs of septicaemia (26.24)? Is he dehydrated?

TREATMENT. **Try to make his mother go on breast-feeding. Give him glucose–salt solution, or salt and sugar water between feeds. If he will not suck from the breast, he can stop having milk for one day. Don't stop breast-feeding for longer than one day. Give him glucose–salt solution, and express his mother's milk. Give him glucose–salt solution in any of the ways in Section 26.18.**

After 24 hours, try to give him breast-milk again. If this makes his diarrhoea worse again, he may have to stop breast-feeding and have glucose–salt solution for another day. Try to make him take breast-milk as soon as possible.

If he has signs of septicaemia, treat it (26.24). If he becomes severely dehydrated, he needs a scalp vein drip, especially if he is vomiting.

26.33 'There is blood in his faeces'

Sometimes, there is blood with a baby's meconium. On the first day after birth this is probably blood which he swallowed during birth. It is not serious. From the second to the fifth day after birth, bleeding may be caused by **haemorrhagic disease of the newborn**.

A baby with haemorrhagic disease cannot stop bleeding, because he lacks vitamin K. He may bleed from his umbilicus (26.38), or into his stomach and vomit blood (26.28). Or he may bleed into his gut and pass blood in his faeces. The blood may be bright red, or it may be partly digested and black. A baby only has one-and-a-half cupfuls of blood in his body, so bleeding more than a few drops of blood is serious.

BLOOD IN VOMIT OR FAECES

PREVENTION. **Give all babies an injection of vitamin K at birth. If you cannot give it to all babies, give it to the very small babies, and to babies who have had a difficult birth.**

Haemorhagic disease

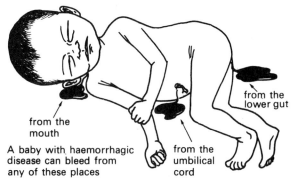

from the mouth

from the lower gut

from the umbilical cord

A baby with haemorrhagic disease can bleed from any of these places

Fig. 26–25 Haemorrhagic disease.

26.30

26.33

26.31

26.28

26.32

26.29

TREATMENT. **How old is the baby?**

One day old. **The blood probably came from his mother. Give him vitamin K and observe him.**

Two to five days old. **Probably haemorrhagic disease, so give vitamin K. Don't give more than 1 mg. It does not help and may cause jaundice.**

**BABIES WHO BLEED BETWEEN
THE SECOND AND THE FIFTH DAY
NEED VITAMIN K**

Diseases of the cord and umbilicus

26.34 'His cord is sticky and smells'

A baby's cord and umbilicus are easily infected. He is in danger of infection until his cord has dropped off and his umbilicus has healed. It usually heals in about a week. Organisms like growing in a wet cord. A dry cord is less easily infected.

UMBILICAL CORD

PREVENTING INFECTION. **Cut a baby's cord with sterile scissors. If a mother is going to deliver her baby at home, give her an envelope for his cord. Put into the envelope a new razor blade to cut the cord, sterile gauze, and some sterile tape or string.**

TREATMENT.

Normal cord. **Keep it dry. Use no dressing so that it can dry in the air. Or use a sterile dry dressing. Never use ointments.**

Infected, 'sticky' cord. **Teach his mother to clean it with spirit. Cover it with a dry dressing.**

EXPLANATION. **Tell his mother not to wet his cord when she washes him. Keep his nappy below the cord. Teach people who deliver babies how to care for cords. DON'T put local medicines, or animal faeces on cords.**

A DRY CORD IS LESS EASILY INFECTED

26.35 'His umbilicus is not healing'

When a baby's cord drops off, it sometimes leaves a red spot which takes several weeks to heal. If you keep the red spot dry, a crust will cover it until it is healed. When it is slow to heal, a red lump may form, but this is not serious. This always goes, but it may last for some months. Gently rub the lump with a crystal of copper sulphate. It will heal faster.

Umbilical sepsis

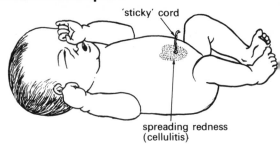

Fig. 26–26 **Red skin round the umbilicus is a danger sign.**

26.36 'The skin round his umbilicus is red'—cellulitis

This is a dangerous sign, because it shows that infection is spreading and causing cellulitis. The baby may get septicaemia and die, so give him penicillin and streptomycin (26.24). Try to send him for help. Sepsis of the umbilicus is infectious, so keep him away from other babies.

**RED SKIN ROUND THE UMBILICUS IS A
DANGEROUS SIGN**

26.37 Tetanus infection of the umbilical cord

A baby's umbilical cord can become infected with tetanus bacteria. They cause tetanus of the newborn (26.42, 18.16). This dangerous disease kills many babies. Tetanus bacteria come from animal faeces and live in the soil and dust. They can grow on a baby's cord and make a toxin (4.2). This toxin goes into his body and makes his muscles contract too strongly. Tetanus usually presents as 'not sucking' (26.20). For prevention and treatment, go to Sections 18.16 and 26.34.

**PREVENT TETANUS—KEEP A CHILD'S CORD
CLEAN**

26.38 'He is bleeding from his umbilicus'

Sometimes, a few drops of blood come from a baby's umbilicus when the crust on it falls off. This is seldom important, but it is sometimes the first sign of haemorrhagic disease of the newborn (26.33). Give him vitamin K (3.38).

Eye disease

26.39 'His eyes are sticky'—conjunctivitis

Examine a newborn baby's eyes while he is feeding at the breast. He will usually open his eyes while he is feeding.

Many babies have a *mild* conjunctivitis which starts after the third day. Sometimes infection causes this. Often there are other causes. There is only a little discharge, and the conjunctiva is not red, or only mildly red. The disease is sometimes called a 'sticky eye'.

MILD CONJUNCTIVITIS

Clean his eyes with wet cotton wool. Pull down his upper eyelids and put some chlortetracycline eye ointment (3.17) onto them.

26.40 'His eyes are red and his eyelids are swollen'—gonococcal conjunctivitis

Gonorrhoea is a venereal (sex) disease of adults. Bacteria called gonococci cause it. These come from a mother's vagina and infect her baby's eyes during birth. She may not know that she is infected. Gonococci cause *severe* purulent inflammation of his conjunctiva with gross swelling of his eyelids *during the first two days of life*. Conjunctivitis which comes later is probably caused by some other organism, especially if it is mild.

Treat gonococcal conjunctivitis quickly, or the baby will become blind. It is a very infectious disease, so don't touch your own eyes with your infected fingers. If the gonococci in your district are resistant to penicillin, use chlortetracycline eye ointment instead of penicillin solution.

GONOCOCCAL CONJUNCTIVITIS

PREVENTION. **Put chlortetracycline eye ointment (or two drops of 1 per cent silver nitrate, or 1 per cent silver proteinate) into the eyes of** *all newborn children*. **Silver nitrate sometimes makes children's eyes mildly red, but they soon recover.**

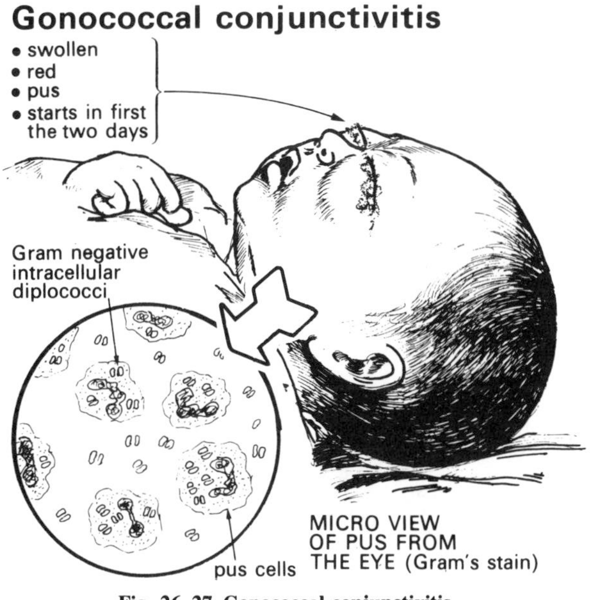

SPECIAL TEST. **Ask the laboratory to look for gonococci (gram negative intracellular diplococci) in a swab of pus from the child's eyes (L 11.5).**

MAKING PENICILLIN SOLUTION 10 000 units/ml.
EITHER (A) Take a clean cup, boil it and let it cool. Fill it half full of sterile saline (or Darrow's solution). If you have not got either of these solutions fill it with cold boiled water and add *half* **a level teaspoonful of salt. You will now have 100 ml of sterile saline.**

Take a sterile syringe and a vial containing 600 mg of *benzyl* **penicillin (3.15). Dissolve the penicillin in the saline, and put it into the cup. You will now have a solution with about 10 000 units of penicillin in each ml.**

OR (B) Dissolve an ampoule of 600 mg of *benzyl* **penicillin in an ampoule of 10 ml of water for injection. Then mix 1 ml of this solution with another 10 ml of water for injection.**

TREATMENT
Give the baby intramuscular penicillin (26.24) for three days.
AND—
(1) Make penicillin solution by method A or B above. Wipe the pus out of the baby's eyes with cotton wool. Use an eye dropper to put a few drops of penicillin solution into each eye every ten minutes for an hour. Then put drops in every hour for the next six hours, and then every three hours for three days. Throw away any penicillin solution you have not used. Wash your hands.

OR (2) Dissolve 600 mg of *benzyl* **penicillin in a quarter of a bottle of sterile saline or Darrow's solution (about 100 ml). Drop the solution into the baby's eyes from a drip set (9–16), as in method (1) above.**

OR (3) Put chlortetracycline eye ointment into the child's eyes every three hours.

EXPLANATION. **Show the baby's mother how to use the penicillin solution. Find a place where other people cannot hear what you say. Explain kindly that her baby has caught this disease from her. Treat her and her husband. Give them each 5 g of procaine penicillin. This is 8 ml into each buttock (16 ml in all). Treat them both on the same day. If you do not treat them at the same time, they may infect one another again. After treatment, examine them both for gonococci (L 11.5) to make sure they are cured.**

SEVERE PURULENT CONJUNCTIVITIS IN THE FIRST TWO DAYS OF LIFE IS USUALLY GONOCOCCAL

26.41 'My baby has a swelling beside his eye'—swollen tear duct

Tears go through ducts (tubes) from each eye to the nose (16–1). You can see the openings (holes) of these ducts

26.40
26.36
26.34
26.37
26.38
26.35
26.41
26.39

Gonococcal conjunctivitis

- swollen
- red
- pus
- starts in first the two days

Gram negative intracellular diplococci

pus cells

MICRO VIEW OF PUS FROM THE EYE (Gram's stain)

Fig. 26–27 Gonococcal conjunctivitis.

at the nose end of the eyelids. Sometimes one of the ducts becomes obstructed. This causes a swelling on the side of the nose near the eye (26–36). Press the swelling gently. You may see a white substance coming out of the duct openings.

SWOLLEN TEAR DUCT

Gently wash out his eye with saline, and put tetracycline eye ointment into it. Tears may come from his eye for several weeks, because the duct is still blocked. But it will open by itself later. Massage (gentle pressing) cures the swelling quicker. Don't put anything into the duct.

Abnormal movements

26.42 Tetanus and fits

Watch normal babies carefully. Learn how they move. Then you will be able to diagnose abnormal movements more easily. A baby's movements are abnormal if he moves too much, too strongly, or too quickly. The spasms of tetanus, or fits can cause abnormal movements.

   Tetanus. The spasms of tetanus (18.16, 26.37) usually start between 4 and 14 days after birth. If spasms start earlier they are more serious. A baby stops sucking (26.20) and crying. He cannot open his mouth, and he passes few stools. His muscles contract strongly and become hypertonic (1.10). Muscle contractions close his jaw, and pull the ends of his lips backwards and upwards. His neck and back bend backwards. His arms and legs become stiff. Sometimes, he has sudden spasms when his muscles contract more strongly. Noise, or moving or touching him, easily starts these spasms.

   Fits. Fits cause short sudden movements. The baby stops breathing for a minute or two, he goes blue, and his eyes look up to the top of his head. Fits are different from the spasms of tetanus. A baby's muscles are normal between fits. If you make a noise or move him, he does not have a fit.

   Birth injuries (26.6) and meningitis (15.6) cause fits. Hypoglycaemia (not enough sugar in the blood) can also cause fits. This is common in small-for-dates babies (26.22). Hypoglycaemia is important, because it can harm a child's brain. You can easily treat it, and prevent it causing harm.

ABNORMAL MOVEMENTS—fits or tetanus?

How old is he? (The fits of brain injury usually start at birth. Hypoglycaemia causes fits in the first three days. Tetanus causes spasms between the 4th and the 14th day. Meningitis causes fits any time after the first two days.)
   Is his body stiff or bent backward between spasms? Does he have a spasm when you touch him or move him?

Are the muscles of his lower jaw stiff, so that he cannot open his mouth to suck? Is his umbilicus 'dirty'? (All these are signs of tetanus.)
   Does he have any upward movement of his eyes (fits)?

TETANUS. **Go to Section 18.16**

FITS. **Try to diagnose which of these four things he has—**

(1) BRAIN INJURY. **Did he have abnormal signs at birth—See Table 26:1. If he did, go to Section 26.6.**

(2) HYPOGLYCAEMIA. **If he is small (less than 2000 g) his body may lack sugar. Mix four heaped teaspoons of glucose, or sugar, in a cupful of water so as to make a 5–10 per cent solution. Give him 25 ml/kg of this by nasogastric drip. If hypoglycaemia is the cause of his fits, glucose will stop them in 15 minutes. If he has hypoglycaemia, he needs energy food often. So feed him every two hours for the next three days. Give him either breast-milk or sugar solution.**

(3) SEPTICAEMIA. **Has he got any of the other signs of septicaemia (26.24)? If he has, treat him for it.**

(4) MENINGITIS. **Has he got a swollen fontanelle (15–9)? If he might have meningitis, he needs a lumbar puncture (15.3).**

MANAGEMENT IF DIAGNOSIS IS DIFFICULT. **Give him sugar and see if his fits stop. If they do not stop, give him paraldehyde or phenobarbitone (3.43), and send him for help. If you cannot send him for help, treat him for septicaemia.**

Skin disease

26.43 Nappy rash

If a baby does not wear nappies, he does not get a nappy rash. But if a baby does wear nappies, he sometimes gets a red rash between his buttocks, and around his genital

Nappy rash

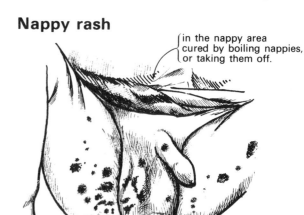

in the nappy area cured by boiling nappies, or taking them off.

Fig. 26–28 A nappy rash.

organs. A baby gets a nappy rash if his mother does not change his nappies often enough. Plastic pants make the rash worse. Organisms live in wet nappies and make a substance (ammonia) which harms a baby's skin. Diarrhoea can also make a baby's buttocks sore.

NAPPY RASH

EXPLANATION. **Tell the baby's mother to wash his nappies and boil them, so that the organisms on his nappies are killed. Wash all the detergent out of them. Leave him with his nappy off, and his buttocks open to the air as much as possible. Put zinc and castor oil ointment, vaseline, or plain ointment onto the rash (3.48).**

26.44 'His skin is peeling.'

A child's skin often peels (comes off in pieces) two or three days after birth. This may happen because he was malnourished in the uterus, or because he was born late. It soon stops.

If a baby possets (regurgitates, 26.27), the acid in his stomach makes the skin on the sides of his face peel. This again is not serious. Tell his mother to clean him as soon as he possets, so he does not lie in the fluid.

26.45 'He has a lot of little red lesions'—erythema neonatorum

Many small red macules (11–3) sometimes come on a baby's skin on the second to the fourth day after birth. In the middle of the macules are small white lesions. These lesions look like pustules, but they are not pustules because they are not infected. This is erythema neonatorum. The rash goes in a week or two and needs no treatment. Although people sometimes call it a 'milk rash', milk does not cause it. So don't stop breast-feeding.

26.46 'There are red–blue marks on his skin'—congenital skin lesions

Many babies have a red–blue lesion at the bottom of their necks, above their noses, or on their upper lips. Enlarged blood vessels cause these lesions, and usually go during the first year of life.

In some districts many children are born with a grey lesion at the bottom of thier backs. This lesion looks like a bruise. These lesions are not serious and go within two years.

26.47 'There are vesicles (or pustules) on his skin'—impetigo of the newborn

Impetigo of the newborn is the most common cause of vesicles. The lesions start as vesicles, and then become pustules and crusts (11–3). If you do not treat the baby quickly, bacteria spread to his blood and cause septicaemia. If a newborn baby has vesicles or any other septic skin lesion, treat him carefully. Put genetian violet

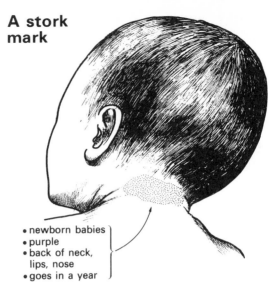

A stork mark

- newborn babies
- purple
- back of neck, lips, nose
- goes in a year

26.44
26.42

Fig. 26–29 A congenital skin lesion.

on the lesions and give him penicillin (26.24). Impetigo is very infectious, so keep him away from other babies.

26.45

VESICLES ON THE SKIN ARE A DANGER SIGN TO BABIES

26.48 'There are sores beside his finger nails'—paronychia

A baby sometimes gets an acute septic infection at the side of his finger nail (paronychia). The skin round his finger nail becomes red, swollen, and tender. There may be pus. Paronychia can cause septicaemia, so give him penicillin (26.24).

26.48
26.43
26.46

Disease of the head

26.49 'His head is the wrong shape'

Sometimes, a baby's skull is a different shape on each side—it is asymmetrical. The kind of asymmetry shown in Figure 26–30 is not serious. It is caused if a baby sleeps more often on one side than the other side. His head will become normal when he starts sitting up.

26.49

26.50 'He has not got a fontanelle'

Mothers often worry about their baby's fontanelles (15–9). In some babies the large fontanelle at the top of the skull is 5 cm across. But sometimes, the fontanelle is so small that you cannot easily feel it. The size of the fontanelle is rarely important. Big ones and small ones both close as a baby grows.

26.47
26.50

A CHILD WITH AN ASYMMETRICAL HEAD

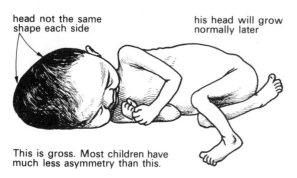

head not the same shape each side

his head will grow normally later

This is gross. Most children have much less asymmetry than this.

Fig. 26–30 A child with an asymmetrical head.

Congenital malformations

26.51 Cleft lip or palate

Malformed means badly made. There are many kinds of congenital malformation, such as skin lesions (26.46), club foot, and the congenital kind of intestinal obstruction. One of the commonest congenital abnormalities is a cleft (cut) in the lip or palate.

Two sides of the face and mouth join together to make the upper lip and palate. If they do not join normally, a baby has a cleft in his lip, or palate, or both. Sometimes, the cleft is mild and is only on one side, or only at the back of the palate. Sometimes there is almost no palate or upper lip. You can easily see a cleft lip. But you cannot see a cleft palate until you look inside a baby's mouth. A surgeon can repair a cleft palate, so send the baby to hospital. Repair a cleft lip at three months, when a baby weighs about $4\frac{1}{2}$kg. Repair a cleft palate at 15 months.

A baby with even a small cleft in his palate has difficulty sucking. Milk comes down his nose. He easily becomes malnourished. We must feed him carefully, so that he is well nourished and strong enough for his operations. Bacteria from his pharynx easily infect his ears, so watch for ear infections (17.9).

FEEDING A BABY WITH A CLEFT PALATE

See if he will suck from the breast. If he will not suck, feed him by cup and spoon.

Observe his weight chart carefully. If necessary, give him expressed breast-milk (26.8) down a tube (26.18). Most of these babies learn to suck better when they grow older.

26.52 'His foot is the wrong shape'—talipes

If there is not enough fluid in the uterus a baby cannot move and kick normally. One or both of his feet may bend into an abnormal shape—talipes (26–33). At birth you can usually bend his feet back into a normal shape very easily. When he is a week old, you will not be able to bend his feet into the right shape so easily. Strap his feet into the right shape *during the first two days of life*. If you strap them later, you may be too late to cure his talipes.

TALIPES

Can you bend his ankle so that the outer side of his foot touches the outer side of his leg? If you *can* he has *not* got true talipes. His feet will grow normally and he needs no treatment.

If you *cannot* bend his ankle so that the outer side of his foot touches his leg, he *has* true talipes. So strap his foot with adhesive strapping (zinc oxide plaster). Each time he kicks the strapping will pull his foot straight. Put benzoin tincture on his leg before you put on the strapping. This will stick the strapping to his leg.

Put pieces of cotton wool over his knee, behind his toes, and on his outer ankle bone (malleolus). The benzoin tincture will stick them to his skin. Put the first long piece of strapping (1) from under his heel up over the cotton wool outside his ankle. Bring it up outside his leg and over the cotton wool on the top of his knee. Bend his ankle straight as you put on this strapping. When the strapping is on, his foot must be in its normal shape.

A CLEFT LIP

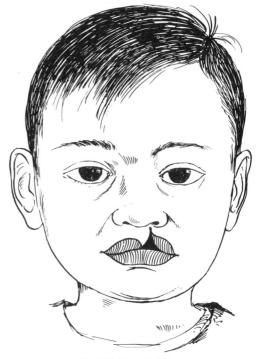

Fig. 26–31 A cleft lip.

280

TREATING TALIPES

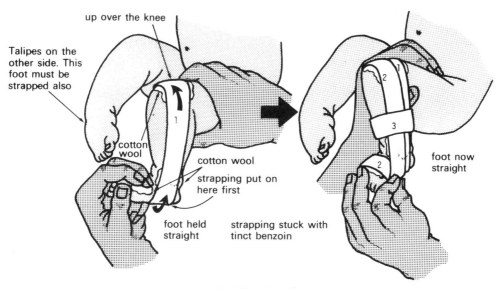

up over the knee

Talipes on the other side. This foot must be strapped also

cotton wool

cotton wool

strapping put on here first

foot held straight

strapping stuck with tinct benzoin

foot now straight

Fig. 26–33 Treating talipes.

26.51

Put on a second piece of strapping (2) round his foot near his toes, up the outside of his leg and his knee.

Put a third piece (3) round his leg. This will keep the two long pieces in place.

Count all his toes and make sure they are pink and warm. If they are blue and cold you have stopped the blood flowing. This is dangerous and his foot might die. Take the strapping off, and put it on looser.

Change the strapping twice a week for a month, then once a week until he is four months old.

We can cure half the children with talipes like this. If the tendon at the back of a child's leg (Achilles tendon) is still too short at four months, he needs an operation.

UNTREATED TALIPES

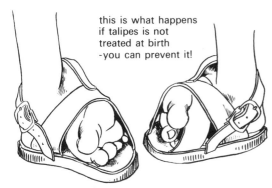

this is what happens if talipes is not treated at birth -you can prevent it!

Fig. 26–34 Untreated talipes.

If you cannot strap his leg or get help, his mother must bend his ankles straight herself. Tell her to bend the outer side of his foot up to touch the outer side of his leg several times a day. This may cure him.

TREAT TALIPES DURING THE FIRST TWO DAYS OF LIFE

26.53 'His tongue is tied'

26.53

A fold of mucosa joins the underneath of the middle of the tongue to the bottom of the mouth. Sometimes, this is very short and a baby's tongue seems to be tied to the bottom of his mouth—'tongue tie'. An operation can be done, but it is rarely needed. Tell his mother that his tongue will grow normally as he grows older. He will be able to speak as well as any other child.

26.54 'He has got an extra finger (or toe)'

26.54

Babies sometimes have an extra finger or toe. Usually, the extra finger or toe is much smaller than the others and has no bone it it. Rarely, it is like a normal finger and contains bone. If you cannot feel any bone in the extra finger, tie a piece of thread soaked in iodine tightly round it. Do this as close to the hand or foot as possible. The extra finger or toe will soon become dry and fall off. But if there is bone in it, the baby needs an operation.

26.52

REMOVING AN EXTRA FINGER

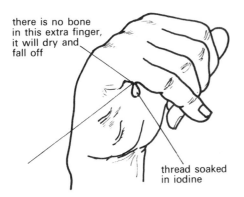

there is no bone in this extra finger, it will dry and fall off

thread soaked in iodine

Fig. 26–35 Removing an extra finger.

Some other problems

26.55 'There are white lesions in his mouth'— thrush

Newborn babies often get a fungus infection of their mouths. We call this thrush (18.5). Their mouths are sore, so they do not want to suck. Thrush sometimes causes mild diarrhoea. Treat thrush with gentian violet (3.48).

26.56 'His breasts are large'

A mother's breasts grow large towards the end of pregnancy and start to make milk. Her baby's breasts may also grow, and both boy and girl babies are sometimes born with large breasts. Occasionally the babies' breasts make milk. This is not serious and large breasts become normal after a few weeks. Tell mothers *not* to squeeze them, because this may cause infection (26.12). If a baby's breast becomes red, swollen, and tender, he has an acute septic infection. Give him penicillin (26.24).

Sometimes a baby girl bleeds from her vagina. This is usually normal and soon stops.

26.57 'He has not passed urine'

A baby often passes urine during birth. If he does this, he may not pass any more urine for the next 48 hours. If he has not passed urine after 48 hours, send him to hospital quickly.

26.58 'His urine is red'

During the first week of a baby's life brown urine is normal.

26.59 'His scrotum is swollen'

There is a cavity (space) round each testicle like the pleural cavity round each lung. One of these cavities in his scrotum sometimes fills with clear fluid, and causes a swelling called a *hydrocoele*. A hydrocoele does not

swell more when a baby coughs or cries. If you shine a torch through a hydrocoele, you can see the light through it. This shows that it is filled with fluid. At one side you will see the testicle. Hydrocoeles usually go by themselves during the first year. If a hydrocoele does not go in a year, send the child for help.

Sometimes, a baby has a swelling which goes down from his groin towards his testicle. It gets larger when he coughs or cries. You cannot see the light from a torch through it. It is an *inguinal hernia* (20–6). These sometimes go by the age of six months. Usually, hernias don't go, and the baby needs an operation when he is older.

26.59b 'He has no testes'

Feel for his testes carefully. There is a muscle which pulls the testis up into the inguinal region. Then you cannot feel it. So, press a baby's inguinal region with your left thumb before you feel for his testis with your right hand.

The testes come down into the scrotum about the time of birth. If they have not come down at birth, they

SOME OTHER PROBLEMS

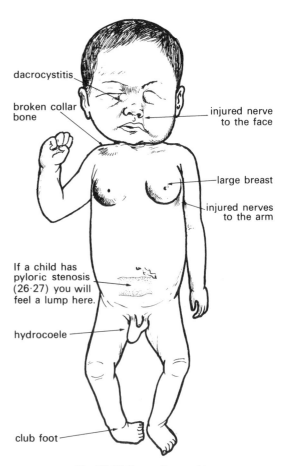

dacrocystitis

broken collar bone

injured nerve to the face

large breast

injured nerves to the arm

If a child has pyloric stenosis (26·27) you will feel a lump here.

hydrocoele

club foot

Fig. 26–36 Some other problems.

usually come down during the next few months. The testes sometimes come down late, especially in preterm babies. The baby's mother must not worry. Testes usually come down by themselves before a child is five. If they have not come down when he is five, send him for help. He may need an operation.

26.60 'He does not move on one side of his face'—facial palsy

The nerves to a baby's face may be injured during birth, especially if forceps have been used. So he cannot move that side of his face. He needs no treatment, and he will recover in a few weeks.

26.61 'His arm is weak'—Erb's paralysis

Sometimes the large nerves under a baby's arm are injured during birth, so that his arm is weak. Unfortunately, there is no treatment. The weakness of the arm does not heal so quickly as weakness of the face. Teach his mother to move his arm to the position shown in Figure 26–37 several times every day. This prevents contractures (1–9).

26.62 'There is a lump on his shoulder'—broken clavicle

A baby's collar bone (clavicle) sometimes breaks during birth. While it heals a hard swelling forms over the break. This swelling goes after some months. It needs no treatment.

26.63 'His arm (or leg) is broken'

Bandage his arm as shown in Figure 26–38. A broken

TREATING A BROKEN ARM

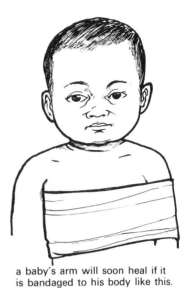

a baby's arm will soon heal if it is bandaged to his body like this.

Fig. 26–38 Treating a broken arm.

leg needs a splint. So fix a splint to the back of his leg with a bandage. Pad it well, and be sure it is not too tight.

26.65 'He cries too much'

All babies cry, because it is the only way they can say that they want something. Babies cry because they are hungry, wet or dirty, or too hot or too cold, or because they want their mother. Babies sometimes cry because they are tired, or because their teeth are coming (teething).

Some babies cry often, and others rarely. Occasionally, a baby cries because he is sick. Most mothers understand normal crying and quickly learn what their baby wants. But some mothers need help, especially with their first babies. Mothers should not leave babies to cry. So we must diagnose why a baby cries. Here are some of the reasons.

He is sick. He cries more than normal. He cries in a different way and *cannot be comforted*. Serious causes are otitis media, meningitis, and tetanus.

He has colic. From the age of about three weeks he cries nearly every day. He cries soon after feeds, he pulls up his legs, and looks as if he has abdominal pain. This kind of pain is called colic. Sometimes it is caused if a baby swallows too much air with his milk. Show a mother how to bring up this air (26–24). Colic usually goes by itself when a baby is about three months old.

Erb's paralysis

Pin his arm to the sheet of his cot in this position

nerves to the arm injured at birth

arm partly paralysed

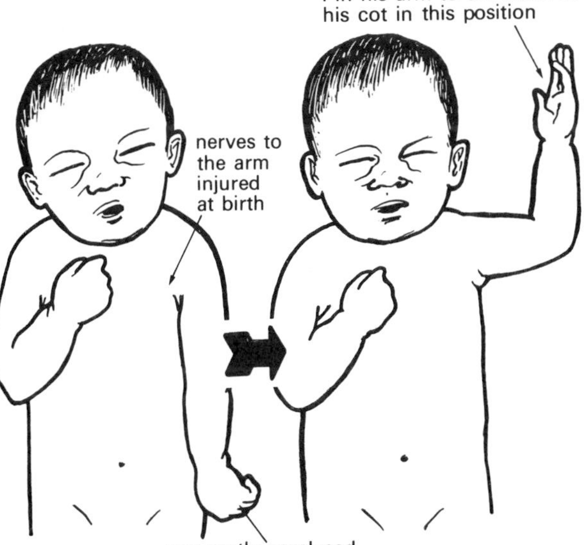

Fig. 26–37 Treating Erb's paralysis.

He wants to suck more. Sometimes a baby cries because he wants to go on sucking. He cries even after he has emptied his mother's breasts and is no longer hungry. If a baby is bottle-fed, a dummy between feeds may help him. Don't teach village mothers who are breast-feeding to use dummies.

He is not getting enough milk. This rarely makes a baby cry too much. But many mothers think that their baby is crying because he is having enough milk. So they start bottle-feeding. This is a bad reason for starting to bottle-feed, so we must prevent it. See Section 26.14.

CRYING

HISTORY. **When did he start crying like this? (If it is a new symptom, he may be ill. If he has been crying for some weeks, it is less likely to be serious.)**
At what times in the day does he cry? (If he only cries at one special time in the day, it is probably not serious.)
Does he go to sleep normally and wake up and cry before feeds (perhaps hunger)?
Does he cry immediately after feeds? Does he pull up his knees as he cries (colic)?
Is he gaining weight normally? (If he is not gaining weight, he may be hungry and need extra food.)
Does his mother put too many clothes on him or too few?

EXAMINATION. **Look for any abnormal signs. Examine his gums (teething) and his ears (otitis media). Is he well nourished?**

DIAGNOSIS. **Teething? Hunger? Colic? Wet? Too hot or too cold? Sick? Otitis media? Meningitis? Tetanus?**

EXPLANATION AND MANAGEMENT. **If you think he is hungry and he is not having enough milk, weigh him. Weigh him again one or two weeks later. If he is not gaining weight go to Section 26.21.**
If you can find a reason, explain it to his mother. If you cannot make a diagnosis and he seems well, comfort her; say that you cannot find anything serious. Tell her to put him to the breast more often. Tell her he will recover in a few months. Teach her how to bring up swallowed air. Put him to sleep on his front, and if necessary, try a dummy. Explain that he must not start bottle-feeding. Ask her to bring him every week, so that you can weigh him, and see if he is growing. Has she any questions to ask?

**IF A BABY CRIES, PUT HIM TO THE
BREAST MORE OFTEN. DON'T
GIVE HIM A BOTTLE**

Disease in the baby's mother

26.66 TB and leprosy

If a baby's mother has infectious TB (13.3), or lepromatous leprosy (12.2), she may infect him. Don't take him away from her, because if he stops breast-feeding he is in much greater danger. He may be badly bottle-fed, and die from marasmus or diarrhoea (9.8). Let him breast-feed, and protect him with isoniazid, or isoniazid and thiacetazone.

HIS MOTHER OR ANYONE ELSE IN THE HOUSE HAS TB. **Treat his mother for TB. Put him on the special care register. Give him isoniazid (3.20) until she is sputum negative.**

**THE CHILDREN OF MOTHERS WITH TB OR
LEPROSY MUST GO ON BREAST-FEEDING**

HIS MOTHER HAS LEPROSY. **Give his mother dapsone (3.24). Some of it will get into her milk and protect him. Give him BCG at birth—dapsone does not kill BCG bacilli. This may give him some protection from leprosy, because the organisms which cause leprosy and TB are very like each other. Put him on the special care register, and observe him carefully. Has she any questions to ask?**

26.67 Some help for the mother of a newborn child

We can help a newborn baby best, if we make sure his mother breast-feeds him. Here are some other ways to help her.

Family planning. His mother should not have another child until her new baby is three years old. So, she should not become pregnant for about 27 months after his birth. Her new baby should be eating all the family's ordinary foods before she becomes pregnant again.
Ask her if she wants any more children. Perhaps she already has a large family. Perhaps feeding and caring for them is difficult. Explain how useful family planning is. Explain that her next child should not be born too soon.

Immunizations and the road to health chart. Give him a weight chart. Tell his mother when to come to the clinic (4.14).

GIVE EVERY NEWBORN BABY A WEIGHT CHART

Vocabulary index

Using this index

Presenting symptoms and the most useful section to go to are in heavy type. Don't forget that a 'dot' is a section (6.3, for example), a 'dash' is a figure (6–3), and a 'two dots' is a table (6:3).

If a child has *more than one presenting symptom*, use these rules.

One If he has *any* of these presenting symptoms, go to the 'Caring for . . .' section for them—Cough (8.20 or 8.21), Fits (15.9), 'Not sucking' (26.20).

Two If he has *mild* diarrhoea and any other symptoms, go to the other symptom. If he has *severe* diarrhoea, go to diarrhoea (9.31 or 9.32).

Three If a child has fever with any other symptoms, go to the *other* symptom.

Four If a child is less than about two months old, look in Chapter 26 on the newborn baby. In this index 'babies' always means Chapter 26.

If a mother uses her own name for a disease, such as 'chiwere' or 'mudulo' (2.9), find out what symptoms it is causing, and look them up.

If you have not used an index before and you have forgotten the alphabet, learn it—ABCDEFGHIJK LMNOPQRSTUVWXYZ. Many words have several meanings. The only meaning we have given is the one we use here.

A

AAFB Acid- and alcohol-fast bacilli. This is the way laboratories report leprosy and TB bacilli in sputum or skin scrapings, 12.3, 13.3.

abdomen The part of the body between the thorax (chest) and the legs, 1.9, **20.1**, examining the abdomen, 20.3.

abdominal pain. 20.11 to **20.13**.

abdominal swelling 20.8 **20.9**; newborn baby, 26.24.

abnormal Anything which should not happen to a healthy child is abnormal, 1.10.

abnormally made or formed See congenital malformation, 26.4, 26.51.

abnormal movements In babies probably tetanus or fits, 26.42.

abscess A space filled with pus, 1.10, 2–3, 2.4, **11.5**.

absorption When food goes into the body through the wall of the gut it is absorbed, 1.9.

accident Injury or death caused by mistake, 2.1, 2:1, 2:2, 2.12, **14.1**.

acidotic breathing A special kind of deep slow breathing seen in dehydration, 8.15, 8:1, 8.21, **9.18**.

acquired resistance If an organism used to be killed by a drug and has now learnt how not to be killed, it has acquired resistance.

acute Short-lasting (hours or days), severe, 2.1.

acute nephritis A kidney disease, 23.7.

acute-on-chronic diarrhoea 9.12.

adaptor The part of a needle which fits a syringe, 3.5, 3–8.

adhesive Sticky, glue. Adhesive strapping is sticking plaster or surgical tape.

adrenaline A drug for treating asthma, 3:1, 3.9, 3–16, **3.40**, 8.13.

allergic If a person is harmed by a drug or other substance which does not harm other people, he is allergic to it, **3.2**, 8.13, 11.24, 16.10.

allergic conjunctivitis 16.10.

alveoli The millions of small air sacs from which the lungs are made, 8.2, 8–2, 8–3.

aminosalicylate ('PAS') A drug used for treating TB, 3–13, 3.19, **3.23**, 13.6.

amoebae, amoebiasis, amoebic dysentery Amoebae are the micro-organisms that cause amoebic dysentery or amoebiasis, 3.26, 9–1, **9.4**.

ampoule A small glass bottle for drugs, 3–4, 3.5.

anaemia Not enough haemoglobin in the blood, 1.10, 5.17, 8:1, 8.21; Chapter Twenty-two, 22.1, **22.9**.

anaesthesia Not being able to feel something, 12.1, 12–2, **12.3**.

angular stomatitis Sores at the corners of the lips, 18.10.

anti- Against, 1.7.

antibiotic A group of antimicrobial drugs, 3.11.

antibodies Special proteins in a child's blood which

help him to fight harmful organisms, 4.2, 4–2.

antihistamine A drug which prevents the harm caused by histamine in the tissues, **3.45**, 8.13.

antimicrobial drug A drug for killing harmful organisms, 2.2b, **3.11**.

antiseptic A substance which can be used for killing harmful organisms on the skin, 1.7, 2.2b, **3.11**.

antitoxin A fluid containing antibodies against the toxins (poisons) made by some bacteria, 4.2; tetanus antitoxin (ATS), 18.16; diphtheria antitoxin, 18.12.

anal fissure A cut or split in the skin of the anus, 25.6.

anus The hole at the bottom end of gut through which faeces leave the body, 1–6, 1.9, 20–1.

anus has fallen out Rectal prolapse, 25.7.

– *itches* Probably threadworms, 21.5.

– *sore* Probably an anal fissure, 25.6.

applicator A metal wire or wooden stick used to hold cotton wool for cleaning out the ear, 3:2, 17–4, 17.5.

areola The brown skin round the nipple, 26–16.

arm broken 14.5; in babies, 26–38, 26.63.

– *circumference* Measuring a child's arm circumference is a way of measuring his nutrition, 5.18, **7.1**, 7.13, N 1.5.

– *painful* 24.7, **25.12**.

– *thin* Probably polio, 24.8.

– *weak* Probably polio, 24.4; in babies, probably Erb's palsy, 26–36, 26.61.

artery A vessel (tube) which takes blood from the heart to other parts of the body.

artificial active immunity The immunity a child gets after being given a vaccine, 4.2.

artifical feeding Feeding children with animal milk, usually from a bottle, 9.8, 26.14. See also bottle-feeding.

Ascaris The roundworm, 3.28, 4.11, 20.8, 20–8, 21.1, **21.3**, 21–3.

asphyxia Not breathing, 26.3.

aspirin A drug for stopping pain, 3–16, **3.41**, 10.3.

asthma A lung disease which causes wheezing, 3.39, 8:1, **8.13**, 8.21.

asymmetrical Different on each side of the body, 1.10, 11.2.

at risk See special care, 6.3.

ATS See tetanus antitoxin, 18.16.

attack (i) To fight. (ii) A sudden illness, 1.10; cyanotic attacks in babies, 26.24.

attendance A visit to a clinic.

auriscope An instrument for examining ears, 3:2, 17–2, 17.3.

average yearly visits per child under five A measure of how much care a clinic is giving to the children of a community, 6.7, **6.10**.

axilla The space under the upper arm between the arm and the body.

B

bacillary dysentery Bloody diarrhoea caused by bacilli, 9.3.

bacilli Long bacteria like pencils, 2–1, 2.2.

back examination of, 24.2, 24–2.

backward A backward child is late walking and talking, 24.9 to 15, **24.16**.

bacteria A kind of micro-organsim, 2–1, **2.2**, 2.3.

barrel The outside part of a syringe.

bathing a newborn baby 26.5.

BCG A vaccine for preventing tuberculosis, 4.3, 4–6, **4.6**, 13.4.

bed-wetting 25.2.

behaviour change When a person changes his behaviour, he does something different, 2.12.

behaviour disease Diseases which show themselves as abnormalities in how a child behaves (what he does), 2.1, 2:1.

beliefs A mother's beliefs about something are what she knows to be true about it, 2.9.

benethamine and benzathine penicillins Penicillins which stay in the body for several days, 3.15.

benzoic acid ointment An ointment for ringworm, also called Whitfield's ointment, 3.48, 11.13.

benzyl benzoate A drug for scabies, 3.48.

benzyl penicillin Also called penicillin G, soluble penicillin, crystalline penicillin, 3.15.

bephenium A drug for treating hookworm infections, 3:1, **3–15, 3.27**, 21.3.

bevel The sharp sloping part for a needle.

bile A yellow green fluid excreted by the liver into the gut.

bile duct A tube that goes from the liver to the small intestine, 1–6.

bilharzia Schistosomiasis, 23.6.

bilirubin The yellow substance that makes a jaundiced child yellow, 22.10, 26.23.

birth 26.1.

birth history The story of what happened to a child at birth, 5.9.

birth injury 24.12, **26.6**, 26.60 to 63.

birth interval The time between a child's birth and the birth of his next brother or sister, 5.25.

birth weight 26.4.

Bitot's spots Lesions in the eye caused by vitamin A deficiency, 16–10, 16.13.

bladder The 'bag' which holds the urine, 1–7, 1.9, examining the bladder, 20.3, 23.1.

blindness blind child, 16.13.

blisters on lip Probably herpes simplex, 18.6.

blisters on skin Perhaps impetigo of the newborn, 26.47.

blocked nose 8.7.

blood, bleeding

– *into the conjunctiva* This sometimes happens in whooping cough, 8–10, 8.17, or in babies at birth, 26.4.

– *from the cord or umbilicus* Perhaps haemorrhagic disease of the newborn 26–25, 26.33, **26.38.**

– *from the mouth* of a newborn baby 26.28.

– *from the nose* 25.10.

– in the sputum In adults this is an important symptom of TB. It is rare in children, 13.3.

– in the stools If the stools are liquid, probably dysentery, 9.3, **9.4**, 9.5, 9.31, **25.7b**; in babies probably haemorrhagic disease 26–25, 26.33.

– in the urine Haematuria, 23.6.

– into the skin A petechial rash, **11.2**.

– from the vagina in babies 26.56.

blood destroying (haemolytic) anaemia 22.3, **22.7**, 22.10.

blood slide A special test in which a drop of blood is put on a piece of glass and examined with a microscope, 5.19.

blood test Ways of examining a child's blood, 5.19.

blood vessel A tube carrying blood round the body, 1.9, 2–3.

blue (cyanosed) lips or skin A serious sign often caused by a lower respiratory infection, 8.2, 8.21; in babies, 26.24, 26.26, 26.42.

boil A septic skin lesion, 2–2, 2.4, 11.3, **11.5**.

bone broken 14.5.

bone painful 25.12.

booster An extra dose of vaccine, 4.4.

borderline leprosy A kind of leprosy which is half way between tuberculoid and lepromatous leprosy, 12.2.

bossing Swellings on the skull in sickle cell anaemia, 22.8.

bottle-feeding 4–10, 7.2, **9.8**; for newborn baby, 26.18.

breast, abscess, breast infection 26.8, **26.12**.

– empty **26.13**, 26.14.

– feeding 2.12, 7.2, 9.2, 9–3, 9.8; newborn baby **26.7 to 21**.

– of baby are large 26–36, 26.56.

– painful Either engorged breasts 26.10, or a septic breast infection, 26.12.

– pump 26.8, 26–11.

breathing difficult 8.9, 8.19, **8.21**; in babies 26.26.

breathing difficult or fast 8.15, **8.21**.

breathing noisily Stridor 8.9, 8.10, **8.21**.

bronchi The large air tubes of the lungs, 8–1, 8.2, 8–2, 8–4.

bronchioles The smallest air tubes in the lungs, 8.2, 8–3.

bronchiolitis A disease of babies in which the bronchioles are infected, 8.14.

bronchitis Inflammation of the bronchi, 2.4, 8.10, 8.11, **8.12**, 8:1, 8.21.

bronchopneumonia See pneumonia, 8.15, babies, 26.26.

bringing up fluid Either posseting or vomiting, 20.15, 26.27.

broad-spectrum antibiotic A drug which can kill many kinds of bacteria, 3.13.

bruise Bleeding into the tissues, 14.5.

burn Skin burn, 14–2, **14.3**; burnt eye, 16.5.

buttocks The parts of our bodies on which we sit, 1.9, 11.21.

C

calamine lotion A symptomatic skin treatment, 3.48.

calcium hypochlorite 3:1, 3.48.

cancrum oris A severe ulcerating disease which destroys the mouth, 18–6, 18.8.

cannot open his mouth Possibly tetanus, 18.16, 18.17.

capillaries Very small blood vessels, 8.2, 8–3.

capsule A way of giving powdered drugs, 3.4, 3–4.

caput succedaneum The swelling on the part of a baby's head which comes first during labour, 26.4.

carbon dioxide A gas made by the body when food is 'burnt' with oxygen to make energy, 8.2, 8–3.

care for To look after, 1.10, 5.27.

caries Holes in the teeth, 18.3, **19.5**.

'Caring for...' section A section telling the reader how to diagnose the disease which is causing a presenting symptom **1.4**.

carrier A healthy person whose body carries harmful organisms, 2.3.

cartilage The hard substance in a child's ears.

case Someone who has a disease is a case of that disease, 1.10.

catheter A rubber or plastic tube 14.6; catheter for newborn babies, 26.4.

causal drugs Drugs which remove the cause of a disease, 3.1.

cavity A space (i) See pleural cavity 8.2, and peritoneal cavity 20.1; (ii) A chronic TB lesion in the lungs of adults, 13–1, 13.3.

cells The very small living 'bricks' from which the body is built, 1.9.

cellulitis An acute spreading septic infection of the tissues, **2.4**, 11.3; cellulitis round the umbilicus, 26.36.

cephalhaematoma Bleeding under the covering of one of a baby's skull bones during labour, 26.4, 26–7.

cerebral malaria Malaria of the brain, 3.25, **10.7**, 15.7, 24.12.

cerebral palsy Paralysis caused by a brain injury at birth, 24–10, 24.15.

cerebrospinal fluid, CSF The fluid over the surface of the brain and spinal cord, 15.2.

chest infection A lower respiratory infection, 8.11, **8.21**.

chickenpox A disease of children causing fever and skin lesions, 11.16.

children's cough mixture 3.46.

children's iron mixture 'Ferrous sulphate mixture paediatric BPC,' an iron medicine, **3.33**, 22.4.

chloramphenicol One of the drugs used for treating septic infections, 3.2, 3:1, 3.9, **3–12, 3.18**, 8.12, 8.13, 8.15, 8.17.

chloroquine A drug for treating malaria, 3–14, 3–17, **3.25**, 5.8, 9.9, 10.3, 10.7, 14.8.

chlortetracycline An antibiotic used to make an eye ointment, **3.17**, 16.9.

choking Unable to breathe because something is obstructing the throat, 25.4.

cholera A severe kind of diarrhoea, **9.7**, 9.31.

chronic   Long lasting (weeks or months), 2.1.

circumcision   Cutting off a boy's foreskin, 23.11.

clavicle (collar bone) broken   In babies, 26–36, 26.62.

cleft   A cut or slit.

cleft lip or palate   A congenital malformation, 26–31, 26.51.

clinic   5.2, 6.12.

clofazimine   A drug used for treating lepromatous leprosy, 3.24b, 12.4.

clothes   10.3, 5–10; clothes and babies, 26.5.

club feet   See talipes 26–33, 26–34, **26.52**.

cocci   Round bacteria like balls, 2–1, **2.2**, 2–3.

cold   (i) 'common cold.' A virus disease of the nose, 2:2, 8.6, **8.7**, 8.20; (ii) Hypothermia, a child who is abnormally cold, 10.4; hypothermia in babies, 26.25.

cold chain   The steps along which a vaccine goes on its journey from a factory to a child, 4.3.

cold sores   Herpes simplex, 11.15.

collar and cuff   A way of holding an injured arm by tying it to the neck, 24–5.

colostrum   The first milk that comes into a breast, 26.7.

coma   A child in coma seems to be asleep but cannot be woken up, 1.10, 5:2, 5.15, 9.18, 14.8.

comforter   A rubber teat that is given to a baby to suck so as to comfort him.

community   The people who live and work together in the same place, 1.7, 2.10.

community diagnosis   2.10, 2.11.

community health action   The people of a community working together to improve their health, 2.13.

complication   A second disease which comes after and complicates the first one, 1.10.

compound fracture   A fracture in which there is a break in the skin over the broken bone, 14.5.

congenital malformation   A mistake in the way a child's body is made or formed while he is growing in the womb, 2.1, 2.2, **26.4**.

– of finger   26.54.

– of foot   Talipes, 26–33, 26–34, 26–36, 26.52.

– skin lesions   26–29, 26.46.

– of lip or palate   Cleft lip or palate, 26–31, 26.51.

– swelling of the testis   Hydrocoele, 26–36, 26.59.

conjunctiva   The thin mucosa over the inside of the eyelids and the sclera, 16–1, 16.2.

conjunctivitis   Inflammation of the conjunctiva, 10.6, 16–6, **16.8**; conjunctivitis in babies, 26–27, 26.39, **26.40**.

conscious   A child who is conscious is awake and interested in what is going on around him, 1.10.

constipation   Not passing faeces often enough, 25.6; in babies, 26.30.

contact   Touching.

contact infections   Infections spread by touching an infected person or thing, 2–6, 2.7.

continuation card   A card for writing a child's records on when the space on his weight chart is used up, 6.2.

continuity of care   Care for a mother or her child which is always given by the same person, 5.2, **5.28**.

contract   When muscles contract they get shorter, 1.10, 8–4.

contracture   A stiff joint which cannot be moved the full amount, **1–9**, 1.10, **24.4**.

convulsions   Fits, Chapter Fifteen, **15.9**.

copper sulphate   A blue chemical used to treat the baby's umbilicus when it does not heal, 26.35.

cord   See umbilical cord.

cornea   The transparent 'window' at the front of the eye, 16–1, 16.2.

corneal ulcer   An ulcer of the transparent part of the eye, 16.7.

corrosive   'Burning' such as that caused by strong acids and alkalis, corrosive poisoning, 14.6, **14.7**.

cot   A child's bed.

cotton wick for feeding baby   26.18.

cough   Chapter Eight, symptomatic treatment, 8.5; ordinary cough, **8.20**; cough with lower respiratory symptoms, 8.21.

– with blood in the sputum   Rare in children, in adults probably TB 13.3.

– at night   Any respiratory disease can make a child cough at night, promethazine will help, 8.5.

– whooping   8.17.

– mixture   3.46, 8.5.

coughed up a worm   Probably *Ascaris*, 21.3.

course   The course of a drug is the length of time for which it must be given, 3.3.

cracked nipple   26.11.

creeping eruption   A skin lesion caused by a worm, 11–15, 11.21.

cretinism   One of the causes of backwardness 24.14.

cross   Angry, 5.15.

cross references   A way of going from one part of a book to another, 1–3, 1.4.

croup   Another word for obstructive laryngitis, 8.11.

crust   The dry yellow-brown top that forms on a septic skin lesion as it heals, 2.4, 11.2, 11–3.

crying abnormally (tantrums)   25.2, **26.65**. *immediately after feed*   26.14.

crystal violet   A coloured drug for the skin, 3.48.

CSF   Cerebrospinal fluid, the fluid around the brain, 15–1, 15.2.

cup and spoon feeding   26.18.

cure   To make a child well again, 1.10, 2.1.

customs   The habits of a people, 2.9.

cuts in the skin   14.4, 14–4.

cyanosed   A cyanosed child has blue lips and mucosae, 5:2, 8.2.

cyanotic attacks   An attack in which a newborn baby suddenly goes blue, 26.24.

D

dactylitis   Swollen painful fingers or toes in sickle cell anaemia, 22.8.

danger signs   Signs which show that a child is seriously ill, 2.12; danger signs for cough, 8.20; danger signs for diarrhoea, 9.31.

dapsone A drug for leprosy, 3.2, 3–13, **3.24**.

Darrow's solution A sterile fluid for intravenous and intraperitoneal rehydration, 9.25.

deaf Unable to hear, examining for deafness, 17.7, 24.16.

decilitre 100 ml or a tenth of a litre.

deficiency A lack or shortage of something, not enough of it.

deformity Part of the body which has grown into an abnormal shape, 1–9, 1.10, 12.1.

dehydration Abnormal dryness of the body, 8:1, 9–8, **9.17**, 9.18, 9.31

- score A way of measuring how dehydrated a child is, 9.18.

delirium, delirious A delirious child talks nonsense, does not know where he is and may be unable to recognize people, 1.10, 5:2, **5.15**, 9.18.

depot penicillin A 'store' of penicillin which stays in the body for several days, 3.15.

dessert spoon The spoon that adults use for eating.

destroy To break or spoil completely, 1.7.

development 24.9.

diagnose, diagnosis To diagnose a child is to find out what disease he has, **1.10**, 5.20.

diaphragm A wall of muscle between the thorax and the abdomen, 1.9, 8–1, 8.2.

diarrhoea A disease in which there are many liquid stools, 2.2, 2.10, 2.12; Chapter Nine, 9.31.

- in babies 26.24, **26.32**.

- bloody **9.5**, 9.31, 25.7b.

- chronic This is often caused by malnutrition, 7.10, **9.12**.

- drugs for 9.30.

- and fits 9.18, 9.29b.

- and vomiting 9.17, **9.31**, 20.14, **20.15**.

difficulty breathing 8.1, 8.21; in babies, **26.26**.

- eating or not eating 7.13, 10.10, 13:1, 13.7, 18.14, **18.15**, 15.3.

- passing urine Dysuria, 1.7, 23.1, 23.5, **23.9**.

- walking Chapter Twenty-four, 24.7, **24.16**.

digestion The breaking down of food in the gut into very small pieces, 1.9.

dilate When one of the tubes in the body, such as a blood vessel, gets wider it dilates, 1.9, **8.4**.

diphtheria A serious bacterial disease of the throat, 8.11, **18.12**, 18–9, 25.10.

disability A child is disabled if he is not able to have normal life, or play, or go to school, 1–9, 1.10, 12.1.

discharge Any abnormal fluid which comes from the body

- from the ear 17.1, **17.14**.

- from the nose 8.7; discharge from one side of the nose only, 25.10.

- from the vulva 23.10.

disease See 1.10.

disinfectants Substances used for killing harmful organisms outside the body, **2.2**, 3.11.

disposable A disposable piece of equipment is used once and thrown away.

dissolve When sugar is mixed with water it can no longer be seen and dissolves, 1.7.

distended Filled up more than normal, 1.10.

dose The amount of a drug that needs to be given each time, 3.3, 3–12 to 3–17.

doubtful Uncertain, not sure, 1.10.

Down's syndrome A disease causing backwardness, 24.13.

DPT A vaccine against diphtheria, pertussis and tetanus, **4.9**, 8.17.

dried skim milk A milk powder from which the fat (cream) has been removed, **7.6**, 7.11.

drinking water 2.7, 9–4, **9.8**; water for babies, 26.16.

drip set A tube and needle through which a child can be given intravenous fluids, 3.7, 9–16, 9.20, **9.27**.

droplet infection An infection in which organisms are spread in very small drops of sputum floating in the air, **2–6**, **2.7**.

drowsy Abnormally sleepy, 5.15, **14.8**, 26.24.

drug(s) 'Medicines' Chapter Three.

– and diarrhoea 9.30.

– and expendable supplies 3:1, 6.8

– jaundice 22.12.

– by mouth 3.4

– poisoning 14.6, **14.7**.

– rash 11.25.

– reaction, sensitivity Serious harm caused by a drug, **3.2**, 3.15, 3.40.

– resistance An organism which cannot be killed by a drug is resistant to it, 3.11, 3.12.

– side effects 3.2.

drum The ear drum is the thin 'wall' between the outer and middle ear, 17.2.

duct A tube, 1.9.

dummy A comforter. A teat given to the child to suck.

dysentery Bloody diarrhoea, 9.3 to **9.5**, 9.31, 25.7b.

dys- Difficult or painful, 1.7.

dyspnoea Difficult breathing, 8.15, 8.21.

dysuria Pain or difficulty passing water, 23.1, 23.3, **23.9**.

E

ear drum The thin 'wall' between the middle and outer ear, 17–1, 17.2, 17–3.

ear pain or discharge Chapter Seventeen, 17.14.

ear-ring causing infection 25.9.

eating badly 5.11, 5.17, 10.10, 18.14, **18.15**, 25.3.

EBM Expressed breast milk 26.8.

eczema A chronic skin lesion, 11.27.

elasticity of the skin Loss of skin elasticity is an important sign of dehydration, 9.18.

elixir A sweet sugary medicine, 3.4.

emergency A disease which will cause death if it is not treated quickly, 1.10, 5.21, 7.10.

empyema Pus in the pleural cavity, 8.16.

energy foods Foods such as rice, maize, sugar and oil which give a child the energy to keep himself warm and run about and play, 1.8.

eneuresis Bed-wetting, 25.2.

engorged breasts Breasts swollen with milk, 26.8, **26.10**, 26–10.

enlarged Larger than normal, see 'swellings', 1.10, Chapter Nineteen, **19.9**.

Enterobius Threadworms, 21.5.

enzymes Digestive enzymes break food down into small pieces, 9.11.

ephedrine A drug used for treating asthma, **3.39**, 3–16, 8.7, 8.13.

epilepsy A chronic disease causing fits, 15.8.

equipment The 'tools' needed by a clinic, such as needles, syringes, or a torch, 3:2, 3.7, 3–18, 3–19, **3.50**, 5.2.

Erb's palsy A special kind of arm paralysis, 26–37, 26.61.

erythema, erythematous Redness of a skin lesion caused by dilated blood vessels, 11.2, 11–2.

Eustachian tube A tube which goes from the pharynx to the middle ear, 17–1, **17.2**, 17–6, 17.9.

evaluate To find out how good or bad something is, 1.7, 2.10.

examination Looking at a child or feeling or listening to him to find out if anything is abnormal, 5–2, 5.15 to 18.

– *for anaemia* 22.1.

– *for skin anaesthesia* 12.3.

– *of the abdomen* 20.2, 20.3.

– *of the back* 24.2, 24–2.

– *for deafness* 17.7.

– *for dehydration* 9.18.

– *for development, milestones* 24.10.

– *of the ears* 17.3.

– *of the eyes* 16.2, 16–2, 16–3.

– *of the legs* 24.2.

– *of the hips* 24–1, 24.2.

– *for thickened nerves in leprosy* 12.3.

– *of the lymph nodes* 2.5, 19–1, 19.1b, 19.2.

– *for meningeal signs* 15.6.

– *of the mouth* 18–1, 18.2.

– *of the newborn baby* 26.4.

– *for night blindness* 16.13.

– *for nutrition, malnutrition* 7.13.

– *of the pulse* 9.18.

– *of the respiratory system* **8.9**, 8.20, 8.21.

– *of the skin* **11.2**, 11.28.

– *of the spleen* **20.3**, 20–3, 20–4.

– *of a swelling* 19.1, 19.9.

– *of the throat* 18–1, 18.2.

– *of the tonsillar lymph nodes* 18–3.

excretion Getting rid of things from the body. Urine is excreted.

expendable supplies Things such as drugs and bandages which are used up by a clinic, 1.3, **3.7**, 6.8.

expire To breathe out, 8.2.

expiry date The date after which a drug or vaccine should not be used because it no longer works or has become dangerous 3.17, 4.3.

explanation Telling a mother about her child in a way she can understand, the 'Eighth step', 5.24.

expressing breast milk Squeezing the milk out of a mother's breasts, 26.8.

eyes, eye disease 2.12, Chapter Sixteen.

– *don't see in the dark* A sign of vitamin A deficiency, 16.13.

– *examination of* 16.2.

– *foreign body* 16.5.

– *injured* 16.4, 16.5.

– *red or sticky* A sign of conjunctivitis, 16.4 to 16.12,

– *red eyes in babies* 26.39 and 40.

– *sunken* A sign of dehydration, 9.18.

– *yellow* A sign of jaundice, 5.17, 22.10, **22.13**; in babies, **26.23**, 26.24.

F

face does not move Probably facial palsy, 26–36, 26.60.

facial palsy Paralysis of the muscles, 26.60.

faeces (stools) The solid waste from the body, 1.10, 9.1, babies faces, 26.29.

– *to mouth infections* 2–6, **2.7**, 9–2, 9.8.

– *to skin infections* 2–6, 2.7, 21.1, 21–1, 21–2.

fainting, 14.2.

falciparum malaria A severe kind of malaria caused by *Plasmodium falciparum*, 9.9, 10.7.

family history The story of what has happened to a child's family, 1–1, 5.12.

family planning Having children only when you want them, the ninth stop in caring for a sick child, 4.12, 5.25.

'Fansidar' See sulphadoxine with pyrimethamine, 3.25.

fast breathing 8.15, **8.21**.

febrile Feverish, having a fever, 10.1.

febrile convulsions Fever fits, 15.5.

feeding a newborn baby 26.7 to 21, 'Seven ways of feeding a newborn baby', 26.18, 26–17, 26–18.

bottle, 5.16, 9.8, 26.14; for newborn baby, 26.18.

feet malformed 26.52.

ferrous sulphate Iron sulphate, a drug for treating iron deficiency anaemia, 22.4.

fever The body becoming too hot, 2.4, 9.18; Chapter Ten, symptomatic treatment, 10.3, **10.10**; sore mouth in fever, 18.4.

fever fits Febrile convulsions, 15.5.

finger malformed 26.54.

born with an extra finger, 26–35, 26.54.

– *nails sore*, 26.48.

firm Half way between hard and soft, 1.10.

fissure A split or tear, anal fissure, 25.6.

fits Convulsions. Sudden abnormal movements and unconsciousness 2.12, 3.43, 5:2, 8.17; Chapter Fifteen, **15.9**, 24.12; in babies, 26.24, 26.42.

flaking paint rash A sign of kwashiorkor, 7.10, 11.22.

flat nipples 26.9, 26–12 to 15.

floppy The arms and legs of a 'floppy' (hypotonic) child hang weakly from him when he is lifted. His muscles have lost their normal tone, 5.15.

flora The organisms that normally live in a place, 2.2, 9.2, 18.7.

flow chart A special 'picture' for showing how things should be done, 9–22.

fluctuant A swelling which feels as if it is full of fluid is fluctuant, 1.10.

fluid Something which flows, such as water or blood, 1.7; needs of a child, 26.15.

fluorescein A yellow stain used to examine the cornea for ulcers, 3.49, 16.7.

folic acid One of the B vitamins, 3.37; folic acid deficiency anaemia, 22.6.

follicles Small round swellings inside the upper eyelid in trachoma, 16.9.

follow up To follow up a child is to see him in the clinic several times, 5–18, 5.28.

fontanelle The soft part of the top of a newborn baby's head.
– *not moving* 9.18, 15.6.
– *not present, or too small* 26.50.
– *sunken* A sign of dehydration, 9.18.
– *swollen* A sign of meningitis, 15.6, 15–9.

food, feeding Chapter Seven, 9.13, 26.18.

food poisoning Diarrhoea and vomiting caused by eating infected food, 9.13.

foreign body Something which gets into an abnormal place in the body, such as a bead into the ear, 1.10.
– *in the bronchus* 8.18, **8.21**, 8–4.
– *in the ear* 17–12, 17.13, **17.14**.
– *in the eye* 16.5.
– *in the nose* 25.11.
– *in the skin* 14.4.
– *swallowed* 25.5.
– *in the throat* 25.4.
– *in the vagina* 23.10.

foreskin The skin on the end of the penis, 23.10, **23.11**.

form To form something is to make it, 1.10.

fracture A broken bone, 14.5.

freeze drying A way of making live liquid vaccines store better, 4.3.

frequency Passing urine often, 1.10, 23.1, **23.9**.

fungus A micro-organism like a very small white plant, 2–1, 2.2; fungi in the skin, 11.13.

G

g Short for gram, see under 'gram'

gammabenzine hexachloride A skin medicine for scabies, 3.48, 11.10.

gastroenteritis Acute diarrhoea often with vomiting. Usually caused by gut infection. See diarrhoea, 9.2, 9.31, 9.17, 20.14, **20.15**.

gauze Thin cotton cloth used for dressing wounds.

general The general signs of disease are the signs that are found all over the body, 1.10.

genital system The sex organs, 23.10.

gentian violet See crystal violet, 3.48.

Giardia, giardiasis An organism called *Giardia lamblia*

causes a kind of diarrhoea called giardiasis, 3.26, 9–1, **9.6**.

gland An organ which makes a juice or secretion.

glucose A special kind of sugar.

– *salt solution* A fluid used for treating dehydration, 3:1, 3.9, 9–10, **9.21**, 9.22, 9.23, 9.24, 9.31 etc.

goitre A swollen thyroid gland, 19–5, 19.6.

gonococcal conjunctivitis 26–27, 26.40.

gonococci The bacteria causing gonorrhoea, 26.40.

gonorrhoea A sexually spread disease, 16.8, 23.10, **26.40**.

graduations The lines on a ruler or on the barrel of a syringe.

gram A small weight. A pencil weighs about 5 grams or 5 g, 3.3.

groin The groin or inguinal region is a fold between the abdomen and the leg, 1–7.

gross Very much, very large, very severe, 1–8, 1.10.

group Several people or things together, 1.7.

group health education Giving health education to several people together, 2.11, 2–11, N 10.1.

growth curve If a child is weighed several times during several months the dots on his weight chart for each weighing can be joined together to make a growth curve, 5.3, 7.1, N 1.3.

growth curve flat or falling. An important sign of malnutrition, 7–7b, 26.21.

grunting The noise a pig makes. An abnormal noise during breathing, 8.9, 26.1.

gums The soft red tissue round the teeth, 1.9.

gut A tube which goes from the mouth to the anus, 1.9, 20–1, 20–5; gut obstruction, 20.2; gut obstruction in babies, 26.27, 26.31.

H

H. nana The dwarf or small tapeworm, 21.4, 21–4.

haematuria Blood in the urine, 23.6.

haemoglobin The substance in the red cells which makes the blood red, 1.9, **22.2**.

– *curve* A record of a child's haemoglobin on his weight chart, 22.2, 22–3.

haemolytic anaemia An anaemia in which red cells are destroyed in the blood vessels, 22.7.

haemorrhage Bleeding.

haemorrhagic disease of the newborn A disease caused by lack of vitamin K, 3.38, 26–25, 26.28, **26.33**.

hair pale, loose, or straight Might be kwashiorkor, 7.10.

hand washing 2.7, 11.28, 26.21.

hard stools Constipation, 25.5; constipation in babies, 26.30.

harm To harm something is to spoil or break it, 1.7.

harmful organisms Very small 'animals' which can cause disease in a child. Also called 'germs', micro-organisms or microbes, 2.2.

hatch A chicken or a worm hatches when it comes out of its egg, 21.1.

head abnormally shaped 26.49.

head between the knees test One of the meningeal signs, 15.6, 15–8.

head lice 11.11.

head swollen Caput, moulding, cephalhaematoma, 26.4.

heal To cure or make healthy again, 1.10.

health education Changing people's behaviour in a way that will make their own health and that of their families better, 2.9 to 13, 4.1.

health education plan A plan that every clinic should have for the health education it does, **2.11**, 6.8, 10.1.

healthy child Chapter Four, 4.12.

heart failure Heart not working normally, 8.2, 18.12.

heat rash 11.26.

helminth A worm.

hepatitis Inflammation of the liver, 3.24, 22.10, **22.11**.

hepatitis virus A and B The two viruses causing hepatitis, 22.11.

hereditary disease A disease which parents give to their children as they are conceived, 2.1, 2:1.

hernia A swelling in which part of the body pushes out through the tissues which cover it, inguinal hernia, 8.17, 20.2, **20.4**, 20.5, 20–6, inguinal hernia in babies, 26.59; umbilical hernia, 20–5, 20.7, 20–7.

herpes simplex Cold sores, **11.15**, 18.6, 11–11.

herpes stomatitis Inflammation of the mouth caused by the herpes simplex virus, 18–5, 18.6.

herpes zoster An infectious skin disease, 11–12, 11.17.

hip The joint at the top of the leg, 24–1, 24.2.

history The story of what has happened to a sick child, 5.4 to 14.

hookworms Small worms that live in the gut and cause anaemia, 2–1, 2–6, 2.7, 3.27, 4.11, 21–1 to 4; hookworm anaemia, 22.5.

hospital letter 5–15.

hotness of the body Fever, 10.1, **10.10**.

hurts, hurting See 'pain' and 'sore'.

hydrocoele A swelling caused by fluid round the testicle, 26–36, 26.59.

hydrogen peroxide A chemical used as a mouthwash, 18.7, 18.8.

hyper- To much, too big, too strong, 1.7.

hypernatraemic dehydration A kind of dehydration in which a child's body lacks water but still has enough or too much salt, 9.18, 26.16.

hyperpyrexia Dangerously high fever, 9.18, 9.31, 10.1, **10.4**, 10–4, 10–5.

hypertonic 'Stiff muscles' or too much muscle tone, 1.7, 1.10.

hypo- Too little, 1.7.

hypochlorite An antiseptic which is also used as a bleach, 3.11.

hypodermic Under the skin.

hypodermic needle A thin short needle (0·45 × 10 mm) used for BCG vaccine, and tuberculin, 3.5, 3–8.

hypoglycaemia Too little sugar in the blood, 7.11, 7.13, 24.12, **26.42**.

hypopigmented Less coloured than normal, 12.3.

hypopyon Pus behind the cornea, 16.7.

hypothermia Abnormal coldness of the body, 10.1, **10.4**, 10–6; newborn baby, 26–23, 26.25.

hypotonic muscles Too little muscle tone 'floppy muscles', 1.7, 1.10, 5.15; newborn baby, 26.1.

I

– iasis Words ending in -iasis are all diseases caused by parasites, for example giardiasis, 9.6.

ill A child who shows the general ('all over the body') signs of not being 'well', 1.10, 2.4, 5:2, 5–7; signs of an 'ill' child, **5.15**.

immunity A child's immunity is how good he is at fighting harmful organisms so that they do not make him ill, **2.3**, 4.2.

immunization To immunize a child is to give a special 'medicine' called a vaccine which will prevent harmful organisms from infecting him, 2.10, **4.2**, 4.10, 13.2, 13.4.

immunization timetable A table showing when vaccines should be given, 4:1, 4.4.

impetigo A septic skin lesion, 11.3, 11.4, 11–4; impetigo of newborn babies, 26.47.

important fifty The fifty most important supplies in a clinic, **3.7**, 3:1, 3.11.

incision A cut. Cutting open an abscess, 11.5, 26.12.

incontinence A child who cannot hold his urine is incontinent, 23.9.

increase To get larger.

incubation period The time between infection and the start of symptoms, 10.6.

indeterminate leprosy An early kind of leprosy, 12–1, 12.2.

individual One thing or person only.

infection When harmful organisms are growing in a child he has an infection, 2.2, **2.4**.

infectious disease A disease caused by harmful organisms which spread from one person to another, 2.2, 2:2.

inflammation The changes that happen in a tissue when harmful organisms grow in it. Inflamed skin is red, **2.4**, 2.6.

inguinal hernia 20.5, 20–5, 20–6; in babies, 26.59.

inguinal region The groin, or the fold between the front of the abdomen and the leg, 1–7, 1.9; swellings of the inguinal region, 20.5.

INH See isoniazid 3.20.

inhale To breathe air (or fluid or vomit) into the respiratory system.

injection abscess An abscess at the place of an injection, **3.6**, 3–10, 3.44.

injections 3.5, 3–9.

injury See accidents. Any harm to the body, 2.12, 24.3.

insect bites 11.9.

insect carried infections 2–6, 2.7.

inspire To breathe in 8.2.

instruments The 'tools' used in the clinic.

insuction (retraction) Sucking in of the skin between

the ribs when a child breathes. Insuction is usually a sign of lower respiratory infection, 8:1, 8–5, 8–6, **8.10**; insuction in a newborn baby, 26.1.

integrated care   Care for well and sick children, maternity care and family planning which can *all* be had at the same time, 5.2, **6.8**.

intestines   The parts of the gut that come after stomach, 1–6, 1.10.

intra-   Inside, 1.7.

intradermal   Into the skin, 3.5.

intramuscular injection   An injection into a muscle, 3.5, 3–9.

intraperitoneal rehydration   Putting fluid into a child's peritoneal cavity, 9–14, 9.20, **9.26**.

intravenous rehydration   Putting fluid into a child through his veins, 9–18 to 9–20, 9.20, 9–22, **9.27**, 9.28.

intussusception   A disease of the gut, 9.15, 25.7.

iodine   (i) A mineral the body needs, 3.34, 4.11, 19.6, 24.14b; (ii) A strong solution of iodine in alcohol is used as an antiseptic, 3:1.

iodine embryopathy   A disease caused by lack of iodine which makes a child backward, 24.14b.

iodized oil   A way of giving iodine by injection, 3.34, 4.11, 19.6, 24.14.

ipecacuanha   A drug for making children vomit, 3.47, 14.6.

iris   The brown or blue part of the eye, 16–1, 16.2.

iron   A mineral used by the body for making haemoglobin, 3.33.

iron deficiency anaemia   Anaemia caused by lack of iron, 22.4.

iron sulphate   A drug used for treating iron deficiency, 3.33

irregular   Happening after different times.

irritable   Easily made cross and angry, an early sign of illness, 1.10, 5:2, 5.15.

isoniazid (INH)   A drug used for treating TB, 3:1, 3–13, 3.19, **3.20**, 13.6, 26.66.

itching   A skin lesion itches if it makes a child scratch, 1.10, 11.2.

itching anus   21.5.

– itis   Words ending in '-itis' are acute infections, 2.4.

J

jaundice   A disease in which the body goes yellow, 5.17, 22–7, 22.10, **22.13**; newborn baby, 26–22, **26.23**, 26.24.

jaws   The bones that hold the teeth, 1.9.

joules   A way of measuring the energy in foods, one calorie is about four joules, 1.8, N 4.1b.

K

keratomalacia   A serious eye disease caused by lack of vitamin A, 3.35, 16–9, 16.13.

Kernig's sign   One of the meningeal signs, 15.6, 15–8.

kerosine (paraffin)   A fuel used for lamps and stoves. A cause of poisoning, 14.6, **14.7**, 14–9.

kidneys   The organs which make urine, 1–7, 1–9, 19.7, 20–5, Chapter Twenty-three.

kindness   One of our objectives, 1.2 and *all* through the book!

Koplik's spots   Lesions seen inside the cheek in measles, 10.6, 10–7.

kwashiorkor   A severe kind of malnutrition in which there is swelling of the ankles and a skin rash, 2.9, **7.10**, 7–10, 8.17, 10.6, 11.22.

L

laboratory methods   Ways of examining specimens of blood, stool, urine etc., 5–12, 5.19.

lacerations   Cuts, see 14.4.

lack of   Missing, not there, not present.

lactose   The sugar in milk.

lactose intolerance   Diarrhoea caused by lactose, 9.29.

large   See 'swollen'.

large liver   7.10, 10.7, **20.3**.

large spleen   See spleen, 10.7, **20.3**.

larva   A young worm, 2.2, 21.1, 21–1, 21–2.

laryngitis   Inflammation of the larynx, 8.11, 8:1.

larynx   A narrow air-filled box at the top of the neck, 1–6, 8–1, 8.2, 8–4, 8.11.

latrine   A special room or house in which urine and stools are passed, 2.12.

learning   1.4, 5–13.

leg thin   **24.8**.

legumes   The family of plants to which peas, beans and groundnuts belong, 7.2.

lens   Part of the eye, 16–1, 16.2.

lepromatous leprosy   A severe kind of leprosy, 12–1, 12.2.

leprosy   A chronic infectious disease, 2.12, 3.24; Chapter Twelve, **12.5**, 24.8; in a baby's mother, 26.66.

lesion   Any diseased or abnormal place in a child's body, 1.10.

lice   Small insects which live on the body (body lice) or head (head lice), 11–9, 11.11.

life cycle   The stages through which an organism goes during its life, 2.3, 21.1.

limping   To limp is to walk painfully or abnormally, 24.1, 24.7.

lip malformed   26.51.

lips, sore   18.10.

liver   A large organ at the top right hand side of the abdomen, 1–6, 1.9; examining the liver, 20.3.

load   A child's worm load is the number of worms that he has inside him, 21.1.

local   In one place only, 1.10.

local events calendar   A list of the dates on which things have happened in a district that can be used for finding out a child's age, N 1.6e, 7.1.

local lesion   The lesion at the place where harmful organisms first get into the body, 2–2, 2.3, 2.4, 2–4.

local medicines   Medicines made in the district which are different from the scientific medicines in this book, **2.9**, 2–10, 5–4.

long case   A child who has a complete history and examination, 5.1, **5.3**.

losing weight   7.13 or 13.7.

lotion   A liquid medicine for the skin, 3.48.

lower line   One of the lines on a weight chart, 7.1, 7–1.

lower respiratory infection   An infection of the larynx, trachea, bronchi, or lungs, 5.17, 8.9 to 8.19, **8.21**.

Luer adaptor   The larger kind of adaptor on a syringe and needle, 3.5.

lumbar puncture   Taking some of a child's CSF for examination, 15–3 to 15–5, **15.3.**

lumbar region   The lower part of the back.

lump   An abnormal swelling which can be felt to be separate from the rest of the body round it, 1.10; see also swelling and swollen.

lungs   The organs with which we breathe, 8–1, 8.2, 8–2, 8.15.

lymph   A clear fluid which is formed in most healthy tissues, 2.4.

lymph nodes   Small bean-shaped organs which filter lymph before it goes back into the blood, **2.4**, 2–2 to 2–4, 2.5, 19–1, 19.1b, 19.2.

lymph vessels   Very small tubes through which lymph flows from the tissues back into the blood, 2.4, 19.1b.

lymphadenitis   Inflammation of the lymph nodes, 2–2, 2.4, 2–4, 2.5, 8–4, 11.3, **19.2**.

lymphangitis   Inflammation of the lymph vessels, 2.4, **2–4**, 11.3.

lysol   An antiseptic, 3.11.

M

macule   A flat skin lesion, which can be seen but not felt, 11.2, 11–3.

magnifying glass   An instrument which makes things look bigger, 16–7.

malaria   A disease caused by a parasite that grows in the red blood cells, 2.7, 3.25, 4.11, 9.9, **10.7**, 10–9, 14.8; anaemia caused by malaria, 22.7.

malformation   A part of the body which has grown in an abnormal way since birth, 26.4, 26.51.

malleus   One of the small bones of the middle ear, 17–1, 17.2, 17–3.

malnutrition   Disease caused by not eating enough of the right food, 2.1, 2.8; Chapter Seven, **7.13**, 9.11, 9.12, 20.8.

malnutrition and infection   **7.5**, 7.11, 7.13, 9.11.

manage, management   To manage a child means to decide what to do for him, 1.10, **5.21**.

marasmic kwashiorkor   A child with this disease has some of the signs of both marasmus and kwashiorkor, 7.10.

marasmus   Starvation, gross wasting, **7.9**, 7–10, 8.17.

mastoid air cells   Small air-filled spaces behind the ear in the bone of the skull, 17.2.

mastoid process   The part of the skull below and behind the ear, 17.2.

mastoiditis   Inflammation of the mastoid air cells, 17.11.

measles   An acute infectious disease caused by a virus, 4.2, 4.8, 8.20, 9.10, **10.6**, 10–8.

meatus   A hole
   (i) The meatus of the ear, 17–1, 17.2.
   (ii) The meatus of the urethra, 23.2, 23.11.

meconium   The first stools of a newborn baby, 1.10, 26.29.

mega-unit   A million units—'M'.

membranes   The thin tissues that cover a child while he is inside the uterus, 26.2.

meningeal signs   Ways of diagnosing meningitis, **15.6**, 15.7, 15–7, 15–8.

meninges   The coverings of the brain, 15–1, 15.2.

meningism   Meningeal signs without meningitis, 15.6.

meningitis   Inflammation of the meninges or coverings of the brain, 15.2, **15.6**, 17.11, 24.12.

mental deficiency   'Lacking in mind', severely backward, 24.9.

mepacrine   A drug used for treating giardiasis, 3–14, **3.26**.

metronidazole   A drug used for treating giardiasis, 3–14, 3.26.

mg   Short for milligram, or a thousandth of a gram, 3.3.

microlitre   A millionth of a litre.

micro-organisms   Any very small organism, or 'germ', 2.2, 4.2.

microplan   See Preface.

microscope   A machine for looking at very small things.

middle ear   The air filled space behind the ear drum, 17.2.

mild   Slightly, a little, 1–8, 1.10.

milestones   Things which a child should begin to do at the right age, such as walking, talking etc., 5.9, **24–8**, 24.9, **24.10**.

miliaria   A heat rash, 11.26.

miliary TB   A severe TB infection which causes millions of small lesions all over the body, 13.2.

milk comes down his nose   Probably cleft palate, 26.51.

– feed for malnutrition   7.11.

– needs of a baby   26.16.

– rash   26.45.

milligram (mg)   A thousandth of a gram, 3.3.

millilitre (ml)   A thousandth of a litre, the same as a 'cc', a large teaspoon holds about 5 ml, there are about 20 drops in 1 ml.

minerals   Substances like salt, or the elements iron and iodine which are needed by the body.

misery, miserable   Unhappiness, a sign of any illness, but especially kwashiorkor, 5.17, **7.10**.

mixture   (i) Anything which is mixed.
   (ii) a fluid containing drugs, 3.4, 3–4.

ml   Short for millilitre.

moderate   Half way between mild and severe, 1–8, 1.10.

molluscum contagiosum   A virus disease of the skin, 11.19.

mongolism   See Down's syndrome, 24.13.

monitoring growth   Observing growth, 7.1.

monosulphiram   A drug for scabies, 3.48, 11.10.

294

monthly check A quick examination given to a child on his monthly visit to a clinic, 4.13.

Moro reflex A sign to see if a newborn baby is normal, 26.6.

moulding The squeezing of the skull during birth, 26.4.

mouth Chapter Eighteen.

– *cannot open* 18.17.

– *has white lesions* Probably thrush, 18.5.

– *sore* 18.9.

'mouth to mouth' resuscitation 26.3, 26–5.

moving nose One of the signs of a lower respiratory infection, 8.9, 8.21.

mucosa The wet red 'skin' covering the inside of the gut and respiratory system etc., 1.9, 8.2, 8–4.

mucus The thick clear sticky liquid that comes from a child's nose when he has a cold, 1.10.

mumps A virus infection of the parotid gland, 19–3, 19.4.

N

nails sore In a newborn baby perhaps paronychia, 26.48.

nappy rash 26.43.

nasal cavities Two air-filled spaces behind the nose, 1–6, 8–1.

nasogastric rehydration Giving a child fluids through a tube down his nose, 9–13, 9.20, **9.24**.

nasogastric tube A tube which goes from a child's nose down into his stomach, 9–13, 9.20, **9.24**.

natural active immunity The immunity a child has after an attack of some infectious disease, 4.2, 4–3.

natural passive immunity The immunity a child is given by his mother, 4.2.

neck stiffness One of the meningeal signs, 15.6, 15–7.

neck swelling 19.9.

nephritis Inflammation of the kidneys, 23.7.

nephrotic syndrome A kidney disease which causes swelling of the face and legs, 19–6, 19.7.

nerve thickening in leprosy 12.3, 12–3.

nettle rash Urticaria, 3.45, 11.24.

newborn baby Chapter Twenty-six.

niclosamide A drug for treating tapeworms, 3.30.

nicotinic acid One of the B vitamins, 11.23.

night blindness A sign of vitamin A deficiency, 16.13.

nipple flat 26.9, 26–12 to 26–15.

– *shield* A glass funnel with a rubber teat which helps a baby to suck from a flat nipple, 26.9, 26–15.

– *sore or cracked* 26.11.

niridazole A drug used for treating schistosomiasis, 3–15, 3.31.

no testis 26.59b.

nodule A small swelling.

noisy breathing See stridor, **8.21**.

noma See cancrum oris, 18.8.

non- Not.

normal Anything which happens in a healthy child is normal, 1.10.

nose bleeding 25.10.

– *blocked* 8.7; in newborn babies, 26.26.

– *discharging* 8.9. If the discharge is bloody or from one side only, see 25.10.

not breathing normally In older children, **8.21**, 25.1; at birth, 26.1, 26.3; in babies a few days old, 26.26, 26.42.

– *eating* 7.13, 13.7, 18.14, **18.15**, 25.3.

– *eating solid food* 25.3.

– *growing, gaining weight* Perhaps an underweight child, 7.8, 7.13; in newborn babies, **26.21**.

– *passing milestones* Perhaps backward, 24.9 to 24.16.

– *passing stools* Constipation, 25.6; in babies, 26.30.

– *passing urine* Retention of urine, babies, 26.57.

– *running about or playing* If for hours or days, any infection, 10.10. If for longer perhaps malnutrition, 7.13, or TB, 13.7.

– *seeing in the dark* Vitamin A deficiency, 16.13.

– *standing* 24.16.

– *sucking* Won't start sucking, 26.19; stopped sucking or sucking weakly, **26.20**, 26.24.

– *talking* 24.16.

– *walking* 24.16.

notice To see something, 1.6.

nutrients The things from which foods are made, such as protein, fats etc., 3.1.

nutrition education Teaching about food, 7.2, 7.4.

– *examination* The signs which show whether a child is well nourished or not, 5.18.

– *history* The history of what a child has been eating, 5.4, 5.11, **7.13**.

O

objectives Things we try to reach, 1.2.

observe To observe a child means to watch him carefully, 1.10, 5.21.

obstruction A block in one of the tubes of the body, respiratory obstruction, 8–4, 8.10; gut obstruction, 20.2.

obstructive laryngitis An inflammatory disease which blocks the larynx, **8.11**, 8.21.

oedema A swelling caused by too much fluid in the tissues, 7.10.

oesophagus A tube which takes food from the pharynx to the stomach, 1–6, 1.9.

ointment A skin medicine which is 'thick' like butter.

opaque Difficult or impossible to see through.

ophthalmia neonatorum See gonococcal conjunctivitis, 26.40.

oral By mouth.

– *rehydration* Putting fluid into a child through his mouth, 9–12, **9.20** and 21.

organ A part of the body such as the brain, heart, lungs, or kidneys, 1.9.

organism Anything which is alive, 2.2.

oralyte See glucose–salt solution, 9.21.

osteomyelitis   An acute septic infection of bone, 24.5.

otitis externa   Inflammation of the outer ear, 17.2, **17.12**, 17.14.

otitis media   Acute infection of the middle ear, 9.10, 10.10, Chapter Seventeen, acute otitis media, 17–7, 17–8, **17.9**; chronic otitis media, 17.10.

otoscope   See auriscope, 17–2.

ova   The eggs of worms, 21.1.

oxygen   One of the gasses in the air, 8.2, 8–3; oxygen for resuscitating newborn babies, 26.3, 26–6.

P

pain   See also 'sore'.

– *in the abdomen*   20.11 to **20.13**.

– *in a bone*   25.12.

– *in the ear*   Perhaps otitis media, **17.14**.

– *passing faeces*   25.6.

– *passing urine*   Dysuria, 23.9.

palate   The roof of the mouth, 1–6, 8–1.

palate malformed   26.51.

pale   White, whiter than normal.

pale hair   Perhaps kwashiorkor, 7.10.

pallor, paleness, pale skin or lips   This is a sign of anaemia, 22.1, **22.9**; septicaemia in babies, 26.24.

palsy   Paralysis, 26.60 and 61.

PAM   Procaine penicillin monostearate, 3.15.

Pandy's test   A test for protein in the CSF, 15.3b, 15–6.

pannus   A lesion in the cornea in trachoma, 16.9.

papule   A raised skin lesion which you can feel with your finger, 11.2.

paracetamol   (acetaminophen) A drug for stopping pain, 3–16, **3.42**.

paraffin   See kerosine, 14.6, **14.7**, 14–9.

paraldehyde   A drug used for treating fits, 3:1, 3.4, 3–16, **3.44**.

paralysed   Not able to move.

parasite   Harmful organisms which cause disease, 2.2; malaria parasite, 10.7.

paronychia   A septic lesion beside a baby's finger nail, 26.48.

PAS   Another name for aminosalicylate which is a drug for TB, 3.23.

pass   To pass urine or stools means to get rid of them from the body.

passes stools too seldom   See constipation, 25.6; in babies, 26.30.

passive immunity   The immunity a child gets when he is given antibodies instead of making them for himself, 4.2.

patch   A large chronic skin lesion, 11.2, 12.3.

path   A small road.

paths of infection   Ways in which harmful organisms spread from one person to another, 2–6, 2.7.

patient   A sick person, 1.10.

patients per worker per day score   A measure of how much each health worker does, 6.7, 6.9.

PCM, PJM   This is now called protein-energy malnutrition or PEM, 7.7.

pellagra   A skin disease caused by lack of nicotinic acid, 11–16, 11.23.

pelvis   The hip bone, a bony basin at the bottom of the abdomen.

PEM   Protein-energy malnutrition, **7.7**, 7–11, 9.11, 24.12.

pemphigus neonatorum   A severe skin infection of babies, 11.4, 26.47.

penicillin   The most useful antibiotic drug, 3.4, 3.9, 3–12, **3.15**, etc.

– *reaction, sensitivity*   Severe symptoms coming on immediately after an injection of penicillin, 3.2, 3.15.

penis abnormal   23.11.

perforation   A hole. Perforated ear drum, **17.9**, 17.10, 17–10.

peritoneal cavity   The space containing the organs of the abdomen, **20.1**, 20–1, 20–5.

peritoneum   A thin sheet of tissue covering the inside of the abdomen, 20.1.

peritonitis   Acute infection in the peritoneal cavity, 20.2.

permanganate   See potassium permanganate, an antiseptic skin wash, 3.48.

pertussis   Whooping cough, 8.17.

petechiae   Dark red lesions caused by bleeding into the skin, 11.2, 11–2.

pharyngitis   Sore throat or upper respiratory infection, 8.6, 9.10, 18.11.

pharynx   The throat, 1–6, 1.9, 8–1, 8.2, **18–2**.

phenobarbitone   A drug for stopping fits, 3:1, 3.4, 3.9, 3–16, **3.43**.

phenol   Carbolic acid. A substance used in Pandy's test, 15.3, 15–6.

phimosis   Too narrow a hole in the foreskin, 23.11.

phlycten, phlyctenular conjunctivitis   13:1, **16.11**.

physiological jaundice   A harmless kind of jaundice in newborn babies, 26.23.

pink   Pale red.

pinworms   See threadworms, 21.5.

piperazine   A drug for treating *Ascaris* (roundworms) and threadworms, 3:1, 3–15, **3.28**, 21.3, 21.5.

pityriasis versicolor   See tinea versicolor, 11.14.

placebo   A harmless medicine which pleases a patient but does not cure his disease or remove his symptoms, **3.1**, 3.5, 3.9, 3.46, 8.5.

plasmodia   The organisms causing malaria, 10.7.

pleura   The thin smooth tissue covering the lungs, 8.2.

pleural cavity   The space round the lungs, 8–1, 8.2, 8–2.

plunger   The inside part of a syringe.

pneumonia   An acute infection of the lungs, 2.2, **8.15**, 8.21, 9.10, 10.6; pneumonia in newborn babies, 26.26.

poisoning   14.6, 14.7.

polio (poliomyelitis)   A virus disease which causes muscle wasting, 2:2; polio immunization, 4.8b, **24.4**, 24–3 to 24–5, 24.7.

porridge Any soft food for young children, 1.8, 2.12, 7.2.

posseting (regurgitation) The harmless bringing up of milk by babies, 26.27.

potassium One of the minerals in the body, 9.17.

potassium permanganate A purple powder used for treating septic skin infections, 3.48, 11–5.

PPF See procaine penicillin forte, 3.15.

prepacked drugs These are drugs put into small packets or bottles ready for a mother to take home with her, 3.4, 3–6.

presenting symptom Something, such as cough or diarrhoea, which makes a mother think her child is ill, 1.4, **5.6**.

pressure cooker A pot for sterilizing instruments in steam, 3:2, 6–9, **6.13**.

preterm Born too early, 24.12, **26.22**.

prevent To prevent a disease is to stop it happening, 2.1.

primary infection When two kinds of organism infect a child, one after the other, the first organism causes a primary infection, **2.6**, 8.3.

primary TB A child's first TB infection, 13.2.

procaine penicillin A kind of penicillin which only needs to be given once a day, 3.15.

procaine penicillin forte or 'PPF' A mixture of procaine penicillin and benzyl penicillin, 3.15.

prolapse To fall out, prolapsed rectum, 25–2, 25.7.

promethazine An antihistamine drug, 3–16, **3.45**, 8.5, 25.8.

protective foods Foods which help to prevent diseases, 2.12, 7.2.

protein The body-building part of some foods. Beans, milk and eggs contain protein, 1.8, 7.2.

protein energy malnutrition A group of diseases caused by lack of protein and energy food, also called PEM, 7.7.

protozoa The group of micro-organisms to which the malaria parasite, amoebae, and *Giardia* belong, 2–1, 2.2.

pulse The beating of the heart and arteries.

pulse rate The speed at which the heart beats, 9.18; newborn baby, 26.1.

pupil The 'hole' in the iris through which light gets inside the eye, 16–1, 16.2.

purge, purgatives Medicine to make a patient pass faeces, 3.30, 25.6, 26.30.

purulent Pus-like, containing pus, 1.10.

pus The yellow liquid in a septic lesion such as a boil, 2–3, 2.4.

pus cells White cells from the blood which have gone into a septic lesion to fight bacteria and pus, 2–3, 2.4.

pustule A small pus-filled abscess in the skin, 11.2.

pyloric stenosis 26.27.

pyoderma A name for several kinds of septic skin infection, 11.3, **11.6**.

pyogenic Septic, 'pus making', 1.10, 2.4.

pyomyositis Abscess in a muscle, 10.10, **24.5b**, 19.9.

pyrimethamine A drug used for preventing malaria, 3–14, **3.25**, 10.7, 14.6.

Q

quality How good something is. Here it means how good the care is that we give, 1.2, **6.7**.

– *control* Measuring how good the work of a clinic is, 6.8.

– *score* A measure of how good the care in a clinic is, 6.7, **6.8**.

quantity How much of something there is. Here it means how much child care we give, 1.2, **6.9**.

R

rash Many lesions on the skin, 1.10, 11.2; drug rash, 11.25, **11.28**.

reaction Sensitivity reaction, severe side effects caused by a drug, 3.2.

recognize To know what something is when you see it, 1.7.

recording Writing down what is found out about a child.

recording and reporting The tenth step in caring for a child, 3.4, 5.26, **6.1** to 6.6.

rectal temperature The temperature as shown by a thermometer in the rectum, 10.1, 10–3.

rectum The last part of the gut before the anus, 1–6, 20–1.

rectum fallen out (prolapse) 25–2, 25.7.

red, cells Blood cells filled with a red substance called haemoglobin, 1.9, 8.2, 8–3.

– *throat* Pharyngitis, 18.11.

– *urine* Probably haematuria, red urine babies, 26.58.

– *eyes* Probably conjunctivitis, 16.8, red eyes in babies, 26.40.

reduce To make something smaller, 1.7.

register A file or book, 6.3.

regurgitation in babies See posseting, 26.27.

rehydration Putting fluid back into a child, 9–9, 9.20 to 9.29.

rehydration outfit A tray containing the equipment for oral rehydration, 9–12.

relax When muscles relax they get longer, 1.10.

report, reporting To report something is to tell it to someone else, 6.1, **6.7 to 6.10**.

resistant An organism which is resistant to a drug cannot be killed by it, 3.11, **3.12**, 3.19.

respiration Breathing.

respiratory rate The speed of breathing, 8.9, **8.15**, 8.1, 8–9; newborn baby, 26.1.

restless Not able to stay still, 1.10.

resuscitation 'Making alive,' resuscitating a newborn baby, 26.3, 26–5.

retention Having a full bladder, but not being able to pass urine, 23.1.

retina The part of the eye which sends messages to the brain, 16–1, 16.2.

retraction See insuction, 8.9.

ribs   The curved bones round the sides of the chest, 8–1, 8.2.

rice water stools   Probably cholera, 9.7.

rigor   Severe shivering during a fever, 10.1.

ringworm   A chronic fungus disease of the skin, 3.48, **11.13.**

road to health chart   The weight chart, 6.2. the road to health is the space between the upper and lower lines on this chart, 7.1.

rooting reflex   A sign to see if a newborn baby is normal, 26.4.

roundworms   See *Ascaris,* 21.3, 21–3.

rules   See rules for good nutrition, 7.2.

running nose   See discharging nose, 8.7, 25.11.

S

saline   A solution made by adding half a level teaspoonful of salt to a cupful of water, 3.48, 10.3.

salt and sugar water   An oral rehydration fluid, 9–11, **9.21**, 9.22.

scabies   A skin infection caused by insects, 2–1, 3.48, 11–7, **11.10.**

scales   (i) A weighing machine.
(ii) Small thin pieces of dry skin that can be scratched off some 'scaly' skin lesions.

scalp   The skin of the head.

scalp vein set   The equipment for scalp vein infusion, **9–16**, 9.27.

scar   The white lesion that is left when a septic lesion or an injury heals, 11.2.

schistosomiasis (bilharzia)   A worm disease of the bladder or gut, 9.5, 23.6, 23–4, **23.8.**

sciatic nerve   A large nerve which runs from the buttock down the back of the leg, 3.5.

sclera   The white part of the eye, 1.9, 16–1, 16.2.

score   The number of marks or points that someone gets in a game or an exam, quality of care score, 6.7 to 6.11; dehydration score, 9.19.

scratching anus   Probably *Enterobius* (threadworm), 21.5, 21–5

– *skin*   Any itching skin lesion, 11.28.

scrotum   The bag containing the testes.

secondary infection   When two kinds of organism infect a child, the organisms which come second cause a secondary infection, 1.7, **2.6**, 8.3, 11.3.

segment   A piece of something, 21.4.

sensitive, sensitivity   (i) Drug sensitivity in a *patient* is a special kind of side effect in which a usually harmless drug causes severe symptoms, **3.2**, 3.40.
(ii) An *organism* which can be killed by a drug is sensitive to it, 3.2, 3.12.

septic, septic infection   Any infection where pus is formed, 2.4, 2–4, 3.13; septic lymphadenitis, 19.2; septic arthritis, 24.5; septic skin infections, 11.3.

septicaemia   A very serious disease in which bacteria grow in the blood ('blood poisoning'), 2.3, 2.4, 2–3, **11.3**; septicaemia in babies, **26.24.**

severe   Much, very large, very serious, 1–8, 1.10.

shivering   Perhaps a rigor caused by a fever, 10.1, 10.10.

shock   A child in shock is severely ill, cold and pale, 5:2, 9.18, **14.2.**

short case   A child who has a short history and examination, 5.27.

short process of the malleus   A part of one of the small bones of the middle ear, 17–3, 17.4.

shorthand   A way of writing something quickly and easily, 6:1.

sick   'Ill', not 'well', 1.10. Caring for a sick child Chapter Five; sick newborn baby, 26.6.

sickle cell anaemia   20.11, 20.12, **22.8.**

side effects   The harm that drugs sometimes cause, **3.2**, 3.14.

sign   Anything which can be seen, felt or heard to be abnormal in a child, such as a rash, a swelling or a cough, 1.10.

silver nitrate solution   Used for preventing gonococcal conjunctivitis in the newborn, 26.2, 26.40.

six rules of good nutrition   7.2, 7–2 to 7, 7.13.

six signs of lower respiratory infection   8.9.

skin, blisters   Skin vesicles, 11.2, 11.28, 14.3; vesicles in babies, 26.47.

– *disease*   Chapter Eleven, **11.28**; skin disease in babies, 26.43 to 48.

– *elasticity*   Examining the skin elasticity is a way of seeing if a child is dehydrated, 9–8, 9.18.

– *peeling*   In babies, 26.44.

rash   Many lesions on the skin, 1.10, 11.2; drug rash, 11.25, **11.28.**

– *sepsis*   Acute septic infections of the skin, 11.3.

– *scraping*   A special test to see if there are leprosy bacilli in the skin, 12.3.

– *sores*   See ulcers, 11.7.

– *ulcers*   11.7.

skull   The box of bones that contains the brain, 1.9.

sleeping   Best way for newborn babies to sleep, 26.5, 26–8.

sleepy   See drowsy. Abnormally sleepy newborn baby. Perhaps septicaemia, 26.24.

slide   A piece of glass on which blood, stool or urine are put so that they can be examined with a microscope, 5.19.

soak   Make wet with water.

small baby   A baby weighing less than 2 kg, 26.22.

sodium chloride   Ordinary salt, **9.17**, 9.21.

sodium thiosulphate   A chemical used to treat tinea versicolor, 11.14.

solution   Substances as salt dissolve in water to make a solution, 1.7.

sore eyes   Perhaps conjunctivitis, 10.6, 16.8; in babies, 26.39, 26.40.

– *lips*   18.10.

– *mouth*   18.9.

– *nipples*   26.11.

– *skin*   11.28.

– *throat*   18.11.

– *tongue*   Perhaps stomatitis, 18.9.

– vulva Vulvovaginitis, 23.10.

'sores' Skin ulcers, 11.7.

spasm (i) Strong sudden muscle contractions, 1.10, 3.44; spasms of tetanus, 18.16.

(ii) A sudden severe attack of coughing, 8.17.

spastic 'Stiff', spastic child, 24.15.

spatula A piece of wood or metal used for examining the throat, 18.2.

special care For small newborn babies, 26.22.

special care card and register A record of children for whom the clinic takes special care, 4.14, **6.3**, 6–3, 6–4, 6.8, 7.13.

special tests Special ways of examining a child or specimens from him, **5.19**.

specimen Blood, stools, urine, or CSF taken from a child for special tests, 5.19.

spectrum See broad spectrum antibiotic, 3.13.

speculum The part of an auriscope which goes into the ear, 17.3.

spine The vertebral column or bones of the back, 1.9, 15.1.

spinal cord A thick 'nerve' which goes down the body inside the bones of the spine, 15–1.

spirochaetes Snake-like bacteria which cause Vincent's stomatitis and yaws, 2–1, 2.2, 18.7.

spirit lamp 17–4.

spit To throw something out of the mouth, 1.9.

spleen An organ at the top left hand side of the abdominal cavity, 1–6, 1.9, 10.10; examining the spleen, **20.3**, 20–3, 20–4, 20–7.

spots on skin See skin rash, 1.10, 11.2; drug rash, 11.25, **11.28**.

spreading septic skin infection 11.3.

sputum Pus or mucus which is coughed up, 1.9, 8–4.

sputum positive A sputum positive patient has TB bacilli in his sputum.

squint Eyes looking in different directions, 24.14b.

stage One of the steps through which something goes, 1.7.

standard faecal smear A way of examining the stools for ova, 21.1, L 10.2.

staple food The most common food of a country, such as rice or cassava, 7.2.

sterile Something is sterile when there are no living organisms on it. 2.2b.

sterilizing needles and syringes 2.7, 3.5, 3.6, 15–3, **6.13**, 22–7.

sticky eyes Perhaps conjunctivitis, 10.6, **16.8**; conjunctivitis in babies, 26.39, **26.40**.

stiff neck A sign of meningitis, 15.6, 15–7.

stitching cuts 14.4, 14–4.

stomach Part of the gut which is widened to form a bag for food, 1–6, 1.9.

stomatitis Sore mouth, 10.6, 11.15, 18.3, **18.11**.

stools (faeces) The solid waste from the body, 1.10.

stools black Probably iron medicines, 3.33; perhaps digested blood in the stools, 26.33.

– red Blood in the stools, **9.3**, 9.4, 9.5, 25.7b; babies, 26.33.

– like rice water Probably cholera, 9.7.

– watery Diarrhoea, 2.10; Chapter Nine, **9.31**; diarrhoea in babies, **26.32**.

stopped breathing, eating, growing etc. See not breathing etc.

strangulated A strangulated hernia cannot be reduced (pushed back), 20.5.

streptomycin A drug used for treating TB, and sometimes for septic infections, 3:1, 3.11, 3.12, 3–13, **3.22**, 8.12, 13.6.

stridor Noisy breathing, 5:2, **8.9**, 8:1, 8–5, 8.21.

Strongyloides A worm which lives in the gut, 3.29, 9.5; creeping eruption, 11.21, **21.6**.

stye An abscess on the eyelid, 16.3, 16–5.

stylet The wire that goes inside a needle, 15–2, 15.3.

substance Something which is the same all through, such as sugar, or water and which can be cut up without being spoilt, 1.7.

sugar water A solution of four heaped teaspoonfuls of glucose or sugar in a cupful of water (5–10 per cent), 26.42. *Not* the same as *salt* and sugar water (SSW), 9.21, or saline, 3.48, 10.3.

sulphadiazine One of the sulphonamide family of drugs, 3.14.

sulphadimidine The most useful of the sulphonamide family of drugs, 3.4, 3.7, 3.8, 3.9, 3–12, **3.14**, 8.13, 8.14, 8.15.

sulphadoxine with pyrimethamine compound tablets A drug for treating chloroquine resistant malaria, 3:1, 3.25, 10.7.

sulphonamides The family of drugs to which sulphadimidine, sulphadiazine and 'triple sulpha' belong, 3.14.

sulphur ointment A drug for scabies, 3.48, 11.10.

sunken eyes A sign of dehydration, 5:2, **9.18**.

sunken fontanelle A sign of dehydration, 9.18.

supplementary food A protein containing food for malnourished children, 7.6.

supplies Things such as drugs and bandages which are used in a clinic.

suppression A way of using drugs to prevent the harmful effects of malaria, **3.25**, 10.7.

swab A piece of gauze or cotton wool used for cleaning.

swabbing Wiping away discharge, swabbing ears, 17–4, 17.5.

swallowed foreign body 25.4.

– poison, pills, kerosine etc. 14.6.

swelling, swollen Enlarged, larger than normal, Chapter Nineteen, **19.9**.

– abdomen 20.8, 20–8, 20.9; babies, 26.24.

– at the anus Probably rectal prolapse, 25.7.

– bone 19.9, 24.5.

– (engorged) breasts 26.10.

– behind the ear Perhaps mastoiditis, 17.11.

– under one or both ears Perhaps mumps, 19.4.

– beside a newborn baby's eye 26.41.

– eyes Perhaps conjunctivitis, 10.6, 16.8; con-

junctivitis in babies, 26.39, 26.40; eyelids, 19.5, 19.8.

– *face* 19.5, 19.8.

– *feet* **19.7**, 19.9.

– *fontanelle* A sign of meningitis, 15.6.

– *hands and fingers* Perhaps the 'hand foot syndrome', 22.8.

– *of hands and feet in newborn* Perhaps hypothermia, 26.25.

– *in inguinal region (groin)* 20.5.

– *injection site (place)* Injection abscess, 3.6.

– *legs or feet* 19.7, **19.8**.

– *lips* 18.10.

– *lymph nodes* 19.2; TB lymph nodes, 19.3; swollen lymph nodes after BCG vaccine, 4.6.

– *neck* 19.9, 19–5.

– *scrotum* Perhaps inguinal hernia, 20.5; swollen scrotum in babies, 26.59.

– *of the skin during birth* Perhaps caput succedaneum, 26.4.

– *umbilicus* Perhaps umbilical hernia, 20.4, 20.7.

symmetrical The same on both sides of the body, 1.10, 11.2.

symptom Something, such as pain or diarrhoea, that a person feels wrong with himself, or that a mother sees as wrong with her child, 1.10.

symptomatic drugs Drugs which stop symptoms, but do not remove the disease which caused them, 3.1, 3.39 to 46.

syndrome A group of signs and symptoms. Nephrotic syndrome, 19.7; Down's syndrome, 24.13.

syringe 3–8, 3.5, 3.6, 22–7.

– *and needle carried infections* 2–6, 2.7.

– *jaundice* A kind of jaundice carried by infected syringes, 22.11.

syringing ears Washing away wax and discharge, 17.6.

syrup A sweet sugary medicine, 3.4.

system Several parts of the body which work together to do the same job. For example, the urinary system makes and stores urine, 1.9.

T

tablet A way of giving solid drugs, 3–4.

Taenia saginata The beef tapeworm; *Taenia solium* is the pork tapeworm, 21.4, 21–4.

talipes 'Club foot' A congenital abnormality of the foot, 26–33, 26.52.

tally A way of counting by making marks and adding them up, 6.4, 6–4.

tantrums 25.2.

tapeworm A long white worm that lives in the gut, 3.30, **21.4**, 21–4.

TB (tuberculosis) A chronic infection, 2:2, 2–6, 8.1, 8–4, 8.16, Chapter 13, treatment, 13.6, **13.7**; TB in a baby's mother, 26.66.

– *of bones and joints* 13–1, 24.6.

– *lymph nodes* TB lymphadenities, 8–4, 13–1, 13.1, 19–2, 19.3.

– *meningitis* 13.1, 13–1, **15.6**.

– *of the spine* 24–7.

TCE (tetrachlorethylene) A clear liquid used for treating hookworm infections, 3:1, 3.9, 3–15, **3.27**.

teaching, mothers 'Explanation and education' the 'eighth step', 5.24.

– *our helpers* 1.5.

– *ourselves* 1.4.

tears coming from a baby's eyes 26.41.

teaspoon A spoon holding about 5 ml, 3–1, 3.4, 3–7.

teething New teeth coming through into the mouth 25.2c, 26.65.

temperature How hot or cold something is, 10.1, 10.2.

ten steps These are the steps or stages in caring for a sick child, 5.1, 5–1.

tender A tender part of the body hurts when it is touched.

testis absent, undescended 26.59b.

– *swollen* In newborn baby, hydrocoele, 26–35, 26.59.

tetanus A disease in which there are abnormal muscle contractions, 3.44, 15.1, 18–10, 18–11, **18.16**; umbilical tetanus, 26.37; tetanus in babies, 26.42.

tetanus antitoxin Antibodies for preventing tetanus, 3.2, 4.2, 18.16.

tetanus toxoid A vaccine for preventing tetanus, **4.3**, 18.16, 26.42.

tetrachlorethylene See TCE, 3.27.

tetracycline A drug used for treating septic infections, 3:1, 3.9, 3–12, **3.17**.

thermometer An instrument measuring temperature, 10.1, 10–1 to 10–3.

thiacetazone A drug used for treating TB, 3–13, 3.19, 3.21, 13.6.

thigh The upper part of the leg.

thin Perhaps an 'underweight child', 7.8, **7.13**, if part of the body only is thin, see 24.8, thin newborn babies, 26.21.

thorax The chest.

threadworms *Enterobius,* small thin worms, 3.28, **21.5**, 21–4, 21–5.

throat Chapter Eighteen, examining the throat, 18.2.

thrush A fungus disease causing white lesions in the mouth, 2–1, 18.3, 18–4, **18.5**; thrush in babies, 26.55.

tiabendazole A drug used for treating some kinds of worm infections, 3–15, 3.29, 11.21.

Tinct. Benzoin Co. BP A sticky fluid used for making adhesive strapping stick to skin, 26.52.

tinea versicolor A harmless fungus disease of the skin, 11.14.

tissues The different pieces from which the body is made, such as liver tissue, muscle tissue, skin tissue, etc.

toe Extra toe in newborn baby, 26.54.

tone The normal contractions (shortening) of muscles, 1.10.

tongue has white lesions Perhaps thrush, 18.15; in babies, 26.55.

tongue tied 26.53.

tonic A useless medicine, 3.9.

tonsils Two special organs like lymph nodes at each side of the back of the mouth, 8.8, **18.2**.

tonsillar lymph nodes The nodes under the angles of the jaw, 5.17, **18.2**, 18–3, 19–1.

tonsillitis Inflammation of the tonsils, 8.6, 8.20, **18.11**, 18.13.

tooth abscess 19–4, 19.5.

total attendances The number of patients coming to the clinic during a month or a year, 6.7.

toxins Poisons, especially those made by bacteria, 2.3, 4.2, 4–2, 18.16.

trachea A tube which takes air from the larynx to the lungs, 1–6, 8–1, 8.2, 8–2, 8–4.

trachoma A chronic virus infection of the conjunctiva, 16.9.

traditional medicines 'Local medicines' made from plants or animals, **2.9**, 2–10, 5–4.

traditional practitioner A person who treats patients in a traditional or local way, and who does not use 'modern medicine', 1.5, 5.8.

transparent Easily seen through, like water or glass.

travel sickness Vomiting, or the feeling of wanting to vomit, caused by travelling in a car or bus, 3.45, 25.8.

treatment Doing things to a child to make him well, 5.23.

triceps The muscle at the back of the upper arm, 7.13.

Trichuris The whipworm, 3.29, 9.5, 21.1, 21–4, **21.7**, 25–2, 25.7.

triple vaccine See DPT vaccine, 4.3, 4.9.

tube feeding In malnutrition, 7.11; passing a nasogastric tube, 9.24; tube feeding newborn babies, 26.18, 26–20.

tuberculoid leprosy A kind of leprosy, 12–1, 12.2.

tuberculosis See TB, Chapter Thirteen.

tumbu fly A fly which lays its eggs in the skin, 11.12.

tumour A disease caused by the abnormal growth of a tissue, 2.1, 2:1.

turbid Cloudy, not clear like clean water.

typhoid fever A serious long lasting fever, 3.18, **10.8**.

U

ulcer Any break in the skin or mucosa so that the tissue under it is no longer covered, 1.9, 11–6, **11.7**.

– after BCG vaccine 4.6.

umbilicus, umbilical bleeding Perhaps haemorrhagic disease, 26.38.

– care at birth 26.2.

– cord The cord which joins a mother to her child, 26.2, 26–2, 26–4.

– hernia A swelling at the umbilicus, 20–5, 20.7, 20–7.

– not healing 26.33.

– red Skin round the umbilicus red. Perhaps septic infection, 26.34, 26–26.

– sticky Probably infected, 26.34.

unconscious An unconscious child seems to be asleep, but cannot be woken up, 1.10, **14.8**.

underweight An underweight child weighs less than he should for his age, and is below the bottom line on his weight chart, **7.8**, 7–8.

undescended testis 26.59b.

unhappy child 7.10, **25.2**.

UNICEF United Nations (International) Children's (Emergency) Fund, 3.10.

upper respiratory infection 'URI', **8.6** to 8.8.

ureters Tubes which take urine from the kidneys to the bladder, 1–7, 1.9.

urethra A tube which takes urine from the bladder outside the body, 1–7, 1.9.

urgency Wanting to pass urine quickly, 23.1, **23.9**.

URI Upper respiratory infection, 8.6; acute 8.7; chronic URI, 8.8; pharyngitis, tonsillitis, **18.11**.

urine, urinary The fluid a child passes. Chapter Twenty-three.

– abnormal colour 23.1.

– examination 23.2.

– infection 9.10, **23.4**.

– none passed or too little passed In rehydration, 9.18; nephritis, 23.7; after birth, 26.57.

– red In older children probably haematuria, 23.9; in babies probably normal, 26.58.

– system The parts of the body which make and store urine, 1.9.

urticaria A raised red itchy rash, 3.45, **11.24**.

uterus The organ in which a child grows while he is inside his mother.

V

vaccine A 'medicine' made from micro-organisms which can be used to prevent infection, 2.8, 3.9, **4.2**, 4–4, 4–5, 4–8.

vaginal bleeding 26.56.

varicella Chickenpox, 11.16.

vertebral column The bones of the back, 1.9.

vertigo A feeling that the world is going round.

vesicles Skin lesions filled with fluid, 11.2, 11–3, **11.28**, 14.3.

– in babies 26.47.

vessel A tube containing blood or lymph, 1.9.

vial A small drug bottle with a rubber cap, 3–4, 3.5.

vicious circle Two things which make one another worse.

– of malnutrition and infection 7.5, 7–8.

– of malnutrition and diarrhoea 9–7, 9.11.

– of too little milk in the breast and a baby who is too weak to suck 26.8, 26–9.

Vincent's stomatitis A severe mouth infection, 18.3, **18.7**.

viruses The smallest micro-organisms, 2–1, 2.2.

visual aids 'Pictures' that are helpful in teaching, 1.3, 2.11.

vitamins Substances which a child needs to eat in very small amounts to keep his body healthy, 1.8, 2.12, 3.35, 4.11, 16.13, 16.14, **16.15**.

vitamin A A vitamin which prevents night blindness,

xerophthalmia and keratomalacia, 3.35, 4.11, 16–10, 16.13, **16.5**.

vitamin B A group of vitamins which prevents pellagra, and some other diseases, 3.36.

vitamin K A vitamin which prevents haemorrhagic disease of the newborn, 3.38.

vomit, vomiting To bring up food out of the mouth, **20.14**.

– *and abdominal pain* 20–9, 20.14.

– *attacks* 20.14.

– *blood* A little blood is common in any kind of vomiting. It is seldom serious.

– *blood in babies* 26–25, 26.28.

– *in the bus* Travel sickness, 25.8.

– *and diarrhoea* **9.31**, 20.14.

– *milk* Perhaps posseting, 26.27.

– *caused by drugs* 3.4.

– *green or yellow*. Or with much force, of bad smelling, or like faeces. Signs that vomiting is serious, 20.14.

– *making a child vomit* 14.6, 14–7, 14–8.

– *newborn baby* 26.24.

– *rehydration fluid* 9.23.

– *worms* 21.3.

vulva The skin around a girl's genital organs, 23.10.

vulvovaginitis Inflammation of the vulva and vagina, 23.10.

W

warts Small chronic thickenings of the skin, 11–14, 11.20.

washing children 11–16.

– *hands* 5.18, 26–22.

wasting Severe thinness of all or part of the body, 1.10; wasting of the whole body, 7.13; wasting of an arm or leg, 1–9, 24.8.

water for washing 5.14, 11.1.

– *needs of a baby* 26.16.

weighing The first of the 'ten steps', 5.1, **5–3**.

scale 3:2, 3.48.

weight chart or road to health chart A special chart for finding out how well a child is growing, 1.8, 2.8, 2.12, 4.1, 6–1, 6.2, 7.1, 7–1; weight chart for recording anaemia, 22.2.

well (i) Thoroughly, good.

(ii) Healthy A 'well' child may have local lesions (2.4), but he does not have the general signs that show he is 'ill', 1.10, **5:2**, 5.15, 5–5, 5–6. Well child Chapter Four.

wheezing The noise that a child with asthma makes when he breathes, 3.2, **8.10**, 8.13, 8.14, 8:1, 8.18.

white cells Cells in the blood which fight bacteria, 1.9, 2–3, 2.4.

Whitfield's ointment See benzoic acid ointment, 11.13.

whooping cough 3.18, 8.10, **8.17**, 8.20.

worm load The number of worms a child has in his body, 21.1.

worms (helminths) 2.2, 3.27 to 31, 4.11; Chapter Twenty-one, 20–8.

worried mother 25.1.

X

xerophthalmia One of the stages in the eye disease caused by lack of vitamin A 3.35, **16.13**.

Y

yellow bubbly diarrhoea stools Perhaps giardiasis, 9.6.

yellow eyes A sign of jaundice, 5.17, 22.10, **22.13**; in a newborn baby, 24.12, **26.23**, 26.24.

yellow teeth These may be caused by tetracycline, 3.17.

Appendix

A long case—the story of Okeke

Okeke, a child of about two, is carried in by his mother.

Step 1—weighing. Okeke's mother carries a weight chart. His chart has been filled in by a helper. It shows the first dot for his weight.

Step 2—history. *'Biku welu oche. Gabaghalu anyi maka ichelu odu. Ginwa bu Nwanyi Obiozo. Unu bi na akuku Ogbete?'* The family are Ibos, and although we cannot speak this language we have learnt enough of it to greet patients. We shall have to take the rest of the history with the help of someone who can speak both our language and Ibo. We have said very politely. *'Please sit down. We are sorry that you have been waiting. (Looking at his mother's name on his weight chart) You are Mrs Obiozo. And you live in house number two in Ogbete?*

'Hullo Okeke, we will soon make you well again. Here is a toy for you to play with.'

'You are his mother? I see that this is the first time that you have come to our clinic. So he weighs 8 kg. Let us fill in his weight chart. How old is he? When is his birthday?'

'Yes, I am his mother. I do not know how old he is. I do not know when his birthday is.'

'Don't worry, Mrs Obiozo, we can easily find out his age.'

We find out his age with a local events calendar (N1.6e) which we have made for our district. We find that Okeke is about two years old, and is below the road to health. There is not time to explain the weight chart to Mrs Obiozo now. We will explain it later.

We have already seen several things about Okeke and his mother. He looks moderately thin and unhappy, and is sucking a comforter (dummy, teat). He is restless and not interested in what is happening around him. He is not completely 'well', or very 'ill' (5.15). He is probably in Stage C in Table 5:2. His clothes and his mother's clothes are old, poor, and clean.

Presenting symptoms. *'What symptoms has he?'*
'Okeke has diarrhoea and his body feels hot.' These are the symptoms he has now, or his presenting symptoms. Section 9.31 is the 'Caring for . . . .' section for a child with diarrhoea, so we turn to this section and keep it open beside us.
'Anything more?'
'Yes, he coughs.' Cough is probably less important to her than diarrhoea or hotness of the body. She did not say anything about it until we asked if there were any other symptoms.
'Anything more?'
'No, that is all.'

Quantity or severity of the presenting symptoms. *'How many stools has he passed today?'* This tells us how serious his diarrhoea is.

'He has had diarrhoea for a long time.' She has answered another question. She has not answered the question we asked her.

'Thank you, I will ask about that in a minute. But, first,

OKEKE BEING BROUGHT TO THE CLINIC

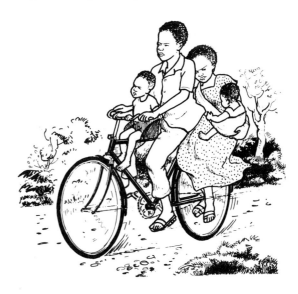

tell me how many stools he has passed today.' We are trying to get the answer to the question we asked, not the answer to another question.

'Sorry, he has already passed three diarrhoea stools this morning already.' Now she has answered our question. His diarrhoea is probably moderate.

Quality of the presenting symptoms. 'What do his stools look like?
'Yellow and liquid.'
'Is there any blood or mucus on them?' The Ibo word for mucus is 'ife naalolo'. Our interpreter uses it. If Okeke has blood in his stools, he may have dysentery (9.5).
'No.'

Time of the presenting symptoms. 'How long has he had diarrhoea?' 'When were his stools last normal?' These are both ways of asking—how long?
'His stools have not been normal since before the harvest last year.' So he must have had diarrhoea for at least a year.
'Does he have diarrhoea all the time?'
'No, his diarrhoea comes and goes.' The chronic diarrhoea of malnutrition (9.12) often does this.
'Is his diarrhoea becoming better or worse?' Knowing this may be important in deciding how to manage him.
'Sometimes his diarrhoea is worse. It has been worse these last two days, especially yesterday. Today it is bad again.' We now know that he has had diarrrhoea for about a year, and it has become worse during the last few days. We already know he is underweight, so we can begin to make a diagnosis. He might have chronic diarrhoea caused by malnutrition, perhaps with acute diarrhoea and dehydration also. Now we can ask about his other symptoms.
'How long has he had hotness of the body?'
'For about two or three days.'
'Tell me Mrs Obiozo, does he wake you up at night with his cough?'
'He does not cough much at night. He coughs in the day sometimes.' So his cough is mild.

Other important symptoms. 'Is he vomiting?' If he is vomiting, oral dehydration may be difficult.
'No.' So he will probably drink fluid. Perhaps he has a gut infection which is causing his fever. We must also look for diseases that can cause both diarrhoea and fever, such as tonsillitis and otitis media (17.9).
'How much urine is he passing, Mrs Obiozo?'
'He passes very little urine now. His urine is very dark.' This is a sign of dehydration. Notice that we are calling Mrs Obiozo by name. Most patients like being called by name. It shows that we are interested in them.

SPEAK TO PATIENTS BY NAME

Past treatment. 'What treatment have you been giving him Mrs Obiozo?'
'I have been giving him as little to eat and drink as I can.' This is the worst thing she could do. Mrs Obiozo will need careful health education.
'Have you given him any medicine for his diarrhoea?'
'Yes, I have been giving him akwukwo achara na manu anu.' This is local mixture of ground herbs and honey.

Birth. 'Mrs Obiozo, was his birth normal?'
'He was very small, but he sucked strongly and quickly soon after birth. He is not growing now.'

Past history. 'Has he been ill before?'
'Yes, about nine months ago he had fever and fits. I took him to hospital. The nurse said that he had malaria of the brain. Since then he has not been the same. He does not walk, or say any words.' Now that she knows that we are interested in Okeke, she is telling us what is worrying her. She is worried because Okeke is two years old and is not walking or saying any words. The milestone for walking is 18 months. The milestone for saying single words is 21 months. He probably had cerebral malaria, and may be backward because of it (10.7).
'Thank you for telling me about that Mrs Obiozo. I hope that you will come and talk to us about it another time, when there are fewer children waiting.' It is useful to ask a mother to come back another day if we need her for more time and her child's illness can wait.

Nutrition history. 'Do you breast-feed Okeke?'
'I stopped breast-feeding him about a year ago.' This is too early. A child who drinks no other kind of milk should breast-feed until he is about two years old.
'What do you give him with his porridge, Mrs Obiozo?'
'Ofe okazi.' This is a thin soup with vegetables. From this we see that Okeke is not fed often enough. He is not given any protein food with his porridge. We have been to the market and found that in our district the 'best protein buy' (N 6.4) is mayi manyi (bean cake). Okeke needs more energy food also, so fried bean cake would be a good food for him.
'Does Okeke like fried bean cake?'
'Yes.' Okeke is not fed often enough, and his mother does not add a protein food to his porridge. We must teach Mrs Obiozo how to feed Okeke when we get to Step 8.

What has happened to his brothers and sisters? 'Where does Okeke come in the family?'
'He is my youngest child, and I don't want to become pregnant again.'
'How many other children have you had Mrs Obiozo?'
'Seven.'
'How many are living?'
'Four.' Now we know that three children have died. But we have not asked her this.
'Let us write the names and ages of all three children on the back of Okeke's weight chart.'

'Has anyone else in the family got diarrhoea, or fever?'
'No.'
'Or a cough?'
'An uncle who came to stay some months ago has a bad cough.' This may be important. Although Okeke's cough does not seem serious, his uncle may have TB (13.3). So we need to observe Okeke carefully. If we had never asked this question about cough, we would not have known about Okeke's uncle.

What kind of family has Okeke got? 'Mrs Obiozo, what is your husband's job?'
'He works on a farm.'
'He is a good man and he gives me all the money he earns.' We know that the family are poor, but not very poor. The family also seems happy.

House, water, and latrine. 'Where do you fetch your water from and what kind of latrine have you got?' Because Okeke has diarrhoea the family's house is less important than the water they have, and the latrine they use.
'I buy clean water in buckets, and we use pit latrines.' So they have some clean water.

Step 3—examination. Early in the history we saw that Okeke was not very 'well', or very 'ill' either. He is thin, but not thin enough to be marasmic (7.9). He is also irritable and not interested in what is going on around him. Now, we see that his eyes are mildly sunken (9.18). His lips and conjunctivae moderately pale (22.1). He is not jaundiced. His breathing is normal. His hair is normal and his neck is not stiff (15.6). He has a few enlarged but not tender lymph nodes under the corners of his jaw, under his arms, and in his groins.

The skin of his abdomen has lost some of its elasticity (9.18). We can just feel his spleen. The skin around his anus is sore. There are some infected scabies lesions on his arms and legs.

His ears and throat are normal, but his mouth is dry. His temperature is 37·5°C. Okeke can stand holding a chair, but he will not walk (24.1).

Step 4—special tests. We get some stool to examine by putting a short piece of plastic tubing into Okeke's anus. A laboratory assistant reports—liquid yellow stools, 4 hookworm ova in a standard stool smear. Haemoglobin 9 g/dl. Blood Slide—*P. falciparum* +.

Step 5—diagnosis. We see that Okeke is nearly two kilos below the road to health. So he is **moderately malnourished**. He is also **moderately dehydrated** and **mildly anaemic**. He has a few **malaria** parasites in his blood and a large spleen. He has infected **scabies** which is causing **chronic septic lymphadenitis**. He has a **mild hookworm infection** (22.1). He has **chronic diarrhoea**. Malnutrition is probably causing his diarrhoea, but he now has **acute diarrhoea** also. He is also **backward**, and there is also someone in his family with a cough which

OKEKE'S RECORDS WRITTEN ON HIS CONTINUATION CARD

things describing a symptom bracketed together

June 30   ×3 today   blood o

C.O   DIARRHOEA ———— 1 year   mucos o

presenting symptoms   comes & goes
in capitals   worse 3/7

'HOTNESS OF BODY — 3 weeks   Vomiting o
             urine ↓

Cough — mild   signs and
            symptoms not

PT   Starved, not given fluids   found are
             also recorded

PH   Fever and fits 9/12 ago ? cerebral malaria
    Not walking or talking

NH   Breast fed until 1 year
    Not given protein foods

FH   Youngest of 7   dehydration
    3 died   signs bracketed
    Father farmer   together
    Uncle has chronic cough

OE   'Ill' +   38.5°C   (eyes sunken
    anaemia ++   mouth dry
    thin +   skin elasticity ↓
    scabies +   drinks well
           haemoglobin
    spleen +   shows him to be
           less anaemic

Lab   Hb 9g   than we thought
    BS P. falciparum +
    Stool 4 HW ova

this is the 'Medical Shorthand' in Table 6.1

D = (1) Acute on chronic diarrhoea
    (2) Malnutrition ++
    (3) Dehydration ++
    (4) Anaemia +
    (5) Malaria   (8) Backward
    (6) Scabies   (9) ?? TB
    (7) Hookworm

              Special care   (S)

R/   SSW
    chloroquine ——no need to say how
             much drug given unless

TCA   July 2   there is some reason to
          sign your records

FP   Next visit   M.H.K.

these records have been spread out to make them easier to read, they should be much closer than this so that paper is saved

305

might be TB. Okeke might seem to be very unfortunate to have so many diseases. But many children have more than one disease. Some children have as many diseases as Okeke.

He comes from a poor family, but a good one. His mother loves him, but she has been giving him the wrong treatment for his diarrhoea—too little fluids, and not enough food.

Step 6—management. Now we can ask ourselves the management questions in Section 5.21.

A *'Are we sure of his diagnosis?'*

'Yes.' We are sure of his diarrhoea and dehydration. We are also sure that treatment of his other diseases can wait.

B *'How ill is he now?'*

'He is moderately ill.'

C *'How far away does he live from the clinic?'*

'He lives about half a kilometre from the clinic.'

D *'If he is not treated, will he recover or become worse quickly or slowly?'*

'His dehydration might become worse quickly.'

E *'Can we treat him?'*

'Yes.'

From this 'Management possibilities 3 and 8' (5.21) would probably be best for Okeke. We can manage him at home by giving him oral fluid (9.20) for his dehydration. We can teach his mother how to feed him. We can suppress his malaria with pyrimethamine. Fortunately, he lives near the clinic, so we can observe him carefully. His mother can bring him back if his dehydration becomes worse. When his growth curve starts climbing he may start walking. He should also come to see Dr Okonkwo, when he next visits our clinic.

Step 7—treatment. Let us give Mrs Obiozo the 'rehydration outfit' shown in Figure 9–12. She makes a cup of salt and sugar water. Okeke drinks it thirstily (9.18), so rehydration is easy.

Step 8—explanation and education. *'Okeke has several troubles, but do not worry. When you go home, make some more "salt and sugar water" in the way you made it here. Let him drink as much as he can. He weighs 8 kilos, so he needs at least eight cups every day until his stools are normal (9.22). Give him plenty of food as soon as he wants to eat. Can you get him any milk?'*

'Yes my sister has a cow. She will give us some milk for a few weeks.'

'Good, give him plenty of milk. Give him porridge three or four times a day, and add some protein food to it. Akara (bean balls) are the 'best buy' in the market this month. Fry them. Oil is a good energy food for him. If you feed Okeke, he may soon start walking and talking. I am very interested in him. Please bring him to the clinic on Monday, July the 2nd when Dr Okonkwo comes. When he is stronger he may need some more treatment. Bring him back quickly if he starts vomiting, or if his diarrhoea gets worse, or if his eyes look sunken. Bring him back at any time, even at night. I live next to the clinic.'

Step 9—family planning. *'One more thing Mrs Obiozo, do you want to know about family planning? We are busy now, let us talk about it when you come again?'*

'Yes, I should like to. I have always been frightened of the clinic before, but I shall not be after today.'

'Have you any more questions Mrs Obiozo?'

'No. Thank you so much. This is the first time that anyone has been so kind to my children. I shall tell all my friends what good health workers have come to help us.'

Step 10—recording and reporting. The figure shows Okeke's continuation card and the records we have made on it. Notice how his presenting symptom 'DIARRHOEA' is in capital letters. The answers to the 'quantity', 'quality', and 'time' questions are in brackets beside it. There is a tick beside the things we have looked for and found normal. There is a '0' beside the symptoms we have asked about and not found. All his diagnoses are listed.

Because Okeke might be backward we have put him on our special care register (6.3).

Epilogue

Each sick child who comes to see us might be our child. We must care for him as if he was our child. This book tells us how we *could* care for him. So we must care for him like this or better. We must learn how to care for children, and we must teach our helpers (1.5). We may not be able to do everything in the book, but we can probably do more than we do now. We may have to change what we do, and do new things. For example, we may have to change the way we give antibiotics (3.13). If we have no special care register (6.3), we must start one. If we have never given nasogastric drips (9.24), we must start giving them. If we don't give integrated care (6.8), we must start giving it. Change is not easy. Often, we don't like it. But we must try to change, so that we can give *good* quality care to the children who need it. We must give some care to *all* our children, and more care to those in special need.

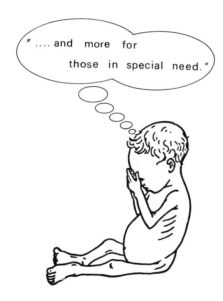

" .... and more for those in special need."

Use this for other drugs

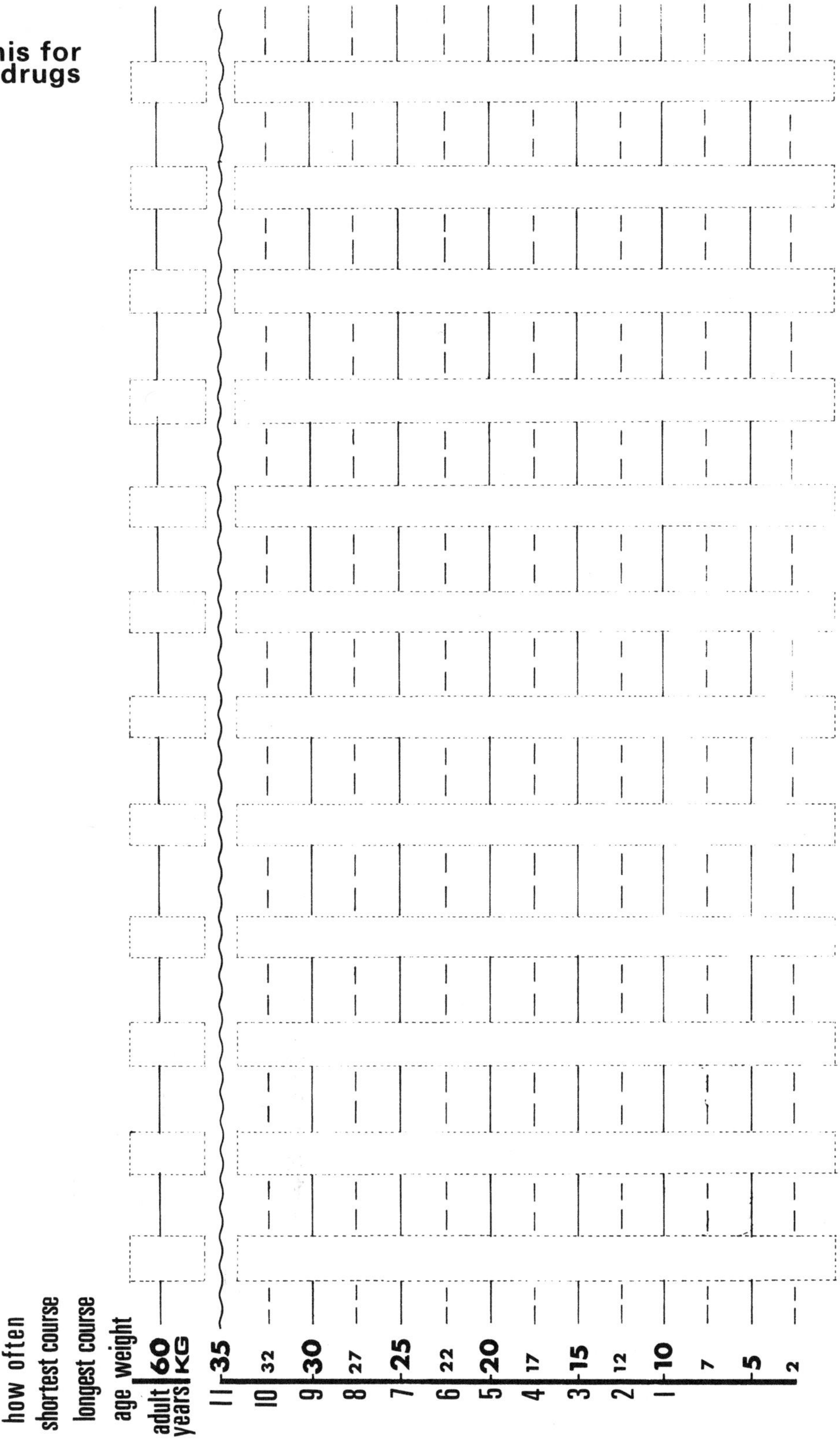

how often
shortest course
longest course
age weight

adult	**60**
	KG
11	**35**
10	32
9	**30**
8	27
7	**25**
6	22
5	**20**
4	17
3	**15**
2	12
1	**10**
	7
	5
	2

309

DRUGS FOR SEPTIC INFECTIONS

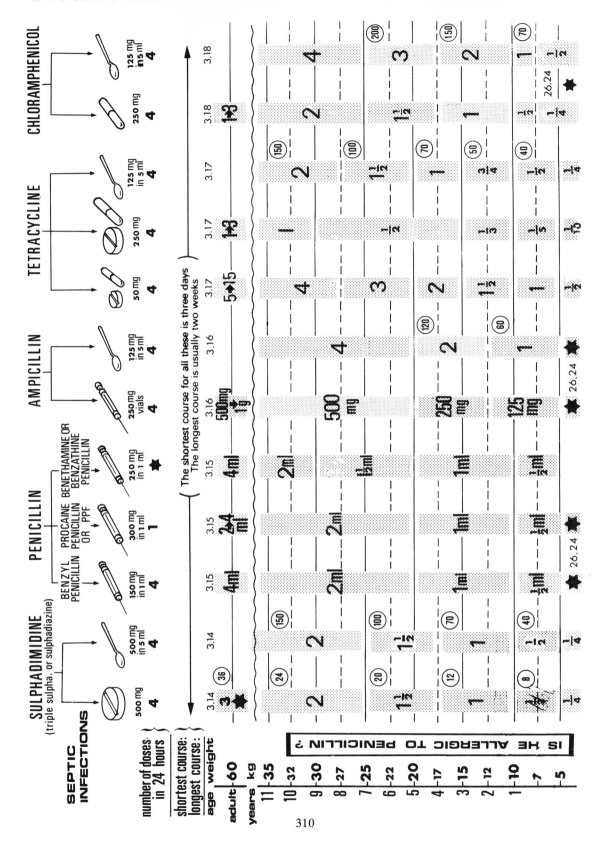

DRUGS FOR TB AND LEPROSY

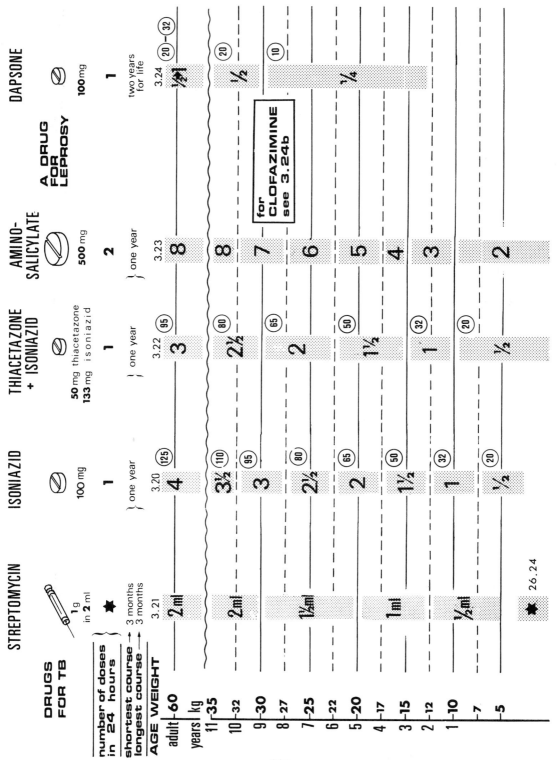

DRUGS FOR MALARIA AMOEBA GIARDIA

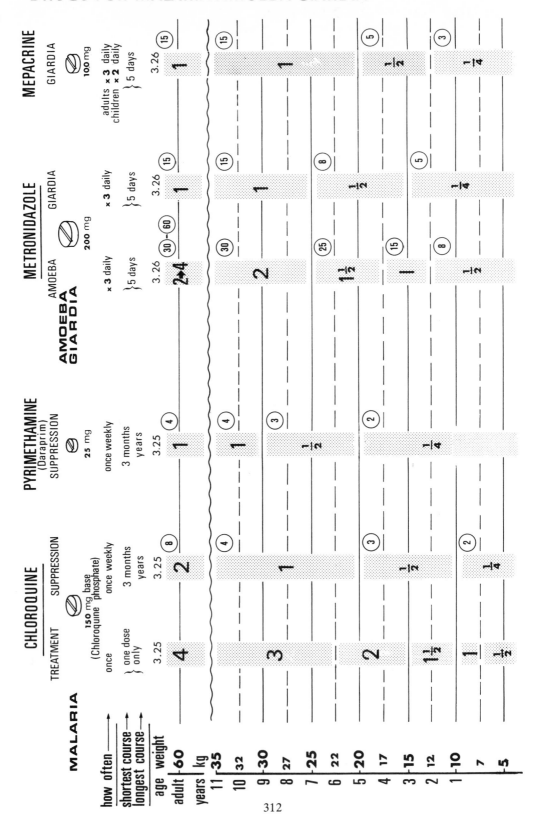

DRUGS FOR WORMS

WORMS	TCE hookworms	BEPHENIUM hookworms	PIPERAZINE Ascaris	PIPERAZINE Ascaris	PIPERAZINE threadworms	PIPERAZINE threadworms	TIA-BENDAZOLE Strongyloides Trichuris	NICLOSAMIDE tapeworms	PYRANTEL PAMOATE	NIRID-AZOLE Schistosomes
form	clear liquid	packet powder 5g	500 mg	500 mg in 5 ml	500 mg	500 mg in 5 ml	500 mg	500 mg	250 mg in 5 ml	500 mg
how often / course	{ one dose only	{ one dose only	{ one dose only	{ one dose only	x 1 daily one week	x 1 daily one week	x 2 daily 3 days	{ one dose only	{ one dose only ★	x 2 daily one week
ref	3.27	3.27	3.28	3.28	3.28	3.28	3.29	3.30	3.30b	3.31
age / weight										
adult 60 / 35 kg	3½ ml	1	8		2→4		3 (18)	4	15 ml	1½ (18)
11 / 35–32	3½ ml		7	7	3 (21)	3	2 (12)	3	7 ml	1 (14)
10 / 32	3 ml									
9 / 30	3 ml									
8 / 27										
7 / 25	2½ ml	1	6	6	2 (14)	2	1½ (10)		6 ml	½ (8)
6 / 22										
5 / 20	2 ml		4	4	1½ (10)	1½	1 (6)	2	5 ml	
4 / 17										
3 / 15	1½ ml	½	3	3	1 (7)	1	½ (4)		4 ml	½ (4)
2 / 12										
1 / 10	1 ml		2	2	½ (5)	½	¼	1	3 ml	¼
/ 7										
5										

SOME SYMPTOMATIC DRUGS

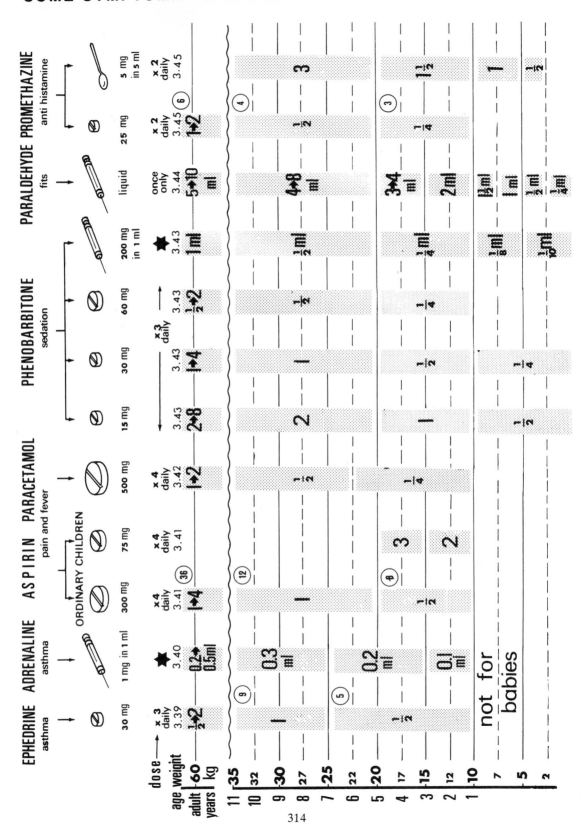

314

INJECTIONS OF CHLOROQUINE AND QUININE

Chloroquine

2 ml
1½
1
½

weight in kg

4 5 6 7 8 9 10 11 12 13 14 15 16 17 18 19 20

CHLOROQUINE
200 mg in 5 ml

Quinine

5 ml
4
3
2
1

weight in kg

4 5 6 7 8 9 10 11 12 13 14 15 16 17 18 19 20 21

CHECK
STRENGTH

QUININE
60 mg in each ml

315

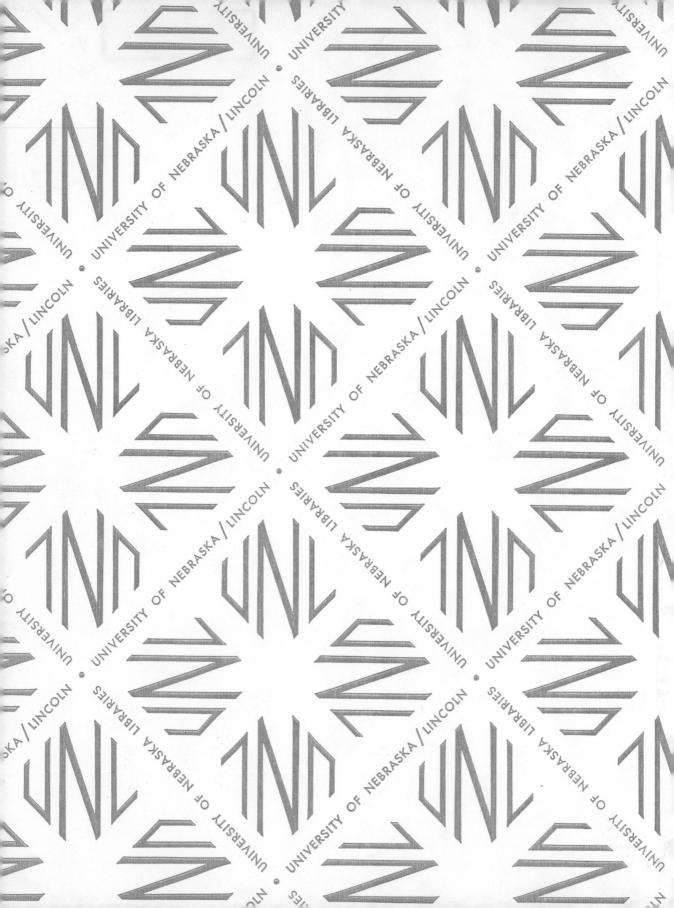